Reflective Practice in Psychotherapy and Counselling

Poornima Bhola · Chetna Duggal · Rathna Isaac

Reflective Practice in Psychotherapy and Counselling

A Practitioner Guide

Springer

Poornima Bhola
Department of Clinical Psychology
National Institute of Mental Health
and Neuro Sciences
Bangalore, Karnataka, India

Chetna Duggal
School of Human Ecology
Tata Institute of Social Sciences
Mumbai, Maharashtra, India

Rathna Isaac
Parivarthan Counselling, Training
and Research Center
Bangalore, Karnataka, India

ISBN 978-981-96-9731-1 ISBN 978-981-96-9732-8 (eBook)
https://doi.org/10.1007/978-981-96-9732-8

This Springer imprint is published by the registered company Springer Nature Singapore Pte Ltd.
The registered company address is: 152 Beach Road, #21-01/04 Gateway East, Singapore 189721, Singapore

Preface

This book has been conceptualized as a companion for psychotherapists and counsellors who wish to embark on a journey of self-discovery and professional growth. For those of us who have thought, "I would like to be more reflective in my work, but I don't know how", this resource offers opportunities to explore reflection as a valuable tool. We aspire to make reflective practice more accessible to thoughtful practitioners, providing a pathway to enhance their personal and professional development. By the end of the book, we hope readers will have gained the knowledge and confidence to incorporate reflective practice into their work, paving the way for a richer, fuller and more meaningful engagement with their therapeutic endeavours.

The terms *therapist(s)* and *counsellor(s)* are used interchangeably throughout the text to ensure relevance for all trained practitioners providing psychotherapy, counselling and psychosocial care to individuals, families and communities. The term *client(s)* has been used throughout the book. *Client* is sometimes preferred as it suggests a more equal relationship, shared power and a shift away from the medical model. However, some practitioners may favour the term *patient(s)*, as it connotes a care relationship and the need for healing, rather than a financial or transactional exchange. As you engage with this text, take a moment to reflect on which term resonates with you and aligns with your own values and approach. Regardless of the terminology we prefer, it is essential that we uphold the core values of the psychotherapeutic relationship and space.

This book is suitable for therapists at all levels of professional development and is framed from an adult learning perspective, assuming self-directedness, active participation and self-paced engagement. While the book is conceived as a psychotherapist's journey and is best read from beginning to end, each chapter can also stand alone. We invite you to follow your inner reflections, allowing yourself to pause, explore and linger on the sections that evoke deeper contemplation.

The chapter topics have been curated to encompass the essential components of reflective practice relevant for mental health practitioners. The focus alternates between the therapist's inner world and their interaction with clients, supporting practitioners across different stages of professional development in navigating their journeys with greater awareness and intentionality. Each chapter situates reflections within the context of scientific research, as well as the broader sociocultural and political landscape. Rather than providing definitive answers, the aim is to open possibilities for reflection and exploration. We invite you to critically examine and personalize ideas that can nurture both personal and professional growth.

Self-reflective exercises, presented as *Pause and reflect* boxes, are integrated throughout the chapters. These exercises invite readers to slow down, engage in introspection and connect new ideas with their existing sense of self. The goal is to support the integration of new knowledge by fostering an expanded experience that lies at the heart of reflective practice. Additionally, these activities can be easily adapted for use in reflective groups or training programmes. *Vignettes* illustrating various therapy and supervision interactions are interwoven throughout the book, grounding the reflective process in real-life experiences, decisions and actions.

Reflective practice is brought alive through narratives, interviews and experiential accounts contributed by psychotherapists, clients, academicians, mental health leaders and advocates, from around the world—including India, the USA, the UK, Japan, Rwanda, Australia and Canada. These narratives, specifically crafted for this book, create a rich tapestry that showcases the diverse ways in which reflective work enriches the field of psychotherapy. Wherever client experiences are referenced, narratives have been thoughtfully crafted with identifying details altered or omitted to safeguard confidentiality.

Each chapter concludes with a section dedicated to *Training and development*, outlining critical issues and recommendations for incorporating reflective practice into psychotherapy training and supervision contexts. This section provides practical suggestions on curriculum design, methodology and pedagogical approaches, addressing key issues essential for nurturing reflective practitioners. Our goal is to create a pathway that encourages trainers and organizations to embrace and integrate a reflective lens more fully into their programmes.

In the first chapter *Getting Ready for Reflective Practice*, we introduce the concepts of reflection, reflexivity and critical reflection, situating the role of reflective practice in the growth and development of psychotherapists. Reflection is presented as a vital tool for analysing experiences, challenging assumptions and deepening our understanding of both ourselves and our clients. The chapter explores how these insights can inform therapeutic work through iterative cycles of reflection and action. A range of models and methods are introduced to guide this process. In setting the frame for the book, we engage with important questions on, who should reflect, what to reflect on, how we reflect and when do we reflect, and contextualize the explorations to follow. The reader is invited to consider their current place in their journey as a therapist and to consider what reflective practice might offer at this stage.

The second chapter, *Tracing Motivations to Become a Therapist*, delves into the question, why do we do what we do? It invites readers to reflect on their personal motivations for entering the profession, encouraging them to consider their own stories and ask, what brought me here?" We explore the notion of the therapist as a *wounded healer* and what becomes possible when therapists engage with their own narratives of pain and healing. The chapter juxtaposes the exploration of overarching motivations with the immediacy of quotidian needs and motives that surface moment to moment in therapy. Recognizing that motivations can change over the life span, we also examine the pushes and pulls that draw individuals towards psychotherapy as a second career. We explore what sustains therapists in their work, enabling them to stay meaningfully engaged with all that psychotherapy has to offer.

Discovering the Self-of-the-Therapist is a chapter that focuses on using reflective capacities for exploring the intersections of our personal and professional selves. Recognizing the centrality of self-awareness to the effective use of self in therapy, we present multiple pathways for self-discovery, including experiential exercises and creative ways of getting in touch with different layers of experience. We discuss how various facets of the self—the personal, relational, collective and the spiritual—come alive in the therapeutic space. By delving into each aspect, we illuminate how the self-of-the-therapist can be harnessed most effectively in the psychotherapy process. The chapter concludes by illustrating how artmaking and movement can provide a unique space for personal exploration, allowing an expression of what may be difficult to articulate through words alone.

Theoretical models provide the framework through which we understand our work and communicate with clients. The chapter on *Adopting a Theoretical Lens* starts with a reflection on how theoretical models are experienced and expressed, both within the self of the therapist and in the therapy room. Readers are encouraged to actively reflect on how their theoretical lens shapes therapeutic work and explore ways of building a closer rapprochement between their beliefs, intentions and actions. Recognizing that therapists' relationships with their theoretical orientations are constantly evolving, we trace the journey of finding a theoretical home, identifying critical moments that guide decisions to integrate different models into practice. The chapter concludes with an in-depth exploration of therapists' individual styles and personal theories of change, highlighting how these elements evolve and align with their therapeutic practice.

In the chapter on *Connecting with Clients and Building a Therapeutic Alliance*, the relational matrix is explored from multiple perspectives. Recognizing the therapeutic relationship as the primary vehicle for change, the chapter reflects on its unfolding, from tentative beginnings to eventual dissolution. The chapter begins by reflecting on how therapists can attune to their clients, creating a space where the client feels truly seen, heard and understood. The therapeutic journey is rarely smooth, and misunderstandings, unmet expectations or emotional disconnection are inevitable. Through learning how to recognise and repair these ruptures, therapists can foster a deeper, more resilient connection with their clients. We also explore the use of countertransference as a mirror to the emotional worlds of both therapist and client. The section on power dynamics addresses the nuances of shifting, sharing and embracing power in therapy spaces and mental healthcare systems. It invites reflection on how paternalism and value imposition can take root, and the ongoing challenge of truly centring the client's autonomy and voice. The chapter concludes with a discussion on the complex emotions of accomplishment and loss that accompany the closure of the therapeutic journey.

With the view that therapy is not value-neutral, the sixth chapter, *Understanding Personal and Professional Values*, centres on engaging with values and contemplating their links with social and professional identities. We examine the dynamic relationship between how values are embodied in the therapeutic work and how this influences the values we uphold. Both therapist and client values come into play within the therapy, with areas of alignment and misalignment both opening an arena for reflection. The chapter explores several territories, including recognizing and understanding client values, prioritizing them when needed and working through value conflicts. In the contemporary context, where social justice and systemic inequalities are increasingly at the forefront of global conversations, engaging with sociopolitical values is more relevant than ever. The chapter brings a focus to both spoken and unspoken sociopolitical values of client and therapist, exploring the potential and possibilities that such dialogue can offer.

The chapter *Engaging with Diversity in the Therapy Room* illuminates how we live in a world that is both shared and divided. Issues of diversity lead us to the edges and margins of experience, where reflection is a tool for understanding and working with the most vulnerable individuals and communities. The chapter introduces a critical examination of the concepts of culture, social location and intersectionality, laying the foundation for a reflexive awareness of self-in-context. The social locations of class, caste, religion and gender are explored in detail as we reflect on their contributions to the experience and expression of psychological distress. Each subsection delves into the therapist's self, beliefs and assumptions, discussing how social location impacts the therapeutic process. The reader is guided to locate themselves through their social identities, unpack notions of privilege and power, and link these reflections to culturally sensitive and affirmative psychotherapeutic practice. The chapter introduces the power wheel as a lens for understanding experiences of marginalization and privilege, which grounds the exploration of diversity-informed approaches, decolonizing perspectives and community-based initiatives.

In *Navigating Therapy Practice in the Digital World*, we examine the many ways technology intersects with the practice of psychotherapy, reshaping relational dynamics, professional identity and the very spaces in which therapy unfolds. Particular attention is given to sustaining the therapeutic alliance in telepsychotherapy through intentional, adaptive and relationally attuned practices. While therapists navigate challenges of managing their personal and professional digital presence, media platforms present new opportunities to shape mental health discourse and curate professional profiles. This also positions them alongside a growing community of mental health influencers, raising questions about authority, authenticity and impact. The chapter also explores the growing role of artificial intelligence and digital mediation in mental health support, from enhancing therapeutic processes to the development of AI-supported platforms. We spotlight evolving professional guidelines on telepsychotherapy, social media use and online research, and pose searching questions about the impact and ethics of technology integration in psychotherapy practice, training and research.

Learning from Clients directs our attention to the other half of the therapy equation—our clients. The chapter explores ways of listening and learning from clients, encouraging us to open ourselves to their narratives and metaphors, attuning to their preferences, eliciting their theories of change and responding to their feedback on the therapeutic process. Historically, client voices have been silenced, and their perspectives systematically overlooked. The chapter raises critical questions about who holds expertise in the room and where power resides within the therapeutic relationship. We advocate for a deliberate and concerted effort to draw on the wisdom and expertise of individuals with lived experiences of mental illness. The collective voice of clients and the consumer/survivor/carer movement can play a pivotal role in re-examining therapeutic practices. Every interaction with our clients moves us and shifts something within us. The chapter offers avenues for therapists to reflect on the enduring, and even transformative, life lessons learned from clients.

In the tenth chapter, the focus is on *Bringing Reflective Practice into Supervision.* It offers a panoramic view of the therapeutic and supervisory landscape, showing how reflection helps supervisors and supervisees navigate this terrain. To begin with, the focus is on how supervisors can set the frame and elicit goals, matching processes to the specific needs of the supervisee. A safe supervisory alliance is essential for self-reflection and exploration, and we reflect on supervisor attitudes and habits that can nurture this safety. The highlight of the chapter is the toolkit for supervisors that brings together a range of methods and interventions that can be used to facilitate reflective dialogue and questions in both one-on-one and group supervision formats. We envisage supervision as a crucial reflective space and a mechanism through which a reflective stance can be internalized. In conclusion, we suggest ways to enhance the skills of supervisors and support their professional development.

The chapter *Being in Personal Therapy* explores the complex world of therapists undergoing their own therapy. It offers insights into the hopes and hesitations around the personal therapy process and considers its deep impact on their therapeutic work with clients. Personal therapy provides a unique opportunity to reflect on the self-of-the-therapist while offering support in attending to and healing the parts of ourselves that require care. The chapter explores several key questions around why therapists seek therapy, how they choose their therapists, which therapeutic orientation works best for them, the appropriate duration and timing for therapy, and the barriers that prevent therapists from using therapy as a space for self-reflection. What matters most is recognizing how being a client and experiencing the therapy process deepens the connection with clients, fosters greater self-awareness and strengthens reflective capacity. Reflective questions guide the reader through the complexities and challenges of providing personal therapy to another therapist. The discussion on mandatory therapy completes the circle of inquiry by addressing the ethical, practical and contextual dimensions of requiring therapeutic experiences for trainees.

The chapter *Investing in Self-Care Through Reflective Practice* highlights the stresses that can arise from working with clients, balancing personal lives and navigating work settings. While therapeutic work can be deeply fulfilling and enriching, caring for clients who have experienced trauma and adversity can also lead to compassion fatigue, vicarious traumatization and burnout among therapists. Self-care becomes crucial, especially in the aftermath of a client's suicide or during personal loss and challenges. We emphasize that responsibility for self-care should not rest solely on the individual, as systemic factors significantly contribute to therapist burnout and overwhelm. Additionally, we advocate for training institutes and workplaces to prioritize well-being and resilience among therapists. This chapter encourages reflective engagement in developing a personal self-care plan that responds to unique needs and emotional experiences, incorporating creative, spiritual and personally meaningful pathways.

The last chapter *The Reflective Path: Integrating Reflection into Psychotherapy Training, Practice, and Research*, encourages readers to draw from the reflective opportunities in the book and articulate the main takeaways that will inform their future work. The chapter goes well beyond simply looking back at the path covered, threading together the sense of accomplishment in having come this far with the anticipation of what might lie ahead. The discussions hold space for the complexities, challenges and paradoxes inherent in reflective work, placing the onus on leaders, trainers, supervisors, researchers and practitioners to create safe and supportive spaces for reflection. We close the book with a set of 'big questions' that call for ongoing reflexive engagement. These questions reflect our commitment as authors to wrestle with difficult, often uncomfortable, issues that matter to us. We explore topics such as the usefulness of diagnosis and the dominance of the biomedical lens, the intersections between the political and the therapeutic, and the risks of siloed thinking in the name of disciplinary purity and apolitical neutrality. The chapter encourages critical thinking about the future of the profession and the relational and ethical dimensions that ground our work. Our hope is that by remaining reflective throughout our individual and collective journeys, we will make possible the work we dream of.

Bangalore, India Poornima Bhola
Mumbai, India Chetna Duggal
Bangalore, India Rathna Isaac

Acknowledgements This book is our way to give back to the profession the gifts of reflection we have received from clients and teachers, supervisors and supervisees, and trainers and trainees. It is a tribute to the transformative power of reflective practice that we have witnessed and experienced in our work. We hope this book serves as a valuable resource for fellow practitioners, offering insights and pathways that can enrich their journeys.

We thank the institutes that we have been part of—the National Institute of Mental Health and Neurosciences (NIMHANS), Bengaluru, the Tata Institute of Social Sciences, Mumbai—for nurturing us and our ideas.

We would like to thank our teachers, Kiran Rao, Ahalya Raguram, Anisha Shah, Malavika Kapur, Rachna Johri and Jayanti Basu, whose work inspired us, ignited our curiosity and deepened our understanding. Your insights into the intricacies of psychotherapy fostered our growth as academicians, practitioners and authors.

Poornima Bhola expresses deep gratitude to David Orlinsky, Helge Rønnestad and the Society for Psychotherapy Research Collaborative Research Network (SPR/CRN) for opening the door to the world of psychotherapist development. Many thanks to friend and collaborator Shveta Kumaria, for our joint research explorations of the experiences and development of psychotherapists in India, conducted as part of the SPR/CRN.

We are grateful to all contributors for bringing the potential of reflective practice to life through their shared personal narratives: Anuja Gupta, Archana Ramanathan, Ashwini Ailawadi, Asiya Niyaz, Brinda Jacob-Janvrin, Deepti Guruprasad, K. Dharani Devi, Grace Gatera, Hargun Ahluwalia, Hiba Siddiqui, Jyothsna Chandur, Jyotsna Agrawal, Kanika Mehrotra, Laura S. Brown, Maliha Ibrahim, Maitri Chand, Malika Verma, Mehak Sikand, Mick Cooper, Muzammil Karim, Nancy McWilliams, Nupur Dhingra Paiva, Pallavi Banerjee, Prabha S. Chandra, Roy Sinai, Shigeru Iwakabe, Simran Chatha, Smriti Joshi, Soumitra Pathare, Suman Bolar, Susan Howard, Tanmoy Goswami and Yashpal Jogdand. We appreciate the time, thought and honesty you dedicated to this process. Your contributions remind us of the collective wisdom within our community and the profound impact we can create when we come together to share our experiences.

Thank you to Denise Defey, George Silberchatz, Harold Chui, Helene A. Nissen-Lie, Jacques P. Barber, James Bennett-Levy, Jamuna Rajeswaran, Kalyani Gopal, Kenneth L. Critchfield, Ladislav Timulak, Mudita Rastogi, Rachna Johri, Shalini Bharat, Thomas Schröder and Ueli Kramer for their generous endorsements, capturing the essence of our work and articulating its significance in the field of psychotherapy.

We appreciate the generosity of Ganga M. Nair, Founder of the Listener's Collective and James Bennett-Levy, Southern Cross University, for their permission to reproduce the two figures used in the book.

Much of our understanding of reflective practice came from facilitating reflecting spaces, very often together. We would like to acknowledge all the trainees and practitioners who have participated in the workshops, seminars and discussions we facilitated. Thank you for your openness and the willingness to share your experiences, which inspired us to approach the writing of this book with greater depth and authenticity.

A special thanks to Anokhi Mehra for the thorough critique and review of all the chapters. Your thoughtful questions and encouraging comments have enriched and strengthened the ideas in the book.

We also thank beta readers, Kanika Mehrotra, Kavvya Sankritik and Nupur Singhal, for proof-reading early versions of the chapters. Arpitha Ravishankar and Madhuri Dugyala were research assistants on a project exploring the personal and professional development trajectories of trainee psychotherapists in India. Your contributions have informed this work and we thank you for your commitment.

We appreciate the support from Mallika Badrinath at the Pen and Mouse for the meticulous artwork on the figures.

Thank you to Satvinder Kaur, Ramya Somasundaram, Princy Sagayam Lasar and the entire team at Springer, for your patience and support through the writing process.

We want to acknowledge the love and deep understanding from our families that anchored us through this journey. Your support and encouragement provided the motivation we needed, during the hours, days, months and years spent discussing ideas, going down rabbit holes, developing concepts and writing late into the night.

Most importantly, we wish to honour our clients. Being witness to your journeys of self-discovery inspired us to be better practitioners and continue to learn and evolve. Each lesson learned and each story shared has contributed to the foundation upon which we built this book.

Writing this book has involved a reflective process of brainstorming and joint writing sessions. Bringing it together has not been a straightforward task—we meandered along till we found *our* voice. This voice belongs to the three of us and emerged from our experiences as practitioners, trainers and supervisors. We have used this opportunity to express our love for our work and stand up for what is important for us. This is also our deliberate attempt to open conversations that are much needed within the professional community, ask questions that might have been avoided and bring to the forefront voices that are often unheard. Through this book, we invite those of us who are ready—to play, explore, be curious, get lost and be found.

Competing Interests The authors have no competing interests to declare that are relevant to the content of this manuscript.

Praise for *Reflective Practice in Psychotherapy and Counselling*

"Occasionally an outstanding book emerges which takes a field to a whole new level. *Reflective Practice in Psychotherapy and Counselling* is one such book. Over the past half-century, many words have been written about reflective practice, but no authors have created such a masterful work as Bhola, Duggal and Isaac have managed. Scholarly, beautifully written, and packed with case studies and stories that bring reflective practice to life, this is essential reading for all clinicians, researchers, and educators with an interest in reflective practice."

—James Bennett-Levy, Ph.D., *Professor, Southern Cross University, Australia, Author,* Experiencing CBT from the Inside Out: A Self-Practice/Self-Reflection Workbook for Therapists

"The authors of *Reflective Practice in Psychotherapy and Counselling: A Practitioner Guide* graciously offer deeply personal and incredibly insightful tales about their journeys into being and working as psychotherapists. This is one of the most beautiful and meaningful books on psychotherapists and psychotherapy that I have read. Read it - you will be inspired."

—Helene A. Nissen-Lie, Ph.D., *Clinical Professor and Psychotherapist, University of Oslo, Norway*

"With *Reflective Practice in Psychotherapy and Counselling: A Practitioner Guide*, Poornima Bhola, Chetna Duggal and Rathna Isaac help us open our eyes, our minds and our hearts to the process of reflectivity. Across twelve beautifully written chapters—interwoven with personal accounts by researchers and practitioners of psychotherapy and lots of hands-on exercises—the reader is invited to take a step back, pause, reflect, become aware and act. A thoughtful tribute to an integrative and a deeply human growth process!"

—Ueli Kramer, Ph.D., *Professor in Psychiatry and Psychotherapy, University of Lausanne, Switzerland, Past President, European Society for Psychotherapy Research and European Society for the Study of Personality Disorders & Editor of* Case Formulation for Personality Disorders: Tailoring Psychotherapy to the Individual Client

"This book is quite a jewel. An extremely valuable resource for therapists looking to enhance their reflective skills, it offers practical guidance, drawing from the insights of therapists, clinicians, patients and researchers. The *Pause and reflect* boxes encourage readers to contemplate the material and apply insights into their own practice. This insightful book is highly recommended for mental health professionals aiming to improve their overall competence, particularly in the area of reflective practice."

—Jacques P. Barber, Ph.D., ABPP, *Professor Emeritus and Dean Emeritus, Gordon F. Derner School of Psychology, Adelphi University, NY, USA, Past President, International Society for Psychotherapy Research & Co-author,* Psychodynamic Therapy: A Guide to Evidence-Based Practice

"Reading this book was an incredibly stimulating and thought-provoking experience. It is extremely rare to come across a book that will be deeply and equally appreciated by experienced psychotherapists, clinical supervisors, early career therapists and students. The focus on reflective practice makes this a book that will be read, re-read and widely discussed. I commend the authors for their excellent contribution."

—George Silberschatz, Ph.D., *Clinical Professor, Department of Psychiatry and Behavioral Sciences, UCSF Weill Institute for Neurosciences, USA, President, San Francisco Psychotherapy Research Group*

"As therapists and counsellors navigate the complexities of human emotions, relationships and therapeutic dynamics, reflective practice is not just advantageous—it is essential. Each chapter contributes unique insights, methodologies and frameworks that illuminate the reflective process. I recommend this book as an indispensable resource, providing trainers with perspectives and tools to nurture these critical capacities in their trainees."

—Jamuna Rajeswaran, M.Phil., Ph.D., *Professor and Head, Department of Clinical Psychology, National Institute of Mental Health and Neuro Sciences, Bangalore, India*

"This thoughtful book speaks to trainees, educators and healers at various stages of their learning and practice. It facilitates a fundamental looking inward through the use of questions, theory, exercises, vignettes and resources. Written by a team of experienced therapists, this book will make you pause, go deeper, grow and hone your craft. I highly recommend it!"

—Mudita Rastogi, Ph.D., *Clinical Professor & Department Chair, Master of Science in Marriage and Family Therapy, The Family Institute at Northwestern University, USA, Editor of* Multicultural Couple Therapy

"Being a reflective practitioner is an aspiration shared by most therapists, but sustaining a reflective stance in pressured healthcare services and busy practices can be difficult. This book will help you maintain and develop your own reflective practice at any stage of your career and in all kinds of settings. It offers a rich array of practical exercises, ensuring that you will find some that chime with you and some that challenge you. The book's greatest strength lies in its plurality of voices, enabling each reader to recognize something that resonates, and much to discover that is new and thought provoking."

—Thomas A Schröder, Ph.D., *Professor of Clinical Psychology and Psychological Therapies, Mental Health and Clinical Neurosciences Unit, School of Medicine, University of Nottingham, UK*

"*Reflective Practice in Psychotherapy and Counselling: A Practitioner Guide* is a lucid, comprehensive and intersectional work that bridges critical gaps in the literature on clinical supervision, practice and self-reflection within mental health. Kudos to the authors."

—Kalyani Gopal, Ph.D., HSPP, *Past President, APA Division 12, Society of Clinical Psychology. USA*

"This excellent book provides potential readers with an extraordinary combination of scientific evidence, theoretically grounded considerations and practical issues to be taken into account in the consultation hour. By featuring seasoned reflections and concepts by the experienced authors, alongside candid and deeply personal narratives from therapists, patients, supervisors and supervisees, the book offers a vivid glimpse into the real challenges of the clinical encounter. Written beautifully, it provides a rich description of the inner side of psychotherapy by approaching therapists' feelings—fears, joys and painful moments—in their work. The chapter on diversity deserves a special mention, since it invites therapists to open their eyes, minds (and hearts...)

to cultural realities so different from their own, transforming their work into an experience of cultural humility."

—Denise Defey, Ph.D., *Professor, University of Uruguay, Montevideo, Uruguay, Former President, Society for Psychotherapy Research—Latin American Chapter*

"The self, with all its entanglements, is the primary resource for members of the therapeutic community. This book will be of enduring value to all those who see therapeutic work as an ongoing process of transformation for themselves and others."

—Rachana Johri, *Distinguished Visiting Professor, School of Liberal Studies, BML Munjal University, Haryana, India*

"Drs. Bhola, Duggal and Isaac's text is rich, comprehensive and accessible. It is also timely and important. Therapists are expertly guided to engage with their own perceptions, identities, values and meaning-making, within a transtheoretical framework. As someone who trains therapists and cares deeply about relational and attachment processes, I know that I will be recommending this book to trainees and colleagues going forward."

—Kenneth L. Critchfield, Ph.D., *Associate Professor of Psychology & Clinical PsyD Program Director, Ferkauf Graduate School of Psychology, Yeshiva University, New York, USA*

"Practitioners, trainees and supervisors are invited to explore reflection as an art, a skill and a pathway to self-discovery. Featuring rich experiential accounts from practitioners with diverse experiences across geographical and cultural contexts, the book opens a window into the inner world of therapeutic practice."

—Shalini Bharat, Ph.D., *Former Vice Chancellor, Tata Institute of Social Sciences, Mumbai, India*

"This book provides actionable insights for trainees and practitioners to reflect on their personal and professional lives and use this self-awareness to enhance therapeutic effectiveness and foster personal growth. Bhola and colleagues take readers on a thought-provoking journey of self-discovery, deepening the understanding of reflective practice and the very essence of being a counsellor and psychotherapist."

—Harold Chui, Ph.D., *Associate Professor, the Chinese University of Hong Kong, President of the Society of Psychotherapy Research - Asian Area Affiliate & Co-author of* Helping Skills: Facilitating Exploration, Insight, and Action *(6th edition)*

"Well-researched and thoughtfully crafted, this book by Bhola, Duggal and Isaac offers a wealth of information and perspectives, making it a remarkable achievement. Congratulations to the authors on this exceptional work!"

—Ladislav Timulak, Ph.D., *Professor in Counselling Psychology, Trinity College Dublin, Ireland & Co-author of* Transdiagnostic Emotion-Focused Therapy

Contents

Personal Narratives

Chapter 2
A Therapist Speaks: Lost and Found
Roy Sinai
A Therapist Speaks: Psychology at the Heart of Social Change
Mick Cooper
Chapter 3
A Therapist Speaks: Meditations on the Self
Jyotsna Agrawal
A Therapist Speaks: Using the POTT-er's Wheel to Shape the Self of the Therapist
Maliha Ibrahim
A Therapist Speaks: My Strength Tree
Deepti Guruprasad
A Therapist Speaks: To Move and be Moved
Brinda Jacob-Janvrin
Chapter 4
A Therapist Speaks: What Feels True
Malika Verma
A Therapist Speaks: My Integrative Journey
Shigeru Iwakabe
Chapter 5
A Therapist Speaks: The Girl in a Locked Room
Poornima Bhola
A Therapist Speaks: Warp and Weft
Susan Howard
A Therapist Speaks: Do you Want to Switch Seats with Me?
Jyothsna Chandur
Interview: Power, Policy and Mental Health Practice
Soumitra Pathare
A Therapist Speaks: On Letting Go
K. Dharani Devi

About the Authors

Poornima Bhola is a psychotherapist, teacher, supervisor and researcher, and Professor in the Department of Clinical Psychology at the National Institute of Mental Health and Neurosciences, Bangalore, India. She leads the MENTEM division, which explores mentalization processes, assessments and interventions. Deeply committed to advancing psychotherapy, she coordinates the department's psychotherapy training programme and serves as Vice-President of the Society for Psychotherapy Research—Asia Affiliate Group. In 2020, she contributed to shaping the *Guidelines for Tele-psychotherapy Services* for clinical psychologists in India. Her research interests encompass psychotherapy processes, training and development, social cognition, personality dimensions and youth mental health.

Chetna Duggal is Associate Professor, School of Human Ecology, Tata Institute of Social Sciences (TISS), Mumbai, India. She is a psychotherapist with over 20 years of experience and teaches courses on psychotherapy, counselling and supervision in the masters and postgraduate diploma programmes and supervises trainee therapists and practitioners. Her research interests include psychotherapy practice, training and supervision, and adolescent and youth mental health. She heads the School Initiative for Mental Health Advocacy (SIMHA), and Rahbar, an initiative for supervision. She has developed the *National Disaster Management Guidelines: Mental Health and Psychosocial Support Services in Disasters* released in 2023 in collaboration with the National Disaster Management Authority, Government of India.

Rathna Isaac is a therapist, supervisor and trainer with over 20 years of experience. She is primarily a private practitioner in Bangalore. She also holds the position of external consultant and supervisor for the Couple and Family Therapy Programme at Parivarthan Counselling, Training and Research Centre, Bangalore, and is on the Board of Studies for the Department of Psychology, St. Joseph's College of Arts and Sciences, Bangalore. She has created and conducted both basic and advanced training programmes on couple therapy as well as training modules for early career therapists. She provides group and one-on-one supervision for both systemic and individual relational therapy and is deeply interested in the psychotherapy process.

List of Figures

Chapter 1
Getting Ready for Reflective Practice

Human beings have always wondered about the world around them.
Why are we here?
Where does the sun go at night?
Why did the apple fall from the tree?

The stories and theories that we have developed in response to questions like these make up much of our knowledge and understanding of our world. They have become the truths that we trust, and that define our perceptions, opinions and actions. This contemplation of the world around us—a serious and committed seeking to make sense of our observations, and to find less obvious patterns and meanings—can be termed *reflection.* While reflection is often deliberate and careful, it can also be unstructured, a sort of musing around rather than delving deep. Whether we are analysing, intuiting or doubting, the central process remains one of learning. We all use reflection in our everyday life, though some of us might be more aware and conscious in our use of it. Reflection helps us build knowledge and awareness of what is, as well as create what could be.

We may turn an open, curious, gaze onto our thoughts, emotions, bodily sensations, memories and experiences. This process of self-reflection is a dynamic and continuous process, and we may catch ourselves dwelling on everyday experiences or asking larger questions about the purpose of life. A disagreement with a partner makes us puzzle over the reasons for our reactions and the ways in which they impact those around us. This can create space for us to wonder about the beliefs and emotions in the mind of our partner and get better at understanding and predicting their actions. In this process of mentalizing, we can see ourselves from the outside and others from the inside and create a shared social world (Allen & Bateman, 2008). As we embrace uncertainty while holding multiple perspectives, this can open possibilities for change. Our reflections on how we respond to relational conflict may eventually strengthen the relationship.

Who we are influences *what* we see (and do not see) and *how* we see it. In her book, *On Looking*, Alexandra Horowitz takes us on a series of walks with eleven

P. Bhola et al., *Reflective Practice in Psychotherapy and Counselling*,
https://doi.org/10.1007/978-981-96-9732-8_1

experts; including an artist, a geologist, a sound designer, a naturalist, a typographer, physician, a wildlife scientist, an urban sociologist, a blind woman, a toddler and a dog. The same neighbourhood is viewed through different lenses, and in this process "the familiar becomes unfamiliar, and the old the new" (Horowitz, 2013, p. 13). While the physician speculates about people's medical conditions from their appearance and gait, the typographer illuminates the city's history through fonts and lettering on signs and buildings, the geologist notices the fossils of sea creatures trapped in building walls, and the dog leads us to explore through smell. Each person takes their unique walk and zooms into the different angles and layers of experience.

Pause and reflect...

Find a spot and sit still for a few minutes. Mark an X to locate yourself on a piece of paper and document all the different sounds you can hear in the space all around you. You may use words, images or colours to map the sounds and the direction they seem to be coming from. The sounds may be loud or faint, close or far, harmonious or discordant, familiar or unfamiliar, and expected or unexpected.

Close your eyes. Does this make a difference to what you hear?

Walk around or shift your location and see how the sounds change.

If you are doing this with another person, or in a group, compare your sound maps.

As we pause to play with sensations and experiences, looking at them from different perspectives, we enter a reflective space that allows us to ask questions about what happened, how we felt and what we did. The therapy room may also be experienced as a transitional space to explore possibilities and take risks with relatedness. Of course, staying with the tensions between the familiar and the unfamiliar, the certain and the uncertain, the spoken and the unspoken, the known and the unknown (and the unthought known), can be deeply uncomfortable. Transitional spaces are like that—neither here nor there, but this is what creates possibility. This third space is seen as linking the inside and outside worlds in the fields of architectural design and mythology. Winnicott reminds us that transitional spaces are spaces of play and creativity (Winnicott, 1971). As therapists, we may retreat into certainty—recreating the trope of the nodding, pensive, all-knowing, even all-empathizing therapist who rushes to say, *I understand*. Perhaps we need to remember to pause, dwell in the in-between spaces and reflect.

In this chapter we introduce a conceptual understanding of reflective practice, locate it in the field of psychotherapy and guide you towards frameworks that can help build and integrate new learning. We invite you to join us in experiencing the value of questioning, learning the art of observation and reflection and discovering how to apply this perspective to enhancing your work with clients.

Reflection, Reflexivity and Critical Reflection

Nina and her supervisor began watching the video recording of her therapy session with her adolescent client, Rohan. As she revisited the session, Nina noticed how frequently he mentioned his parents' critical attitude toward him—something she had completely missed during the session! Her supervisor gently encouraged her to reflect on what had gone unheard. Nina allowed her thoughts to drift through her feelings and beliefs about parenting. She realized how much she relied on her own parents and valued their guidance. Discovering how these beliefs might connect with her lack of response to Rohan's concerns allowed her to stay more attentive and attuned in the next therapy session. In later supervision sessions, Nina deepened her reflections, asking herself, "Where do these ideas come from? Whom do they serve, and whom do they silence?" She became more aware of how much she might have internalized the dominant discourse about being a 'good child', the expectations around respect and gratitude toward parents, and the norm of not disclosing family matters to outsiders. This lens seemed to have shaped both how she related to her parents and how she viewed her adolescent client's concerns around parental criticality.

In this vignette, Nina begins reflecting about her session experiences along with her supervisor. As her attention turns towards how her personal experiences might have influenced what she missed and what she noticed, she is engaging in a more reflexive process. Markham (2017, para 6) describes *reflexivity* as "trying to look at yourself looking in the mirror". This involves us owning our involvement and actively becoming aware of how our personal values and beliefs create the lens through which we reflect. It is a process that challenges us to examine our assumptions, ideas and emotions and how they influence what we reflect on and how we reflect. Our beliefs and ideas are also shaped by the sociocultural-economic-political milieu we belong to and have grown up in. *Critical reflexivity* is the process of becoming aware of the beliefs that influence how we reflect, linking these beliefs to our sociocultural context, and critiquing the assumptions that they are based on (Morley, 2015). Unpacking this can visibilize the power that societal beliefs carry and the ways in which they impinge on our interactions inside and outside the therapy room. Through this book, we have conceptualized reflective practice to include reflection, moving to reflexivity and critical reflexivity.

Reflection and the Profession of Psychotherapy

So, what is the relevance of reflection and reflexivity for professionals? With the formalization of education systems and easy access to information through books, the internet and emerging artificial intelligence applications, knowledge comes ready-made and packaged to us. While such accessible information saves both time and personal effort, it can also lead to a blind acceptance of external systems and book learning, leaving less scope for new thinking (Schön, 1983). In his classic book *The Reflective Practitioner*, Schön (1983) opined that a complete and unquestioning reliance on what is taught was one of the main reasons for the erosion of professional standards. His solution was what he called *reflective practice*—a process of thinking about what we are doing, before, during and after the act. This is done with the aim of understanding why we make the choices we do, evaluating how these choices work and how they impact our practice. It is only through constant reflection that one can continue to improve and evolve professional work quality and respond appropriately to newer challenges.

The practice of reflection seems particularly relevant to the profession of psychotherapy. Many of the concepts underpinning reflection, such as looking into oneself, searching for deeper meanings and underlying structures, or understanding motivations, have been key to the development of the discipline of psychology. Psychology and psychotherapy have always emphasized the necessity of reflection and introspection for growth and understanding of both the self and the discipline. The purpose of therapy itself is to help clients reflect on their lives in new ways. All schools of therapy encourage self-reflection and self-awareness as the path to progress in therapy. So, in many ways, as psychotherapists, we are already comfortable with the idea of learning through reflection.

We use reflection to make sense of our clients' difficulties and ask, *Why this client, with this problem, at this time?* This leads us to develop an individualized approach that recognizes the uniqueness of each client. Culture, location, gender and socio-economic status, all these factors (and more) influence the trajectory of therapy. Practising clinicians may question these frames of understanding and realize that readymade, one-size-fits-all responses are limited in their efficacy. While we need formal systems of research and theory development to base our profession on, dependence on these alone cannot help us work with our clients. In our work as therapists, we often encounter situations that call for a creative and flexible response, and it is here that reflective practice becomes particularly relevant. These zones of indeterminate practice, events or moments characterized by difference, unexpectedness and inherent value conflicts call for a critical engagement with our beliefs, feelings, values and motives (Schön, 1983).

Johns and Burnie (2013) discuss the continuum between doing reflection, which addresses the more behavioural aspects (tools, how to, reflection in and on action), and being reflective, which involves asking questions about who I am rather than what I do. Such explorations may be particularly relevant for helping professions, which demand the use of the therapist self as an instrument. Reflective practice integrates the reflective and scientific facets of the discipline and integrates the rigours of science with the artistry of reflection (Stedmon et al., 2003). The therapist who gains the most is the one who can use both positions to critically throw a spotlight on each other. This position has been validated with the inclusion of reflective practice as a core competency by mainstream professional organizations. However, there is limited consensus or conversation around how to operationalize, inculcate and embed reflective processes within training and practice contexts.

The declarative–procedural–reflective (DPR) model (Bennett-Levy, 2006; Chaddock et al., 2014) provides a framework for understanding how psychotherapists learn and apply therapy skills and describes the intersections between three paths to learning (Fig. 1.1).

The *declarative* system consists of information about therapy and psychological theories—the kind of material we find in a good textbook or learn through lectures. The *procedural* system involves the practical application of declarative knowledge about conceptual, technical and interpersonal relational aspects of therapy. These are the skills we use in the therapy room and involve both clinical decision-making and subsequent actions. They are usually learnt through role-plays, demonstrations and practice. Finally, the *reflective* system involves observing, interpreting and evaluating output from our declarative and procedural systems. As we re-experience and reflect on our thoughts, feelings and behaviours in the session, and their outcomes, we may develop new insights about both theory and procedural skills.

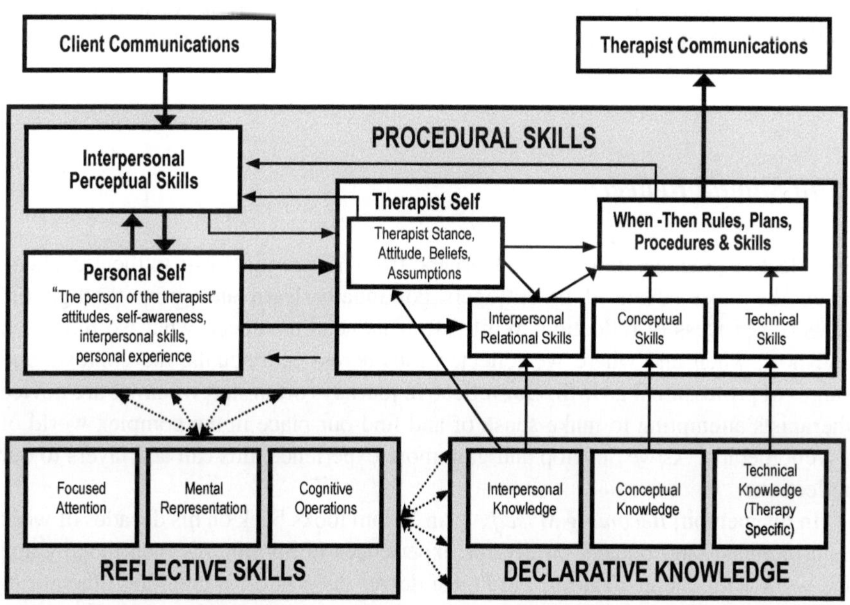

Fig. 1.1 Declarative-procedural-reflective model of therapist skill development (reproduced with permission from James Bennett-Levy, 2024)

The role of a reflective system is a comparative one: to hold and analyse past, current or future experience; compare and contrast it with stored information; identify a plan of action; and either maintain or change encoded information in the light of the analysis. The DPR model emphasizes the central role of the reflective system in our development as psychotherapy practitioners. It is this system that enables us to make fine distinctions, sense when to sit in silence or when to seek connection and when to slow down or when to move faster, as well as develop our sensitivity as therapists. As our therapist identity develops, the use of therapeutic skills is inevitably influenced by the person of the therapist (e.g., personal experiences, attitudes and interpersonal skills) and in return the therapist self also impacts the personal self (Chaddock et al., 2014). Reflection helps knowledge flow between these two sources of information and experience, ultimately building a bridge between our personal and professional selves. It is not our years of experience alone that lead to growth but how much we reflect on, learn from and incorporate this experience into our practice (Skovholt et al., 1997).

Reflective Practice: Asking the Right Questions

The best way to learn is to ask questions, and we discuss some key questions around reflective practice. Understanding what areas of practice to focus on, increasing awareness of useful reflective methods and models, as well as considering where and when reflection occurs, can open new pathways to learning and professional growth.

Who Should Reflect?

In reflective practice, *all* of us are learners, from trainee therapists to their teachers. Even the most advanced practitioners continually learn and grow through the powerful process of reflection. While all of us need to reflect, what we reflect on and how, when and where we reflect, varies across individuals, the contexts and stages of professional growth. Our reflective journeys often start when we are novice therapists attempting to make sense of and find our place in the complex world of psychotherapy. As we develop and gain more experience, this can add layers to our reflections.

In his memoir, *Becoming Myself*, Irvin Yalom looks back on his decades of work as a therapist, and reflects on diverse experiences in his life, his own therapy and his work with clients (Yalom, 2017). He delves deep into his childhood memories to share how he learnt the key lesson of empathy. He interrogates his life, shares his experiences with clients, family and professional colleagues, and explores the intersections between his personal and professional selves. He creates imaginary conversations between young Irvin and the much older Professor Yalom to revisit and reflect on his learnings from therapy and life. Yalom alerts us that exploring and confronting the self often takes us closer to our fears, anxieties and painful realizations. Why then open this Pandora's box? Perhaps because this continuous process of reflection can also bring rewards—of healing, a deeper understanding of our relationships, and an enriched engagement with our lives. As Yalom chronicles his life and experiences with clients, we can see how these reflections are interwoven with the development and growth of the ideas in his existential approach to therapy.

As psychotherapists, we often learn and work within educational institutions or organizations that provide therapy services. When we ask the question, who should reflect?, it seems to put the onus on the individual and shifts the responsibility away from the systems we function within. Our concern here is that without adequate institutional scaffolding and support, the individual therapist cannot find the time or skills to engage in reflective practice. If we want to embed this ethos in our training and work environments, it calls for review and deep reflections on processes, values and spaces within these systems. All organizations have a culture and have their own legacy of training or work processes which do not necessarily privilege reflection. It can be challenging to step away from what seems to be working and reflect critically on how learning occurs or how services are organized and experienced. Building in a culture of reflection does not mean dismantling existing structures, it is more about leveraging and expanding existing pockets of reflective space. These may exist in the form of case discussions, supervision groups and even formal teaching programmes that nourish the reflective capabilities of trainees. The organization itself can initiate reflective practice groups to review its own functioning; for instance, to explore and question decision-making processes, training methodologies or therapeutic services, and their underlying philosophies related to power, participation and dialogue. Such approaches can help strengthen pathways to care for our clients and develop innovative models for intervention. They also provide direction in setting academic curricula, examining supervision processes and identifying needs for staff training or areas of research. Well-being can be promoted through the integration of organizational policies for self-care and support for trainees. An organization with a strong reflective culture is more likely to create a more reflective ethos among staff and students. We recommend that newer organizations, even smaller ones like psychotherapy group practices, consider how they can build reflective practices into their vision, structure and processes, so that they can grow intentionally and responsively, and remain relevant and flexible.

What Do We Reflect On?

In the *Invisible Gorilla experiment*, people were asked to focus on a video in which six people, half in white shirts and half in black shirts, passed basketballs around. They were asked to look out for and count the number of passes made by the people in white shirts. At some point, a person in a gorilla suit walked in and out of the scene, thumping its chest. Would you have noticed the gorilla? Although it seems hard to imagine anyone missing this, Chabris and Simons (2010) demonstrated that about *half* of the watchers did not see the gorilla. This unexpected finding shows us how selective attention operates; if we are not looking out for something, it is easier to miss it. Even when therapists decide to reflect, there are multiple targets and catalysts for reflection; on the therapists' personal and professional self, on critical incidents that arise in the therapeutic process, and a range of complex contextual influences. It can be challenging to attend to all these moving targets and see the array of feelings, memories and sensations that are evoked during, after or before a therapy session.

Pause and reflect...
What aspects of the therapy experience do you tend to notice and reflect on?

Could there be parts of the therapeutic process that you tend not to question?

Entering the reflective space with a broad question or focus is always useful, as it ensures that reflective practice remains purposeful. The psychotherapist has rich areas of exploration for reflection, both inside and outside the self and at their intersection. This includes reflections on practice, employing *general reflective skills* where the focus is on examining therapeutic material such as the therapeutic stance, formulation, goals and approaches, as well as the reconstruction and exploration of therapy events, processes and progress. *Self-reflective skills,* on the other hand, use reflection for a deeper exploration of therapists' personal and professional selves, developmental experiences, relational styles, motivations, feelings, thoughts, attitudes and preferences (Thwaites et al, 2014). We can set aside some time to think about these aspects of ourselves, our strengths and limitations and how they manifest in our practice. Reflecting on who we are and the work we do are closely interlinked, and it is when these two areas are integrated in our awareness that the greatest learning may take place. Although both skills are essential, it is possible to be competent at one form of reflection and uncomfortable or avoidant of the other. Another important sphere of reflection is the *socio-economic-political context* in which both the therapist and client are situated, as this is a context that impacts both. Reflecting on our social positions and contextual realities and how they influence the values, biases, assumptions and attitudes we hold, and might bring into the therapy situation, is also critical. This might be easily missed, unless deliberately integrated into personal and interpersonal reflective spaces.

Reflections on the Therapy Process

Imagine a scenario where a usually stoic client bursts into tears during a session. This can take us by surprise, evoking a range of thoughts, memories, metaphors, visual images, feelings and sensations. Often, it is such unexpected events, moments of uncertainty, stuckness or crisis, and challenges to our skills and knowledge, that operate as signals for us to direct our reflections. However, it is also useful to consider significant moments of success; like an a-ha moment with a client, a time when a client makes a disclosure, a reluctant client agrees to come for another session or shares how things are finally beginning to make sense to them. Focusing on what is going well (rather than just on what is going badly) can help us build and crystallize skills and create our own database of good practice. It is not only stand-out moments that merit reflection. We can also reflect on events that seem innocuous, routine or expected, on our yawns of occasional boredom and unexplained drowsiness during sessions, or perhaps the twinge of loss when a long-term client terminates sessions. All these can also help expand our awareness. While events that bring out strong or unusual emotions may more easily stimulate reflection, thinking back on other experiences may have to be deliberately built into our practice.

The *critical incident* framework (Lister & Crisp, 2007) can be useful in identifying which events to reconstruct and explore, and how to analyse and synthesize that learning. Identifying the critical incident is what opens the door to this structured process of questioning and reflecting. There is no list of critical incidents, and indeed they "are not 'things' that exist independently of an observer and are awaiting discovery like gold nuggets or desert islands, but like all data, critical incidents are created" (Tripp, 1993; pg. 8). A client ending a session saying that they felt heard and understood, or a therapist tearing up on hearing a narrative of personal loss; could both be critical incidents if therapist and/or client attribute significance to the moment. When we pause to view an experience from different angles, expand our view to include what led up to this experience and the meaning it holds for future interactions, we create the potential to transform the therapeutic relationship and process.

Pause and reflect...

Take some time to remember any critical incident from your own practice - an event which made you stop and think, or one that raised questions for you.

Do you think that your client also experienced it as important and meaningful?

Did your response to the experience change anything in the therapeutic process?

What would have been lost if you hadn't noticed it?

Reflections on the Therapist Self

Whatever model of psychotherapy we use, we are people with histories, experiences, strengths and vulnerabilities. These emerge in any social interaction, and therapy is no exception. The inward focus on the self of the therapist reflects the recognition that the therapist factor can influence change processes and outcomes, both positively and negatively, much beyond the tools and techniques used (Orlinsky et al., 2004). Social and neurocognitive research illustrates how the ability to examine and understand ourselves is closely connected to the ability to think about others' thoughts and emotions (DiMaggio et al., 2008), suggesting that a critical reflection on one's own life narratives can lead to a more nuanced understanding of the thoughts and emotions of others, making us more empathetic therapists.

The journey of self-discovery is not without challenges; our travels through this inner landscape may uncover hidden selves that are difficult to accept and integrate. The mirror has been used as a powerful metaphor for self-awareness, described by Sylvia Plath as "silver and exact" and with "no preconceptions" (Plath, 1989, p.173). However, as we search for truth and clarity in the mirror, our own interpretations may colour what is seen. What happens in the therapy room may also resonate with or trigger emotions and memories of our private and personal experiences. In our efforts to sharply demarcate our personal and professional selves and identities, we may not recognise the permeability of these boundaried spaces.

Rober (2017) speaks of the need for an *inner conversation* that parallels the outer conversation between the therapist and the client. Here, the therapist pays attention to the images, moods, associations, etc., which may be evoked by session content and uses these inner experiences to understand what might be happening in the interaction between therapist and client. The Satir model (Satir, 2000), Person-of-the-Therapist (POTT) model (Aponte et al., 2009) and Self-practice/Self-reflection (SP/SR) model (Bennett-Levy, 2019; Thwaites et al., 2014) emphasize how therapists must know themselves and actively use this knowledge to work more effectively with clients along with engaging in their own personal journeys of growth and change. These frameworks require a deep commitment to self-scrutiny as therapists uncover and explore their emotional and interpersonal styles, psychological and family histories, motivations, values and personal challenges. Clearly, as therapists, we must walk the talk as we work towards self-awareness and reflection with our clients.

Reflections on Context

The interwoven tapestry of sociocultural-economic-political influences on the therapist, client and therapeutic process are assumed to be outside the therapy room. The reality is that they enter the therapy space even when unvoiced or unaddressed as explicit agendas. Our clients come from diverse backgrounds; we may begin the day by seeing someone from a minority religious community who has migrated to the city for work and end in a session with an adolescent whose parents are going through a divorce. Therapists need to recognize and reflect on these intersections within the client as well as their own ability to connect with these contextual influences.

Sometimes, the therapist and client have little in common in their social locations, and yet they are supposed to work within the intimate context of a therapeutic relationship. If a therapist is disconnected from the experiences of a client who has experienced caste discrimination, who belongs to a matriarchal community or who identifies as bisexual, how then do they engage meaningfully with their client's fears, wishes and realities? As we locate ourselves and look inwards at our own culturally based templates, we can identify our own assumptions, biases and stereotypes. This awareness can help build empathic connections with clients and find a shared language to work together.

This reflexive stance might lead us to question the dominant sociocultural framework in which psychotherapy itself is embedded. Are the theories, techniques, ethical paradigms and underlying assumptions relevant across cultures? Do they need to be translated? Or do we need newer paradigms and discourses? Reflective dialogues on the applicability of Eurocentric psychotherapy frameworks across cultures can help examine their content, assumptions and methodologies more closely. Psychotherapy itself is a social construction, and its tenets and practices have morphed over time. A critical perspective is essential to locate and interrogate our therapeutic work and the role of psychotherapy in the world. At its highest level, reflective practice goes beyond the therapy room, to understanding and challenging the political and social structures that create clients, therapists and the therapy space (Fook & Gardener, 2007). In our quest to expand and deepen our reflections, we need to engage with persons and perspectives beyond the mental health community—with anthropologists, economists, poets, climate change activists, war correspondents and stand-up comics.

How Do We Reflect?

Models of Reflection

Models of reflection offer templates for practitioners to go deeper into the process of reflection. One of the most straightforward models of reflection was proposed by Borton in 1970 and later extended by both Rolfe et al. (2001) and Driscoll (2007). It is based on three questions: *What, So what* and *Now what*? The beauty of this model lies in the fact that while it provides simple guidelines for reflection, it offers the promise of depth. It begins with *What,* which is the descriptive phase, and involves asking questions like What happened? What did I do? What did the other do? What was I trying to achieve? or What was good or bad about the experiences? This is usually a good starting point to understand an experience or event. Once we understand the *What*, it is followed by the reflective phase, *So what?* This is the phase of analysis and comparison. Here, we ask questions like So what is the importance of this? What more do I need to know about this? or What have I learnt about this? After a thorough analysis, it is followed by the emancipator phase, *Now what?* This is the phase to consider what steps need to be taken to improve practice, learn and change from this experience. Here you can ask Now what could I do? Now what do I need to do? or Now what might be the consequences of this action? (Borton, 1970).

In their experiential learning model, Kolb and Fry (1975) describe a four-step process, which involves identifying a *concrete experience* of doing or experiencing something, followed by *reflective observation* which involves reflecting on and reviewing the experience. This helps us build an *abstract conceptualization* of what we can conclude or learn from the experience, finally leading to *active experimentation* where we can plan and apply the new learning. Based on our concrete experience of trying out the new learning, the reflective cycle can start again.

Another popular model for reflection was proposed by Gibbs (1988) and described as a cycle involving six stages. The first stage involves the *description* of the event, including the context, setting, time and purpose along with one's own response and the response of others. Once the event is described, the focus is to identify *feelings* and thoughts, which is followed by the next stage of *evaluation* of the event, including considering what went well and what went badly. The *analysis* stage is the meaning-making stage where sense is made of the data gleaned, which is followed by the *conclusion* stage, to consider what one could have done differently. This finally leads to an *action* plan which involves making a concrete plan of action about what could be done in future if the event is encountered again.

While these models offer structured frameworks, they do not guide the psychotherapist about the specific areas to explore and there is little designated space for critically reflexive questions and perspectives. Each of us may approach reflective practice differently and also have our favourite ways to apply these models to our psychotherapy practice. We do recommend that all reflective exercises begin with a deep dive into a particular experience, whether internal or interpersonal, and that they end with an attempt to crystallize learning that can be applied back to therapy sessions. In between these two processes however, individual variation may be more the norm than the exception. Each of us may have different questions to ask ourselves—perhaps about the therapeutic alliance, progress in therapy or the meaning of an emotional experience. John's model for structured reflection (2004) suggests specific areas for reflection and introduces a series of questions to aid in reflection. The questions can be personal, like Why did I feel the way I did in this situation?; or related to therapy process like What was I trying to achieve?; or even ethical issues like Did I act for the best for my client? While asking the right questions can open up new areas of experience, asking too many unfocused questions can muddy the waters leaving the therapist more confused. Starting the reflective activity with at least partially defined goals can make it more productive.

There are times where new information can jolt us into questioning our implicit and explicit beliefs, values and assumptions. When we experience such a *disorienting dilemma* in the therapy process, we can use a reflective practice model to guide us deeper into that experience. Mezirow (1991) proposed three dimensions of reflection in his transformational learning theory, starting with content reflection which involves reflecting on *what* we do, feel and think. This is followed by process reflection where the focus is on *how* we do what we do, and *how* we think and feel. Finally, there is premise reflection which involves the *why* and focuses on the foundational assumptions that underlie what and how we think, act and feel. Our internal dialogue helps us examine and contrast our immediate thoughts and feelings during that event, with our current reflections. As we make meaning of the experience by considering alternate perspectives, we use that to guide our next course of action. It is the development of a new perspective, a new understanding or learning that lies at the end of a reflective exercise, which spurs further action. This process goes beyond guiding the next therapy session with the client, or when we encounter a similar event again. It extends to critical evaluation of our belief systems and our ways of knowing and learning. Subjecting our experiences and reflections to persistent self-questioning adds another layer of understanding, a meta-cognitive view on what we experience and why. Most importantly, this deep and layered reflective process creates commitment to act in new and often more creative and effective ways.

One of the better-known and researched reflective practice models is the SP/SR model developed by Bennett-Levy and colleagues (Bennett-Levy, 2019; Thwaites et al., 2014). In this model, trainee therapists work through a CBT workbook that guides them in practising techniques on themselves (self-practice). They then pause to reflect on what they learnt from this experience, first alone through completing written reflective exercises in the workbook and afterwards by discussing their insights in a supportive forum with peers and supervisors (self-reflection). Through this, trainees have reported that they realize a concept, rather than just knowing it. The SP/SR method offers the advantage of the structured process where trainees are scaffolded in their explorations using various participative and experiential methods. The creation of detailed manuals and a steadily expanding evidence base have been instrumental in embedding the SP/SR model within diverse training programmes. However, the focus on acquiring CBT competencies limits the applicability of the SP/SR model to other therapeutic modalities and broader clinical contexts.

Continued growth in reflective capacities can be nurtured through thoughtful supervision processes. Reflective supervision focuses on building the ability to critically examine the therapy process, the self of the therapist and even the supervision process, all in the context of a supportive relationship. For instance, Ladany et al. (2005) proposed an events-based pantheoretical process model of supervision, with three phases: the marker, task environment and resolution, that are embedded within the supervisor–supervisee relationship context. This model explores how specific critical events such as those related to countertransference, multicultural awareness or role conflicts, can be identified by the supervisor and supervisee. As supervisor and supervisee sit together to understand the reasons behind a client's decision to drop out, they can use this critical event as a launchpad for reflective explorations. The reflective stance encourages a close examination of interactions in the last session, subtle signs of an alliance rupture, possible transference and countertransference reactions, the use and timing of interventions, and a host of other experiences. This process deepens the understanding of the critical event itself but that is not all it does. This new learning can inform work with future clients and identify themes that need to come back into supervision.

While being extremely helpful in guiding the reflection process, these models should not be considered as fixed input–output systems for reflection. The atheoretical nature of many of the models has also left them open to over-simplification, as though we just need to pause to think a little before acting in a rational step-by-step process (Thompson & Pascal, 2012). We wonder if this captures the subjectivity of human experience, the artistry of the therapeutic process and the alchemy in the therapy room. A blind following of the steps of any model, ticking off the boxes as it were, can inhibit our creativity and make reflective practice less reflective. It is valuable to regularly consult oneself, trusted peers, mentors and relevant literature when exploring effective ways to reflect. When we use reflective models to support our sense of curiosity and create comfort with uncertainty, this creates a space to play with perspectives and possibilities. This approach deepens our engagement with therapeutic work and supports ongoing professional development.

Methods and Tools

Carl Jung kept a personal journal of his feelings, fantasies, dreams and visions during the most difficult period of his life, after his break with Sigmund Freud. This calligraphed journal has evocative images that accompany imaginative writing, documenting his process of self-exploration and self-discovery, and has been published as the *Red Book*. He drew and painted images from his own dreams, using the therapeutic technique of *active imagination* to connect with his unconscious. This process helped Jung develop his ideas and exemplifies how journaling can be a powerful and rewarding way to explore and draw from one's inner life. Interestingly, the Red Book ends with an incomplete sentence, and the last word is *moglichkeit*—a German word that means possibility.

Writing a journal can help make space for possibilities—for clarifying thoughts, identifying feelings and developing more congruence in therapy sessions. We can pick from a range of creative forms of writing such as stream of consciousness writing, dialoguing, unsent letters, writing from different people's perspectives and writing about a memory (Johns & Burnie, 2013). Digital photo and video diaries, accompanied by written narratives, allow for an immersive engagement with multiple senses and are likely to be the more relatable methods of free expression in contemporary times.

Creative and non-verbal ways of accessing and processing deeper experiences can help therapists access different parts of themselves. These can also feel lighter and be more attractive and engaging for busy therapists. Projective exercises like responding to images or movie clips can help the therapist peep into their own unconscious. Graphical exercises like using timelines, mind maps or algorithms can help organize and make sense of large amounts of information, making them digestible and available for analysis, consideration and reflection. Art expressions are another reflective pathway, where therapists use visual journaling through painting, doodling, sculpting and other exercises to facilitate self-transformation, self-care and learning. Other experiential and body-based exercises that use role-plays, movement and theatre might also facilitate a connection with our immediate experiences and emotional world. This here-and-now awareness can build a more dynamic sense of relating with the self and the other that does not rely solely on verbal expression.

Contemplative practices that encourage tuning inwards, sitting with silence and witnessing our thoughts offer another pathway to foster change and growth in learning environments. Mindfulness practices, meditation and yoga all encourage a stance of openness, allowing us to reflect on our thoughts, sensations and feelings as they emerge in each moment. Through mindfulness practices it may become possible to sit with difficult moments, clear space to think more deeply about ourselves and our work and connect more fully with our clients, without rushing to find quick resolutions (Nugent et al., 2011).

Reflection and critical thinking can be integrated into all our professional activities whether it is the way we write session notes, think and speak about our clients, what we take to supervision and even how we engage with research literature. Searching for larger patterns, looking for underlying meanings and connecting with deeper experiences are all integral aspects of our daily reflection.

When to Reflect?

Reflection can happen spontaneously or deliberately, but it is always useful to set aside time for reflection, whether daily or weekly. Schön (1983) addressed the question of when to reflect, by distinguishing between reflection-in-action and reflection-on-action. Reflection-in-action refers to the process of reflecting on what one is doing while doing it (Lavender, 2003), much like "the hovering hawk in the mind" (Bolton & Delderfield, 2018, p. 66). For the psychotherapist, this implies holding a reflective position during the therapy session. It involves becoming aware of one's own body and emotional reactions and interpreting them to understand what is happening and then using this to guide immediate action. Reflection-on-action, on the other hand, happens after the action is over (or before it starts). It includes analysing one's reactions to experiences in the therapy session and exploring reasons for and consequences of our responses. Here, the focus is more on developing awareness and conceptualizing about the client and the self and connecting this with theory and research. Immediately after the session, when we are still flush with thoughts and feelings, and before defences take over, is an ideal time to ask ourselves, What am I feeling? What am I thinking? or What happened to make me think or feel this way? We are often more open to ourselves when stirred up, so this is the best time to access our experience. Where others might seek to soothe themselves, the reflective therapist seeks to learn.

Information from during and after session, both spontaneous or intuitive and planned or deliberate, is ideally integrated in planning interventions. Taking from the concept of *deliberate practice,* working towards specific goals in a planned and repetitive manner, periodically reviewing progress and sustaining efforts over an extended period, can enhance the effectiveness of reflection (Ericsson & Lehmann, 1996; Rousmaniere, 2017). What appears to distinguish more effective therapists from less effective ones is the amount of time dedicated to reflective activities, such as reviewing challenging cases independently or contemplating past and future sessions (Chow et al., 2015). Giving time to return to an experience repeatedly, in a process of *cyclical reflection,* can enable the therapist to access new nuances and new learning (Turpin & Fitzgerald, 2006).

Reflection in Different Phases of Professional Development

Reflective practice has become an integral part of many training programmes, stemming from the recognition that it offers an opportunity for experiential learning and a deeper understanding of concepts and techniques that conventional training methods cannot provide. While reflection is useful through all phases of professional development, the what, where, how and how much we reflect is also influenced by where we are in our careers.

Before formal training, we often rely on our intelligence, instinct and conventional wisdom to address psychological issues. Theoretical knowledge about what helps and the skills needed to assist may still be nascent and amorphous. Early in the training phase, we begin learning about various psychological and psychotherapeutic perspectives on the self. We may be excited but also overwhelmed by huge amounts of new information. We are also likely to have our first encounters with actual clients. This can lead to anxieties about the self and competence as a therapist and our focus may be more on learning than on reflection. At this stage, mastering step-by-step approaches in the context of supportive supervisory or teaching relationships is typically most helpful.

As we approach the end of our training, it is an ideal time to start reflecting more deeply on different models and theories, considering both their applications and limitations. This can take place through classroom discussions and assignments, as well as through initial experiences of being a therapist. Even as we grow more comfortable in the therapy room, we are often acutely aware of all we do not know yet and continue to rely heavily on supervision. Reflection often takes place within supervision and may be triggered by moments of being stuck in therapy, self-doubt or challenging client responses. At this stage, the desire for certainty and clarity might go counter to the essential uncertainty inherent in the reflective process. Supervisors who balance support and confirmation with challenge and exploration make reflection stimulating rather than overwhelming.

As we advance and become more comfortable with the basic tenets of therapy, we may feel an increased readiness to deepen an awareness of 'self'. At this phase, reflection often focuses on boundaries between self and other, so we learn to stay separate from the client while offering empathy. Reflection on psychological theories coupled with a deeper understanding of the self enables trainees to develop a unique stance or style and gravitate towards or away from particular theoretical orientation(s). We may also wish to reflect on the central role of the therapeutic relationship and what we can do to enhance it. This includes getting more comfortable expressing aspects of the self in the therapy room and asking deeper questions about the therapy process and human psychology.

In the face of real-world challenges, we may look to validate the ideas learned during training, and at times feel disillusioned by them. This often leads to a more intense exploration of the self and the professional environment, as we work to resolve personal and professional tensions and shape our identity as therapists (Rønnestad & Skovholt, 2003). As early career professionals, we are often intrinsically motivated and eager to experience our autonomy. During this phase, we may choose to learn and reflect independently through reading, workshops and other avenues, before seeking formal supervision again.

As our understanding of theory becomes more nuanced, our reflections may begin to centre more on interactions with clients, life experiences, other professions, the arts or spirituality, rather than solely on textbook material. Of course, having these experiences is not enough, it is reflecting on them that converts them into a rich understanding of human nature, self and the process of change in therapy. This allows us to develop greater congruence between our personality and the theoretical orientation we follow, helping us to be more authentic in our sessions. As we come to understand the rules and processes of therapy better, we learn how to modify and adapt them, even questioning the notion of rules. We do grow in both competence and confidence, blending our personal and professional selves, but there can be unexpected challenges at any stage of our career. Even as experienced practitioners, we may find ourselves doubting our abilities or feeling disturbed by negative reactions from clients. These moments can signal the need for a reflective retreat.

As we move further along in our careers and take on roles as teachers, mentors and supervisors, reflection often shifts to include not only our own clinical work but also the therapeutic journeys of our supervisees. In this later phase of professional life, reflection becomes a powerful tool to guard against stagnation, sustain a sense of purpose and cultivate a wisdom worth sharing. Over time, the skilled reflective practitioner weaves together the personal and professional self, bringing insight into their own responses, how these shape therapeutic interactions, and anchoring it in a layered understanding of theory and research.

It could be an interesting exercise to have conversations between our professional selves at different stages of development. What might your novice therapist self feel about the way you maintain session notes now? What advice would your expert therapist self give your student self about asserting boundaries? What might your future therapist self say about your experiences of self-doubt today? As we connect to our growth across different phases of development, we can become more aware of the perspectives and processes that have got stamped in and those that we have left along the way and replaced with new learning. Such reflections can create a feeling of a continuously evolving identity as a psychotherapist.

While reflection is a key pathway for professional growth, too much unsupervised reflection too early can be overwhelming for therapists. Fauth and Williams (2005) warn that particularly for novice therapists, attempts to manage the self during sessions can interfere with the therapy process. Bennett-Levy (2006) echoes this idea, noting that beginner trainees do better at reflecting *on* action rather than reflecting *in* action. As trainees and novice practitioners, we may be more focused on how to respond to the verbal content of sessions—what we hear and speak. Gradually, we may be more able to note and respond to non-verbal content in sessions as they happen. However, we may need the distance and safety that supervision provides, allowing us to go beyond the client's verbal and non-verbal communication and integrate what the session evoked in us.

Pause and reflect…

Think about the phase of professional development you are in now. Perhaps you are a confident trainee, an anxious mid-career practitioner, or transitioning between phases.

What are the primary challenges you are facing as a therapist?

Where Do We Reflect?

While reflection can occur anywhere, it can help to carve out a reflective corner, a space and time that is set apart from busy schedules and commitments. Eventually, just going to this quiet, undisturbed, comfortable and safe space could cue a reflective state. While the image of a solitary thinker is intuitively appealing, learning about ourselves is not always a solo endeavour, as captured in the phrase—it takes two to know one (Culbert, 1970). Being open to learning from peers and supervisors and from our clients can all throw light on aspects of ourselves that we do not otherwise have access to. Trainers, supervisors and mentors who partner in our journey and lead by example are essential in this process. We can learn not only through the way others mirror our psychological realities but also through reflecting on our impact on those around us (Lavender, 2003).

Personal development programmes exclusively focus on the self-of-the-therapist and create opportunities for building self-awareness (McMahon & Rodillas, 2020). These programmes may be structured with specific curriculum and activities or unstructured and exploratory activities such as role-plays and reflective journals. Most times they are facilitated and conducted in groups, especially when they are integral to a training programme. The goal is to create a safe space for reflective practice that fosters personal growth and development for the therapist. An atmosphere of trust and psychological safety is crucial within the group to support the exploration of attachment styles, defences and relational patterns that may influence the therapist's work with clients. Group processes can be challenging and unpredictable, especially as participants delve into intimate and anxiety-provoking experiences. Facilitators will need adequate training and support as they venture into supporting participants.

Other professional activities, such as attending conferences, participating in workshops or engaging in psychotherapy research, can also stimulate reflection. We learn outside the therapy room and draw from our repertoire of life experiences and relationships, and from our engagement with art and literature. A sculpture, painting or theatre performance can evoke deep emotional responses and reveal aspects of human experience in ways that differ from academic texts. Setting aside time to actively reflect on and connect these experiences to therapeutic work is highly recommended.

If we reflect on and engage with our work and selves assiduously, we can develop what Casement (1985) calls the internal supervisor an observing ego which enables the recognition of patterns within ourselves and the client. Our background knowledge including self-awareness, life experience, culture, theory and experiences with clients, all help the therapist make clinical decisions in the foreground of a therapy session. We learn to consult our reflective self while also remaining present and immersed in the therapeutic interaction. Our personal and professional selves come together to create a more unified experience, and we carry our supervisors and reflective spaces within us wherever we go.

Conclusion

We hope that engaging with the ideas in this book supports your continued growth as a practitioner. Reflect on what aspects of your practice you would like to explore further and what you hope to gain from a more reflective approach. As our levels of reflection deepen, we are also better able to support our clients in their reflective journeys. However, it should be noted that reflection alone cannot solve all therapeutic dilemmas and needs to be balanced with practice and theory.

To be effective, the reflective space needs to be playful and creative. It requires both commitment and the belief that it is worth the effort. There is a personal challenge in being open and vulnerable and examining the limitations both within ourselves and in the theories that we deify and love. An experimental approach that focuses on the process of discovery can make the reflective leap a joyous one.

References

Allen, J. G., Fonagy, P., & Bateman, A. W. (2008). What is mentalizing and why do it? In J. G. Allen, P. Fonagy, & A. Bateman (Eds.), *Mentalizing in clinical practice* (pp. 311–322). APPI.

Aponte, H. J., Powell, F. D., Brooks, S., Watson, M. F., Litzke, C., Lawless, J., & Johnson, E. (2009). Training the person of the therapist in an academic setting. *Journal of Marital and Family Therapy, 35*(4), 381–394.

Bennett-Levy, J. (2006). Therapist skills: A cognitive model of their acquisition and refinement. *Behavioural and Cognitive Psychotherapy, 34*, 57–78.

Bennett-Levy, J. (2019). Why therapists should walk the talk: The theoretical and empirical case for personal practice in therapist training and professional development. *Journal of Behavior Therapy and Experimental Psychiatry, 62*, 133–145.

Bolton, G., & Delderfield, R. (2018). *Reflective practice: Writing and professional development*. Sage Publications.

Borton, T. (1970). *Reach, teach and touch: Student concerns and process education*. McGraw Hill.

Casement, P. (1985). *On learning from the patient*. Tavistock/Routledge.

Chabris, C., & Simons, D. (2010). *The invisible gorilla: And other ways our intuitions deceive us*. Crown.

Chaddock, A., Thwaites, R., Bennett-Levy, J., & Freeston, M. (2014). Understanding individual differences in response to Self-Practice and Self-Reflection (SP/SR) during CBT training. *The Cognitive Behaviour Therapist, 7*, Article e14. https://doi.org/10.1017/S1754470X14000142

Chow, D. L., Miller, S. D., Seidel, J. A., Kane, R. T., Thornton, J. A., & Andrews, W. P. (2015). The role of deliberate practice in the development of highly effective psychotherapists. *Psychotherapy, 52*, 337–345.

Culbert, S. (1970). The interpersonal process of self-disclosure: It takes two to know one. In J. Hart & T. Tomlinson (Eds.), *New directions in client-centered therapy.* Houghton Mifflin.

Dimaggio, G., Lysaker, P. H., Carcione, A., Nicolo, G., & Semerari, A. (2008). Know yourself and you shall know the other… to a certain extent: Multiple paths of influence of self-reflection on mindreading. *Consciousness and Cognition, 17*, 778–789.

Driscoll, J. J. (2007). Supported reflective learning: The essence of clinical supervision? In J. Driscoll (Ed.), *Practising clinical supervision: A reflective approach for healthcare professionals* (2nd ed., pp. 27–50). Bailliere Tindall.

Ericsson, K. A., & Lehmann, A. C. (1996). Expert and exceptional performance: Evidence of maximal adaptation to task constraints. *Annual Review of Psychology, 47*, 273–305.

Fauth, J., & Williams, E. (2005). The in-session self-awareness of therapist-trainees: Hindering or helpful? *Journal of Counseling Psychology, 52*, 443–447.

Fook, J., & Gardener, F. (2007). Clarifying our approach to critical reflection. In J. Fook & F. Gardener (Eds.), *Practicing critical reflection: A resource handbook* (pp. 12–21). Open University Press.

Gibbs, G. (1988). *Learning by doing: A guide to teaching and learning methods.* Further Educational Unit, Oxford Polytechnic.

Horowitz, A. (2013). *On looking: Eleven walks with expert eyes.* Scribner.

Johns, C. (2004). *Becoming a reflective practitioner* (2nd ed.). Blackwell.

Johns, C., & Burnie, S. (2013). *Becoming a reflective practitioner* (4th ed.). Wiley.

Kolb, D. A., & Fry, R. (1975). Towards an applied theory of experiential learning. In C. Cooper (Ed.), *Theories of group process* (pp. 33–57). Wiley.

Ladany, N., Friedlander, M. L., & Nelson, M. L. (2005). Towards an event-based understanding of the supervisory process. In N. Ladany, M. L. Friedlander, & M. L. Nelson (Eds.), *Critical events in psychotherapy supervision: An interpersonal approach* (pp. 3–22). American Psychological Association.

Lavender, T. (2003). Redressing the balance: The place, history and future of reflective practice in clinical training. *Clinical Psychology, 27*, 11–19.

Lister, P. G., & Crisp, B. R. (2007). Critical incident analyses: A practice learning tool for students and practitioners. *Practice, 19*, 47–60.

Markham, A. (2017). *Reflexivity: Some techniques for interpretive researchers.* Retrieved from https://annettemarkham.com/2017/02/reflexivity-for-interpretive-researchers/

McMahon, A., & Rodillas, R. R. (2020). Personal development groups during psychotherapy training: Irish students' expectations and experiences of vulnerability, safety and growth. *Counselling Psychology Quarterly, 33*(2), 163–186.

Mezirow, J. (1991). *Transformative dimensions of adult learning.* Jossey-Bass.

Morley, C. (2015). Critical reflexivity and social work practice. In J. D. Wright (Ed.), *International encyclopedia of the social & behavioral sciences* (2nd ed., pp. 281–286). Elsevier.

Nugent, P., Moss, D., Barnes, R., & Wilks, J. (2011). Clear(ing) space: Mindfulness-based reflective practice. *Reflective Practice, 12*(1), 1–13.

Orlinsky, D. E., Rønnestad, M. H., & Willutzki, U. (2004). Fifty years of psychotherapy process-outcome research: Continuity and change. In M. J. Lambert (Ed.), *Bergin and Garfield's handbook of psychotherapy and behavior change* (pp. 307–391). Wiley.

Plath, S. (1989). *Collected poems* (5th ed.). Faber and Faber.

Rober, P. (2017). Addressing the person of the therapist in supervision: The therapist's inner conversation method. *Family Process, 56*(2), 487–500.

Rolfe, G., Freshwater, D., & Jasper, M. (2001). *Critical reflection in nursing and the helping professions: A user's guide*. Palgrave Macmillan.
Rønnestad, M. H., & Skovholt, T. M. (2003). The journey of the counselor and therapist: Research findings and perspectives on professional development. *Journal of Career Development, 30*, 5–44.
Rousmaniere, T. (2017). *Deliberate practice for psychotherapists: A guide to improving clinical effectiveness*. Routledge.
Satir, V. (2000). The therapist story. In M. Baldwin (Ed.), *The use of self in therapy* (2nd ed., pp. 17–28). Haworth.
Schön, D. A. (1983). *The reflective practitioner*. Basic Books.
Skovholt, T. M., Rønnestad, M. H., & Jennings, L. (1997). Searching for expertise in counseling, psychotherapy, and professional psychology. *Educational Psychology Review, 9*, 361–369.
Stedmon, J., Mitchell, A., Johnstone, L., & Staite, S. (2003). Making reflective practice real: Problems and solutions in the South West. *Clinical Psychology, 27*, 30–33.
Thompson, N., & Pascal, J. (2012). Developing critically reflective practice. *Reflective Practice: International and Multidisciplinary Perspectives, 13*(2), 311–325.
Thwaites, R., Bennett-Levy, J., Davis, M., & Chaddock, A. (2014). Using self-practice and self-reflection (SP/SR) to enhance CBT competence and metacompetence. In A. Whittington & N. Grey (Eds.), *How to become a more effective CBT therapist: Mastering metacompetence in clinical practice* (pp. 241–254). Wiley Blackwell.
Tripp, D. (1993). *Critical incidents in teaching: Developing professional judgment*. Routledge.
Turpin, M., & Fitzgerald, C. (2006). *Clinical reasoning and reflective practice*. The University of Queensland, St. Lucia.
Winnicott, D. W. (1971). *Playing and reality*. Tavistock Publications.
Yalom, I. D. (2017). *Becoming myself: A psychiatrist's memoir*. Basic Books.

Chapter 2
Tracing Motivations to Become a Therapist

We belong to a profession that seeks to understand the motivation for everything. We have explanations for why artists paint pictures, why astrophysicists seek to understand the universe, or what inspires social media influencers to build a following. However, how often do we step back and reflect on what motivates us to do the work we do? Understanding motivations is relevant whether one has dreamt of becoming a therapist their whole life or found it as part of a mid-life career change. The meaning we get from work can change and evolve with different factors coming to the fore at each stage of the career path. Motives are not always in our conscious awareness, and even if they are, we may not have actively articulated them. As we reflect on ourselves as therapists, or as clients in our personal therapy, we become more aware of the myriad influences that drew us towards therapy as a profession and continue to keep us invested today.

Not many therapists would describe their choice of profession as just a job. Most are passionate about their work, feeling grateful and privileged at being able to play the role of a healer. The satisfaction of being able to make a difference in someone's life, the thrill of navigating a complex client presentation or the joy from the deep connections formed, can all contribute to the layered, complex and unique meaning attributed to being a therapist. Work can become an integral part of personal identity and add meaning to the therapist's sense of self, often sustaining them through challenging experiences. This profession presents many opportunities for self-discovery and growth. As therapists walk along with clients through their inner landscapes, there is an increasing acceptance of both the light and shadow within. Yet, the very qualities of empathy and openness that enrich therapeutic work also bring therapists into regular contact with the more difficult dimensions of human experience. In bearing witness to losses that might remain ambiguous and questions that resist easy answers, therapists often find that outcomes unfold slowly, with success presenting in subtle and unexpected forms. Loneliness and isolation can be part of the territory, leaving therapists vulnerable to emotionally exhaustion, disillusionment or even hopelessness. The earning potential of this profession can also be variable

P. Bhola et al., *Reflective Practice in Psychotherapy and Counselling*,
https://doi.org/10.1007/978-981-96-9732-8_2

and uncertain, particularly for early career practitioners or those who live and work in certain settings or in majority-world contexts. Despite these challenges, the idea of psychotherapy and examining the self as a means to a more authentic life has captured the imaginations of many people across the world. Film, television and social media are flooded with images of therapists at work, and psychotherapy is increasingly valued as a career option. As we navigate the pushes and pulls and the highs and lows of being a therapist, getting and staying in touch with our motivations can be very useful.

Perhaps just as therapists ask clients what has brought them to therapy, they need to ask themselves what has brought them to the profession (Sussman, 2007). We can explore which aspect of being a therapist feels most fulfilling or ponder on which of our needs it meets. Such musings may surface in the midst of an intense session with a client, during supervision or a job interview, in times of professional crisis, or even when introducing ourselves in personal or professional settings. While some answers can be found more easily, a deeper understanding of underlying motivations tends to emerge gradually. Multiple motivators can simultaneously influence and interact with each other, resulting in a more complex experience. Understanding how these motivators influence one another and pinpointing which are most significant at a given moment calls for thoughtful analysis.

Continued reflection helps illuminate how these factors shape the kind of therapist one becomes, the clients one gravitates toward, and the therapeutic models that resonate best. In this chapter, we explore possible motivations for entering and remaining with the profession of psychotherapy and counselling. We delve into revelatory therapist narratives and share reflective activities that can guide you to locate your motivations. The chapter concludes with an exploration of the ways in which motivations colour therapeutic interactions and processes.

Peeling the Onion: Exploring Therapist Motivations

In her book *Strangers Drowning: Grappling with Impossible Idealism, Drastic Choices, and the Overpowering Urge to Help,* Larissa MacFarquhar (2015) explores the concept of extreme altruism. While it is true that all human beings are interconnected and feel empathy for each other, there are only some who would donate a kidney to a stranger, adopt several children or, like social activist Baba Amte, eschew privilege to live with and work for the welfare of persons with leprosy. Reading essays from this book provokes reflections about people who place giving and goodness at the centre of their lives. MacFarquhar delves into the motivations for their extraordinary commitments and discusses the layer of narcissism that can lie beneath extreme moral positions. As therapists, we can be stimulated to question what makes such giving meaningful and what one stands to gain or lose through such choices. This can also open a line of questioning about our own accepted motives.

Therapists often cite altruism as a primary motivator to choose their profession, sharing how they feel rewarded by making a difference in another human being's life

(McBeath, 2019). The feeling of being able to alleviate suffering, promote growth and make a valuable contribution to society can be a very warm and affirming one. This can increase self-esteem and a general sense of well-being, giving a *helper's high* (Luks, 1988). Altruism also tends to be recognized and celebrated by others and it can be tempting to see ourselves in the prosocial and powerful roles of solvers, protectors or rescuers. If therapists find it difficult to relinquish this image, it can leave less space for clients to use their own strengths and resources (Rober & Seltzer, 2010). Driven by a strong desire to help, a therapist can slip into advice-giving and persuasion, ultimately hindering our clients' psychological growth. The determination to see clients get better can sometimes manifest as disappointment over the slowness of change, possibly leaving the client feeling inadequate.

Condensing all our motivations into the overarching theme of altruism can result in an incomplete understanding of the self. The awareness of deeper layers of motivation often emerges through reflections on smaller moments in therapy. When we ask ourselves, Why did I just agree to schedule that extra session?, we might recognize how our personal needs, perhaps for validation, achievement or even domination, have come into play. A therapist's reflections on a sharp emotional response to an 'ungrateful' client might get them in touch with their deep need for appreciation (Gabbard, 2000). Therapists can also reflect on patterns that become evident over time. For instance, noting that, I find myself being more directly helpful with older clients, could guide the therapist to explore their relationship with authority figures and their need to care for them or get their approval. Patterns that emerge from the therapist's personal lives can spill over into their professional roles. Someone with unresolved grief may find themselves particularly affected by clients who are processing loss. Another therapist might feel an urge to rescue a client who reminds them of a younger sibling or friend they were once unable to help. A quiet sense of vicarious fulfilment could be experienced while working with a client who makes a life change that the therapist has long desired for themselves.

Motivations that are less socially or personally acceptable are often obscured beneath more palatable narratives. Statements like I want to help those in need, can come more easily to our minds than, I can only be truly myself when I am with my clients. Even when we do not recognize, acknowledge or articulate our more complex drivers, they can quietly shape therapeutic choices, including the kind of clients one gravitates towards, the emotional tone of the work and the boundaries one holds, or fails to hold. Critically, these dynamics are not inherently pathological or disqualifying. Rather, they are part of the human complexity that therapists bring into the room and call for awareness and reflective scrutiny.

Pause and reflect...

When you think about what motivated you to be a therapist, what is the first thought that springs to your mind?

As you reflect on your interactions with clients, can you identify any personal needs that frequently make themselves felt? These could be needs for connection and intimacy, validation, control and power, safety and healing, or the search for a sense of purpose…

We do not always take the time to pause and mull over the full range and depth of motivations that drive us in our work. It might be a transformational moment when we engage with the question: "Why did you train to become a therapist? Why did you *really* train to become a therapist?" (Adams, 2014, p. 10). In exploring how this complex web of motivations enters the therapy room, it becomes essential to integrate positive attributes, experiences and strengths alongside vulnerabilities and wounds. There is no single ideal motivation. Rather, the most valuable ideal may be the capacity for honest awareness and acceptance of actual motivations. A coherent story that links past and present experiences to what drives therapists in the therapy room can pave the way for this deeper self-awareness and understanding.

The Storied Lives of Therapists

The best understanding of the motivations to become therapists comes from the deeply personal autobiographical accounts that several therapists have shared. These evocative narratives involve a process of looking within, looking back and also looking forward and illuminate a complex mingling of chance, choice and circumstance in the process of becoming a psychotherapist. Engaging with such stories can stimulate reflections about our own narratives as well.

As we embark on a journey of self-exploration, it is helpful to start at the beginning through reflections on the various reasons that led us to *choose* this identity and profession. For some, the initial impetus to enter the profession may have been availability and access to a training programme, or even just chance. Others may have drawn inspiration from significant others, teachers, mentors or even a family member who in the profession. Personal attributes and interests such as intellectual curiosity, patience, fascination with the inner world, an early interest in reading and an inclination towards the humanities often play a formative role (Duggal & Sriram, 2016). These early motivations eventually meet the lived experience of the work itself, where therapists find resonance and reward in drawing on their empathic abilities, relational skills and communicative strengths. A therapist's inner world, complete with flaws, vulnerabilities and inner conflicts, contributes to their presence in the therapy room. This is a rare space where all our experiences, successes, failures, gifts and weaknesses can be used intentionally and meaningfully for the benefit of others. And this can be deeply validating for us as human beings.

It is through this lens that we begin to understand how the diverse and layered experiences of our lives have contributed to who we are and quietly guided us towards this profession. Positive family experiences can draw individuals closer to this career by shaping their capabilities as well as their vision of a therapist's role and identity. For example, a therapist raised in an environment that encouraged open dialogue may feel more comfortable sharing their emotions, even difficult ones. This ease can translate into their therapeutic practice, where they empower clients to express their emotions, thoughts and experiences more freely. Reflecting on why she became a psychotherapist, McCullough (2005) spoke of family members who were models of generosity and compassion and of deeply held family values about helping those in need. The sense of being loved and cared for in environments which fostered independence and self-expression has been a powerful theme across several therapist narratives (e.g., Orlinsky, 2005).

Therapists' recollections of their childhood and adult lives also encompass experiences of struggles, unmet needs and trauma. Feelings of invalidation and loneliness arising from difficult family contexts involving parental marital conflict, parental mental illness, loss and separations from loved ones, and experiences with illness or disability have been noted as critical influences (Duggal & Sriram, 2016; McBeath, 2019). Speaking of the impact of her mother's depressive illness, Brown (2005) shared how she became acutely sensitive to interpersonal and emotional nuance as a young child, constantly alert to the emotions and needs of her family members. Quite early on, she took on the role of putting the "familial Humpty Dumpty back together again" (p. 952). These experiences, coupled with her feelings of being an outsider at school, led her to become a psychotherapist—a relational space where she felt at home with herself. Some therapists' narratives contain evocative descriptions of themselves as the *parentified child* or the *white knight,* seeking to process their own difficult childhood experiences and rescue others in similar situations (Bryce et al, 2023; Street, 2014). A sense of disconnection can also arise from personal experiences of social exclusion and displacement. Living through such difficult experiences could lend a sharply attuned sensitivity to the pain of others and those who are othered. The continual opportunities for attuned and authentic connection in the therapy room can offer a salve for subjective feelings of loneliness and disconnection. These trajectories suggest that some therapists have professionalized their early experiences by becoming psychotherapists in their adult lives.

Sometimes, it is a personal journey of healing and resilience rather than early family influences, that charts the route to a helping profession. Personal experiences of being in therapy, whether during childhood or adulthood, frequently emerge as pivotal moments in therapist narratives. For some, these experiences reveal the transformative potential of psychotherapy, inspiring a desire to offer the same to others (Bager-Charleson, 2010). For others, a negative encounter with therapy may fuel a commitment to doing things differently and contributing to change within the field (Hill et al., 2013). Additionally, some individuals aspire to provide others with therapeutic support they felt was lacking in their own lives (Mahoney & Eiseman, 2014). Such personal experiences, whether affirming or challenging, can bring home the value of the therapeutic endeavour, inspiring individuals to pursue a career in psychotherapy.

The impact extends beyond the decision to enter the profession; it also influences the kind of therapist one chooses to become. For instance, a preference for long-term engagement or a belief in the transformational power of groups can evolve from a recognition of what was personally helpful. Difficult childhood experiences, such as having a mother who suffered from postnatal depression, might lead a therapist to work directly with children or to focus on the systemic factors contributing to depression in adult women. Legacies of early experiences can manifest in subtle ways, as illustrated by a therapist who felt helpless in childhood and now tends to assert more control during sessions (Bager-Charleson, 2010).

Our stories are interwoven with strands that connect across generations and are linked to familial and historical events that might have occurred even before we were born. Gaps, silences and disconnections punctuate this narrative and joining all the echoes and fragments is not easy. As we begin to understand the complex amalgamation of all these influences, it becomes clear that our stories are not entirely our own. In a deeply reflective account, Hammer (2020) shared a moment of epiphany when he uncovered a family secret and realized that he was a transgenerational Holocaust survivor. His grandfather's revelation brought to awareness how feelings of unspoken grief about losses had reverberated across generations and informed his own world view and life choices. Both past and present contexts seem to have intertwined to influence his motivations to become a therapist, his involvement in civil resistance protests against nuclear weapons and his commitment to social justice work.

Current experiences or contexts usually intersect with past experiences, combining to create a larger narrative about why we do what we do. As each of us constructs our stories, it is useful to consider all possible influences to build an awareness of the needs and motivations they engender.

Pause and reflect...

Use the *Life Story* approach (McAdams, 2001) to trace the strands of motivations that coalesced to lead you towards the profession of psychotherapy. Begin by thinking about your life as if it were a book or novel, with the phases of your life as chapters. Then pause and focus on some key memorable scenes. These could include *high points* (e.g. winning the college scholarship), *low points* (e.g. a lingering childhood illness), a *turning point* (e.g. migrating to another country), both positive and negative *childhood memories* (e.g. summers with doting grandparents, the time father left home), and vivid *adult memories* (e.g. birth of a child). As the story unfolds, trace a *wisdom event*, one in which you acted in a wise way or provided wise counsel to others. You can also search for *religious, spiritual or mystical experiences*, where you felt a sense of transcendence or oneness.

As you construct your life story, reflect on what happened, where and when, who was involved, and what you remember thinking and feeling. Identifying your key values and beliefs and situating the challenges in your journey, can guide you towards a new understanding of their reverberations through your story. A central life theme can emerge from this immersive exploration, linking your important motivators in a meaningful and personally relevant way.

The process of looking back at our life can be emotionally charged, and as we encounter the unknown within ourselves, we may not always like what we discover. It is important to engage in this exercise with self-compassion, giving time for reflections and meanings to emerge. As the awareness of our own stories grows, it can enhance the understanding of interactions with clients. Interestingly, it can also help us map how our identity as a therapist interweaves with this story, and the paths that lie ahead of us. It seems that we are indeed our stories.

The Wound is Where the Light Comes in

Marsha Linehan is known for developing dialectical behaviour therapy, a pioneering treatment for individuals with concerns of self-harm and personality vulnerabilities. In an interview in 2011, she decided to reveal her personal struggles with mental health during her adolescent years, after a patient asked her—Are you one of us? "I honestly didn't realize at the time that I was dealing with myself, she said. But I suppose it's true that I developed a therapy that provides the things I needed for so many years and never got" (Carey, 2011). Linehan's journey from being wounded to becoming a healer embodies the motif of resilience and transformation embedded in the wounded healer archetype.

The archetype of the *wounded healer* (Jung, 1963) connects closely with the idea that it is their vulnerabilities that may lead therapists to this profession. Speaking about wounds, the poet Rumi (1997, p. 142) says, "That is where the light enters you". These words exemplify the positioning of the wounded healer motif in the therapeutic process. Experiences of pain and vulnerability are often seen as conferring an advantage to therapists, who can use them to build an empathic bridge with their clients. For instance, a therapist hurt by parental neglect in childhood could be sensitive to subtle or disguised signs of similar wounds in her client, something a person with a more secure childhood might miss. The therapist may demonstrate skills and commitment in reaching out to her client and in turn could learn new perspectives and solutions that she can then apply to herself. This can create a cycle of shared healing where we heal ourselves as we help others heal. The sense of woundedness among therapists can range from being a core part of their identity to something seen as peripheral to their current life. It is through reflection that personal experiences of woundedness can be harnessed and used as strengths. Reflections on the spaces that wounds occupy in our minds and relationships, and how they are soothed within ourselves and in our interactions, can help make meaning of how they might be guiding our lives and our work. As we connect with our own healing journeys and understand how we deal with our emotions, mentalize our selves and our relationships and try new behaviours, we gain a very personal understanding of our clients' journeys. The possibilities that have emerged in our own lives can help us convey a sense of hope to clients who despair of ever feeling differently.

Therapists may feel compelled to bring their learnings into their work with individuals who seem to have similar experiences and wounds. A therapist who is a survivor of child sexual abuse could choose to work with and build services for other survivors. This can become the cornerstone of how she identifies professionally, through becoming a spokesperson, engaging with advocacy or supporting research and training in the area. Here, the wound fuels passion for the work, adding a depth that might otherwise be difficult to achieve. Conversely, wounds can sometimes be detrimental to therapeutic work, notably when they dominate the therapist's perspective but remain unaddressed. A wound that is hidden, compartmentalized or even forgotten often enters the room in disguise.

While we are always available to hear our clients' stories, there may be less openness to reflecting on and resolving our own disappointments, anxieties and pain, even as we realize how this is connected to our work and well-being. Both therapists and clients may share the belief that individuals in helping professions should be invulnerable and in perfect mental health. The image of the therapist as a *guru* or a benevolent dispenser of wisdom predominates in certain cultures and contexts (Neki, 1973), and this could encourage therapists to represent themselves as well adjusted or even flawless. Clients who put the therapist on a pedestal, feeling that I can never be as good as you, can hesitate to disclose their vulnerabilities and feel inadequate or discouraged in their struggles. Therapists who feel that I must be perfect for you, can end up setting unrealistic standards for clients and themselves, ultimately jeopardizing the authenticity of the therapeutic relationship. Therapists who need to hide from their own shortcomings are less likely to challenge such perceptions. Instead, we recommend modelling humility, self-acceptance or self-compassion, as this can be more inspiring for clients along their journey of change. When we are genuinely comfortable with our flaws and seek an equal relationship with clients, this attitude is communicated through both verbal and non-verbal behaviours. For example, a subtle gesture like a raised eyebrow in response to excessive praise can signal to the client that we might not fully agree with them. Using humour to draw the client's attention to their idealizing stance can be effective, sometimes leading to a deeper conversation about how the client views themselves vis-à-vis others in their world.

Psychological wounds, while holding significant potential for therapeutic growth, can become an Achilles' heel when working with specific clients who trigger those vulnerabilities (Zerubavel & Wright, 2012). In such situations, there is the risk of overidentifying with clients and being blindsided by intense countertransferential reactions. The process of stepping into the client's shoes while keeping one foot in their own can be disrupted if therapists stay immersed in their own emotions and memories. At times, therapists may feel that their important truths and solutions must be imparted to clients for them to follow or emulate. Alternatively, therapists may wish to use their experience as a cautionary tale, becoming too directive in urging clients to take a different path. Either approach can serve the therapist's needs rather than the client's, hindering the ability to be truly present and attuned to client distress. At the same time, an excessive focus on the client can hinder therapists from recognizing their own distress, leading to the neglect of legitimate self-care needs even as their inner resources become increasingly depleted. We bring a critical lens to the wounded-healed binary and the implicit assumption that only the *completely* healed therapist can be effective. Not every story needs a redemption arc; rather, healing and change are nonlinear, ongoing processes that are integral to the human experience. As therapists, we can operate from both positions and identities—being wounded and being a healer—and these are not fixed but mutable. The ways in which we experience and use our woundedness can also vary across situations—sometimes working as a strength and at other times adversely impacting the therapeutic process.

Pause and reflect...

Has there been a moment in therapy when a client's narrative brought an old wound alive for you?

In what way did it impact therapy process?

How did you care for yourself in that moment?

For some like British psychiatrist Ahmed Hankir (2022), the identity of wounded healer is a central motif in their relationship with the profession. Through *The Wounded Healer Project,* he shares his personal story of mental health struggles, dislocation due to civil war in Lebanon and experiences of marginalization and discrimination associated with his religious beliefs. He uses storytelling and film to power his mission to reduce stigma and advocate for practitioners with mental health vulnerabilities. More and more therapists are speaking about their mental health journeys, for example, identifying themselves as neurodivergent on their social media handles. This sends out a message about their own positionality and may also influence which clients seek them, how they are seen by clients, and the processes and interactions in the therapy room.

There are many complexities related to therapists' disclosure of personal struggles and wounds to clients, members of the professional community and the public. While understanding the wounded healer duality facilitates deeper sharing and growth for clients, it is important to assess whether the therapist is in a place to discuss personal narratives without losing emotional control or requiring clients to provide support. The therapist can sometimes feel like they have unwittingly opened a Pandora's box inviting more curiosity and concern from the client than they are ready for. Therapists who choose to open their personal lives to clients also need to respectfully negotiate boundaries, clarifying how much they are willing to share and why. Clients may be made uncomfortable by such disclosures, necessitating careful reflection on the degree and timing of sharing, as well as whose needs are being prioritized. The dilemma of whether to conceal or reveal becomes more complex when mental health vulnerabilities, such as schizophrenia, bipolar disorder or experiences in inpatient psychiatric care, carry significant public stigma (Cvetovac & Adame, 2017). This challenge arises not only from fears of negative and discriminatory attitudes from others but also from internalized stigma and shame, both of which can impede the willingness to share lived experiences.

While many wounds are psychological and internal, others cannot be masked as easily. The decision here is not whether to reveal or not, but whether to conceal or not. In her evocative autoethnography, Stirling (2020) courageously explores the journey from concealment to visibility of her self-harm scars within the therapeutic setting. She shares the struggles with feelings of fear and shame about being seen as different, weak and less competent by peers, supervisors and others in professional spaces. Stirling navigates this complex emotional and ethical terrain to reach a place of deliberate vulnerability. The turning point comes when she stops wearing long-sleeved shirts and chooses to show her scars during sessions with a client for the first time. This gradual progression is marked by a greater self-acceptance, a reclaiming of her body and possibilities for closer connection with her client. In essence, Stirling's experience provides a reflexive framework for therapists to negotiate these complex decisions. The eventual decision may vary across therapists, and choosing to keep vulnerabilities and wounds off the table is also a valid choice.

Woundedness, healing and the profession of psychotherapy seem to be yoked together in many ways. We must be careful before concluding that therapists are more likely to have experienced pain and trauma than others. Perhaps therapists tend to remember and respond to their life experiences differently—holding on to them as they delve into their possible meaning and impact (Farber et al., 2005). We might also ponder whether it is essential to acknowledge ourselves as wounded healers in order to be effective therapists. Many therapists, both trainees and practitioners, do make a connection between their career choice and their motivations to explore and resolve their personal problems (Bhola et al., 2017; Orlinsky & Rønnestad, 2005). But this is not everyone's story. In fact, Hoyt (2005) argues that seeing therapists solely through the wounded healer lens may overly pathologize motivations and the commitment to being psychotherapists. There are, of course, many more dimensions to our experience—the people we meet, the books we read, the places we travel to, the events we participate in and what is happening in the world—that collectively shape our sensitivities and inclinations. By delving deeper, we can enhance our awareness of the complex web of motivations that lead us to enter and remain in the profession and impact how we approach our work.

How Our Motivations Enter the Therapy Room

Entering and staying in this profession are driven by many conscious and unconscious motivations. These motivations are often brought into play at decision-making junctures in a therapist's professional career. As an undercurrent through the psychotherapy process, they can also have an impact in terms of both moment-to-moment therapist–client interactions and overall psychotherapeutic outcomes. For instance, an altruistically motivated therapist who takes pride in being able to help their clients may find it easier to temporarily tune out their own life and needs and be there for the client. A wounded healer who has found a path out of their own troubles might find it easier to be patient or hopeful in the face of their client's struggles. A therapist who retains their curiosity and fascination for the vagaries of human nature may find it easier to stay invested with clients along the ups and downs of their journeys. Therapists are ideally aware of their needs and able to separate them from what their clients are looking for. Straight off the bat, we need to appreciate that what we most want for ourselves from our work—whether a sense of accomplished control or an intimate connection with another—may not be what our clients need from us.

Annie was an experienced therapist, known for being gentle and empathic. She had experienced conflict with her mother, who wanted her to get married rather than become a professional. Annie had stuck to her path and later married a man of her choice. She now had a beautiful home, a teenage daughter, a happy marriage and had made peace with her mother. Her only concern was about her daughter who seemed disinterested in a career, instead shifting from one short- term course to another. Noor was a young woman seeking therapeutic support to manage her low mood. Her parents were divorced and continued to be inconsistent in their parenting—sometimes offering love and possessions and at other times being critical. They were particularly concerned about her use of cannabis and her relationship with a controlling boyfriend. Both her mother and boyfriend disapproved of her ambition to build a career through her artistic talent. Annie and Noor hit it off instantly. Over the course of therapy, there were significant changes in Noor's ability to contain her emotions and negotiate her relationships. Annie felt very deeply for her client and really wanted to support her desire to be financially independent as an artist. She was conscious of an occasional stab of outrage and anger at Noor's parents, particularly her mother, who did not seem to appreciate how courageous her daughter was.

Annie is a therapist who finds joy in being able to help others find happiness, as she has managed to find it for herself. She does not give up on her clients, and this is a huge part of her success as a therapist. However, these altruistic feelings could also play out in complicated ways. What might happen to Annie's feelings towards Noor if she stops improving? What if Noor gives up on her art or does not want to break up with her abusive boyfriend? A therapist whose sense of self depends a little too much on their ability to help may experience distress and discomfort with clients who do not change or heal as their therapist desires them to. This distress can manifest itself in annoyance, withdrawal from or rejection of the client. This in turn can impact the therapeutic relationship and therefore client progress—a vicious cycle that can trap both the well-meaning therapist and the frustrated client. Some therapists may try to help too much by offering extra sessions, free sessions, home visits and personal resources, so that they can be there for the client *every* time they need it, even at a personal cost. As they become more experienced, therapists may stay clear of such dangerous waters, but can still find themselves emotionally giving more, spending more time thinking about this one client or searching even harder for ways and means to help.

Therapist in-session behaviour could be motivated by their personal needs, desires and conflicts which may lead to over-identification or under-identification with the client's experience. Occasionally, we may find ourselves trying to relive certain experiences through our client in the hope of achieving a different outcome. Such an experience can come in the way of the therapeutic alliance, goals and processes in therapy. We may limit explorations of our clients' feelings and responses to align with our own or even push for the same resolution in our clients' stories. In a deeply personal account, Adams (2014) shared how her client's struggles with a night shift resonated with her own previous experience. She recalled having to quit a difficult job and choosing a career shift to begin training as a psychotherapist. During sessions, she found herself repeatedly encouraging her client to reflect on the purpose and meaning behind his work. Finally, her client shared that he was invested in his work and only wanted a change in timings—it seemed that it was the *therapist* who wanted him to leave his job.

Fears of not being good enough, not being respected or failing can leave therapists feeling very vulnerable in sessions. They may address these fears by trying to be more structured, exerting control over interactions and outcomes or aiming for perfection in themselves and their clients. For instance, being liked, valued and accepted by her clients could act as a balm for Annie which soothed her from her mother's initial rejection. But this can also leave her overly sensitive to perceived rejection. Anything less than the perfect response from Noor, even a slight disconnection or dissatisfaction, might make Annie evaluate herself and her therapeutic skill negatively.

Therapists' awareness and reflection on their needs, drives, wishes and fears enable a working through of these issues, keeping them from interfering with the process of psychotherapy. For instance, Annie's struggle with her own daughter might be pushing her to at least achieve success with Noor, by persuading her to take up a more stable profession. If Annie is aware of this, she can keep it from interfering with her client's choices and goals. In fact, therapists need not just put away their motives but can use them to bring a deeper and more nuanced understanding to the session. Annie's experience with difficult career choices both within herself and with her daughter can increase her sensitivity to Noor's internal struggles. Therapy is in essence a very intimate enterprise, and as therapists, our needs for intimacy can also get expressed in sessions. Emotional neediness or dependency can be a significant personal contributor for therapists who fail to maintain adequate boundaries in therapy. For instance, therapists who have more difficult and complex relationships in their real lives can seek the safe and controlled intimacy of the therapeutic space. Noor can never threaten Annie as her own daughter can. Annie can pour all her tenderness into Noor while remaining in control of the encounter. She can terminate or taper sessions, prescribe topics for discussion and subtly stay away from material that is threatening to herself. Time spent with clients can start to feel more rewarding than time in personal relationships, keeping therapists vested in their client's appreciation. Thus, Annie may miss opportunities to challenge Noor and might be scared to confront her on her drug use. If Annie hesitates to bring her own reactions and emotions into the session, she could be less authentic in the session. She may want to hide her vulnerabilities and confusions from Noor and so retreat into an expert position when Noor might need her warmth.

Addressing one's motivations in sessions can be built into regular practice. If Annie had reflected on her work with Noor, she might have asked herself why she was having such strong reactions. She might want to explore where her empathy ends, and her control of the session begins. She could become more aware of her own needs and take steps to meet them outside the session, by improving her relationship with her daughter, for instance. She may decide to start supervision to help keep her needs for altruism, narcissism or intimacy in check. If she recognizes that while she has come far, she still has areas of insecurity or times when she shuts down, she may decide to seek personal therapy.

Annie has many strengths as a therapist, not the least of which is her relatively successful negotiation of her life hurdles and the confidence this has brought her, as well as her empathy, curiosity and desire to help. But we all have buttons, and we all have blind spots. A willingness to become aware of and reflect on them, and act on our learnings, is critical to our growth as therapists. Everybody brings something of themselves and their life experience into therapy. It is how we understand, acknowledge, deal with and actively use them that counts.

The Second Act: Psychotherapy as a Second Career

A Therapist Speaks: Lost and Found

Roy Sinai

I've worn several hats: banker, corporate leader, photographer, performer, mentor, counsellor. A 'people person' – this is what connects the dots across these diverse identities. I had never imagined that I would eventually be a certified counsellor. Or that becoming a therapist relatively later in life would feel so profoundly right. Digging deeper to uncover my motivation and resonance with counselling reveals a very personal healing journey. Perhaps because it has only now begun to reveal itself to me, through the work. The wounds and scars are both physical and psychological. The journey of awareness, recognition and change remains a work in progress.

Unlike some who know their dream and follow it with single-minded focus, I did not know what I wanted to do when I graduated from college. A bank was the first company to offer me a job. I took it. I spent the first eighteen years of my working life, from 22 to 40, as a corporate man. Despite the success and growth, the visibility and spotlight, I felt trapped and unhappy. I read the signals as an opportunity to step off the track I was on and as a chance to manifest my inner artist. In hindsight, true self-care was ignored. Instead, I spent the next two decades in re-inventions that still focused on what was outside: status, fame, reputation, external approval and validation.

This untraveled road was not a walk in the park. It twisted and turned. I tried new things and found myself exploring new vistas. Sometimes, I ended up stuck. Outcomes - not always 'as planned' or hoped for - created situations that I was not prepared for and mishandled. Instead of a litany of victorious milestones, this period resembles a graveyard, littered with loss and disappointment. Changes and transitions create trade-offs: they are a 'Lost & Found'. I had lost status and money and a way of life. I had lost an identity, and power. I had found freedom. I had found time to explore. This was energizing as it was confusing and messy. I was somehow living the worst of possible outcomes rather than the best ones I had imagined.

It took a series of major personal losses – of relationships, friends, health, and parts of myself – to truly wake me up to the need for a much more radical, inside-out, reinvention of self. That journey brings me to today. Among the most difficult of these losses was while caregiving for several friends who found themselves diagnosed with a scary, chronic medical condition; but who could not face themselves or their families with this news, due to stigma. Instead, they came to me for advice and care. One of them passed away – leaving me shocked, grieving, and bereft. This toll on my emotional and physical health was followed by my own diagnosis with a life-threatening illness. A surgical intervention and the loss of a couple of organs pronounced me free of illness, and I finally started paying serious attention to wellness and self-care.

Friends urged me to see a psychiatrist. I reluctantly got an evaluation done. Our session snowballed into a long free-wheeling conversation of nearly two hours, during which he told me he would not be prescribing any pills and suggested that I should seriously consider becoming a counsellor myself. This doctor's visit turned out to be a turning point for me. It confirmed what I vaguely knew about myself and validated me in a way that I needed to hear and absorb.

Starting over again, I enrolled in a yearlong certification program as a counsellor. I also experienced first-hand the power of the mind–body connection in my own healing journey. Being trained as a counsellor has provided me with theoretical frameworks and structures through which I revisit, reinforce, and build on my experiences. It has opened the door for me to continue ongoing inner work and offers me a new lens through which to see myself, and through which I may be seen.

In this 'Lost & Found', I've understood that I am always learning the steps to my life's rhythm. My motivation is personal healing. The vast subject of psychology sustains me. It keeps me growing. I am integrating my many identities and seeing myself afresh.

My reward is to be a mirror to others on their journeys, so that they too may see themselves.

And now, I am a keeper of stories.

Roy Sinai *follows an integrative approach in his therapy work. He works with adults, couples, families and adolescents in his practice in India. He started his academic journey with a BA in Economics from Harvard University in 1987 and is currently pursuing a master's degree in psychology.*

Not all of us begin our careers as therapists. Part-way through other careers, some of us might have found ourselves looking around for something more. This desire could have arisen from a mid-life review that highlighted dissatisfaction with the current path. Alternatively, it might have been sparked by a disruptive life event that compelled a search for greater meaning and connection within uncharted waters. We speculate that a willingness to examine life choices and make changes represents a certain openness about both the self and life. Whatever the underlying reasons, individuals who enter psychotherapy as a second career are often more conscious and intentional about what they seek from the profession and why. Much like those who joined the profession early, mid-career change therapists can also be influenced by the long shadow of childhood experiences, altruistic zeal or a search for meaning. Deeper reasons for such a shift can emerge over time, as more parts of the self are acknowledged and understood.

Previous professional experiences can interact with current ones in varied ways. Some individuals transition from careers that differ significantly from therapy, seeking to move away from that past self as they reinvent themselves. For those who found their jobs empty of connection or very routine in nature, everything about being a therapist may feel entirely new—both exciting and unfamiliar at the same time. At the same time, there may be a growing appreciation for the wisdom and experience carried forward, and for the value of having inhabited more than one world. For therapists who have worked in other professions, it is important to recognize that elements of a previous role can remain deeply embedded. They can remain watchful for old behaviours and patterns, especially those that do not align well with their new professional role. For instance, the former teacher may need to let go of his habit of instruction and the former lawyer may need to let go of her goal of winning the argument.

While still on the outside looking in, one might form a picture of what therapy is and what therapists do. It is often this image that captivates, influencing both the choice of orientation and the setting in which work takes place. It is only when practice begins that there is a true sense of what being a therapist really means. What a therapist actually enjoys about being in the therapy room may be very different from their previous expectations. Motivations for entering the profession often evolve alongside experience, making it essential to keep a constantly reflective finger on the pulse of this process.

Joining a profession late also comes with certain challenges. Therapists need to consider what kind of training is accessible and affordable. Shorter programmes can vary in quality and offer glimpses into the world of psychology and therapy rather than allowing for immersion. Finding a course that provides both theoretical grounding and process training can be challenging, and a readiness to invest the time and resources needed is important. Despite their training, second-career therapists can feel one step behind colleagues who started sooner, experiencing more self-doubt or a sense of constantly playing catch-up. At some point in this journey, they may find that they no longer feel like outsiders and instead have found a new home.

Does the second act always have a happy ending? Some may miss the perks of previous jobs while others may wake up every day, feeling satisfied with their choice. It is important to remain in touch with all these feelings. For those who have chosen to be therapists as a second career, there may be a lot to reflect on and much richness to be gained through these musings.

What Sustains Us

It is a continuous and evolving reflective process to understand our allegiance to therapeutic work and our appreciation for the meaning this work brings to our lives. Engagement with therapy can be quite self-sustaining, and when we feel enriched by deep relational experiences with our clients and inspired by the effectiveness of the psychotherapeutic process, this helps us stay connected to our therapist identity and our purpose. This reinforces commitment, driving us to be even better at our work and know ourselves better. As we experience changes and transitions in our lives, we may come to value the things that helped perhaps a perspective or a practice, and bring this into our work.

Pause and reflect...
We invite you to close your eyes, take a deep breath and visualize your role as a therapist. Reflect on what guides, sustains, and anchors you as you support others in their healing and growth, allowing the image(s) to form in your mind's eye. These could be people, places, objects, or anything else you see. As you engage in this process of visualization, make a note or draw what emerges, so you can stay connected with the symbols of your sustenance.

As you reflect on what you are doing and why it feels meaningful, new drivers may emerge that deepen your work in a specific area or explore new avenues. For instance, a deeper sense of meaning could emerge while working with a specific client group or type of presentation. An expansion into other domains, such as research to stimulate the intellect or teaching to meet a desire for generativity, could sustain therapists through difficult or frustrating times. The decision to make shifts can also be a practical one, as therapists with growing children or increasing financial responsibilities prioritize paths that offer greater financial rewards. Finally, it is useful to note that all motivations and needs cannot (and should not) be met only through work. A meaningful life outside the therapy room provides balance and perspective and works to sustain the motivation to remain a therapist.

Therapists can reflect on whether they have stayed close to the motivations that brought them to the profession. Have earlier motivations remained the same, evolved or been lost over time? Checking in on whether they feel they are building on their motivations can help therapists consider whether they need to change anything about their professional lives. Therapists can ask themselves, What else do I need from my career? Is there a part of me that is not finding the room for expression? Looking at a typical workday to see what resonates and what might feel at odds with one's motivations can be a window into underlying concerns. When we feel like the therapist role feels not just with what we do but with who we are, it is likely that our motivations are congruent with our career choices and can continue to nourish us.

A Therapist Speaks: Psychology at the Heart of Social Change

Mick Cooper

I was always very interested in social change and social justice and really wanted to develop some of my thinking on it. It was a journey that I kept wanting to take for over twenty years, but it was difficult to find the time and the focus. I would keep coming to the idea, touch on it, but then get busy with something else. I initially began with person-centered counselling and then I got involved in psychotherapy research and existential therapy and moved more into the clinical side of things. There was always something that was interesting that kept me involved.

A few years ago, when I went through a really difficult time, I thought I have to get on with writing. So, I planned a book which was going to be at the interface between social justice and therapy and focused on exploring that. I really wanted to write and say all the things I wanted to say and do the thing I passionately cared about.

I was always very interested in social change, and I think my family was the underlying driver. I come from a family of activists, where the core value is about making a difference in the world. My parents are very progressive, their underlying value is very much about making a positive difference. My father's family were Jewish immigrants from Ukraine: his family came to Britain in the 1890s and he was a young man involved in anti-fascist demonstrations. My mother came from Germany: she just escaped the Holocaust. So, there was a very raw sense of how terrible injustice can be, the violence that it can lead to. It was really important for me in terms of having a sense of meaning and purpose to do something that felt we are making things socially better in some way.

It was really life-changing finishing my book. There is something about having said something in your own words that nobody else could do – that is a really powerful feeling. It felt like a real weight off, like I was doing what I wanted to. Of course, I would love it if everybody read the book and it changed the world immediately, but that feels less critical. There is a process of actualising one's potential and expressing that is really deeply fulfilling in itself. You feel real, you feel authentic, you feel you are in the world in a way that is true to yourself without any masks. In humanistic therapies we think that well-being comes through being in the world in an authentic way. So, I guess writing is the same, it can leave us with feeling whole and complete. And I do really feel that psychology has the potential to help make a better world: by helping people to be more understanding, empathic, and compassionate towards each other; by helping us understand the value of cooperative ways of relating; and by teaching us skills in nonviolent, effective communication.

Mick Cooper *is an internationally recognised author, trainer, and consultant in the field of humanistic, existential, and pluralistic therapies. He is a Chartered Psychologist, and Professor of Counselling Psychology at the University of Roehampton, UK. His latest book is Psychology at the Heart of Social Change: Towards a Progressive Vision for Society.*

Therapists are also motivated by things that are happening outside the therapy room. The choice of being a therapist, the kind of therapist they wish to be and the way they engage with the profession on the whole, can be shaped by how they wish to position ourselves vis-à-vis the larger cultural and political issues in the world around. Whether our motivation is more internal and personal or more external and contextual—finding a reason or purpose for our work is like finding a pot of gold. It can sustain us through our careers.

Perspectives on Training and Development

Selection Processes in Psychotherapy Training Programmes

While the selection process for psychotherapy training programmes varies, some centres invite potential applicants to share reflections about their personal motivations for their career choice. This approach represents a commitment to inclusivity, where the entire life experience of the therapist-in-the-making is valued, rather than evaluating them solely through an academic lens. While this is commendable, there are concerns that applicants may feel pressured to share in ways they are not ready for. Applicants might be concerned about their chances of selection if they identify no specific challenges, too many difficult experiences and vulnerabilities or present a positive picture of overcoming all adversity. This can lead applicants to tailor their responses based on what they believe selection committees desire.

In the selection process, the focus is ideally on identifying candidates who demonstrate the skills and emotional resilience necessary for effective therapeutic practice. Research has raised concerns that trainees who are perceived as too vulnerable or still navigating their own emotional wounds may be unfairly excluded from training programmes. Ivey and Partington (2014) argue that these arbitrary decisions can discourage openness about personal motivations and life experiences and limit the diversity and richness of the therapeutic community. Selection for psychotherapy training is ideally based on present abilities and future potential rather than past difficulties.

Developing Trainee Awareness of Their Motivations

We recommend that training institutes keep space for reflections and conversations around motivations and the positive and negative life experiences that may have brought a student to the course. As trainers and supervisors, we have used a personal timeline exercise to initiate trainees' reflections on links between their life experiences, their choice of profession and the potential impact on practice. In this activity, trainees are asked to place important positive and negative events, experiences and people along the trajectory, beginning in childhood up until the present time. As they put their experiences together, they can be encouraged to reflect on the personal meaning of these markers and link them with the possible reasons they chose to become therapists. The pace of trainee exploration can be modulated based on their readiness to look within themselves and their comfort in sharing parts of what they find. Training programmes should be flexible in how they approach personal exploration, understanding that some trainees may be less willing to share due to cultural norms around vulnerability. In some cultures, heightened shame proneness and the pressure to maintain family secrets could constrain individuals from acknowledging difficult childhood experiences or personal struggles (Sommers, 2012). Providing options for private reflection, as well as encouraging group discussion, allows trainees to participate in ways that feel comfortable to them.

The sharing of personal vulnerabilities and growth by experienced and respected practitioners can facilitate a cultural shift within training institutes. We have been inspired by the collective account of eleven psychologists who have come out proud, to publicly acknowledge their lived experience of mental health vulnerabilities (Victor, Schleider et al., 2022). They share how they have experienced, witnessed or feared negative reactions during their training and work lives and advocate for more inclusive professional spaces. We also recommend powerful lived experience accounts of non-suicidal self-injury by three clinical psychologists whose research also centres on this often-stigmatized behaviour (Victor, Lewis et al., 2022). When practising professionals share their experiences and vulnerabilities, including what it means to be so open within their professional community, it legitimizes these for trainees and early career therapists. Most importantly, it encourages the profession to create space for so many among us who are wounded. Their recommendations include open discussions on lived experience and an engagement with complex issues around disclosure in training and work contexts. Most importantly, they urge a sensitivity to the use of language that differentiates persons with lived experiences from professionals in the field of mental health. This us-them distinction serves to reinforce misconceptions about the invulnerability of mental health professionals, making open and honest dialogue even more challenging.

In our experience, it is beneficial to embed various opportunities to build awareness of motivations throughout the training phase. Motivations and needs are not always easy to identify, and some connections come to light only after engaging with clinical work. As training progresses, continued explorations can help trainees identify their strengths and build focal interests.

Professional and Systemic Responses to Therapist Vulnerabilities

We hope for a growing recognition that the distance between the couch and the chair is not as far as some might imagine. The idea of a shared humanity means that all of us can be vulnerable and also have the potential for ongoing healing, change and growth. This understanding can strengthen sensitive, non-judgmental and non-pathologizing approaches in training and supervision spaces and within the professional community at large. One where motives of wanting to help, care and connect are given primacy rather than real motivations or dysfunctional family issues that must first be discovered, explored and resolved. Our attention needs to be directed towards building resilience, a critical attribute of an effective therapist.

An institutional ethos that encourages sharing and has transparent non-discrimination policies in place can leave trainees feeling safe enough to seek help for mental health challenges. Difficulties with disclosure also reflect the inconsistent response of the professional community to therapist vulnerabilities. While compassion and empathy form the bedrock of this profession, therapists often anticipate negative reactions from their colleagues and supervisors and may conceal their struggles (Cvetovac & Adame, 2017). Even when the responses are not obviously negative or well intentioned, they can be experienced as intrusive or invalidating. The ethos also percolates to peer relationships. If we hear about the psychological difficulties of another therapist, we need to respond sensitively protect their privacy, unless it is directly harmful to clients.

When trainees encounter clients' narratives of trauma and injustice, this can be particularly triggering for some and might uncover their vulnerabilities. Supervision is one of the training spaces that presents opportunities to anticipate and observe any such emergent difficulties quite closely. As supervisors, we may need to take a call on how far to push our understanding. While supervisees must know that the door is open for conversations and support, they also need to feel free to share, grow and change at their pace (Wheeler, 2007). When supervisors observe heightened psychological distress or noticeable impairments in functioning, they can proactively facilitate help-seeking and arrange additional support. Clear policies about confidentiality, leave, and accommodations, and support for return after a leave of absence are all essential to expedite help-seeking and comprehensive care. Even when there are safety risks, sensitive response protocols can provide anticipatory guidance about the process of sharing relevant information.

It is also undeniable that there are trainees whose emotional vulnerabilities impede the acquisition and use of therapeutic skills. Even as they remain committed to their profession, the therapeutic work and academic tasks could be too triggering or challenging to sustain. Offering individualized support plans including additional supervision and mentoring, therapeutic support, and the option for breaks or extensions in line with policies, is important. Care must be taken to avoid gatekeeping through premature exclusion, ensuring a balance between upholding standards and supporting trainee well-being. Protection of clients from inadequate care or harm through ethical violation remains a priority throughout the process. When trainees cannot meet competence and attendance standards despite supportive measures, they may be counselled out of the programme, thereby protecting the integrity of both the programme and the profession.

Conclusion

Like Masuji Ono, the protagonist in *An Artist of the Floating World* (Ishiguro, 1986), therapists must cross the bridge of hesitation, a metaphor for those moments when they reflect on their past and link this what lies ahead. For Ono, this bridge signifies a reckoning with his past choices and their consequences. Similarly, for therapists, it represents the critical examination of their personal histories and motivations, and the ways in which they shape their therapeutic practice. Crossing this bridge requires courage, as it involves confronting vulnerabilities and unexamined motivations.

As we re-examine ourselves and our life stories, this understanding can help us see how our motivations inform, support, enrich or impede our therapeutic work. We may return to this exploration at different times in our professional journey; the reasons that pushed or pulled us to become a therapist and the motivations to remain a therapist may not be one and the same thing. As we get familiar with and grow in our careers and lives, it is natural that our motives also evolve. As the field of psychotherapy itself evolves and changes, the dominant motivations to enter the profession might also shift. As you engaged with the ideas in this chapter, did you discover anything new about yourself and your motivations?

References

Adams, M. (2014). *The myth of the untroubled therapist: Private life, professional practice.* Routledge.

Bager-Charleson, S. (2010). *Why therapists choose to become therapists.* Karnac Books.

Bhola, P., Raguram, A., Dugyala, M., & Ravishankar, A. (2017). Learning in the crucible of supervision: Experiences of trainee psychotherapists in India. *The Clinical Supervisor, 36*, 182–202.

Brown, L. S. (2005). Don't be a sheep: How this eldest daughter became a feminist therapist. *Journal of Clinical Psychology, 61*, 949–995.

Bryce, I., Pye, D., Beccaria, G., McIlveen, P., & Du Preez, J. (2023). A systematic literature review of the career choice of helping professionals who have experienced cumulative harm as a result of adverse childhood experiences. *Trauma, Violence, & Abuse, 24*(1), 72–85.

Carey, B. (2011). Expert on mental illness reveals her own fight. New York Times. Retrieved from http://archive.nytimes.com/www.nytimes.com/2011/06/23/health/23lives.html

Cvetovac, M. E., & Adame, A. L. (2017). The wounded therapist: Understanding the relationship between personal suffering and clinical practice. *The Humanistic Psychologist, 45*(4), 348–366.

Duggal, C., & Sriram, S. (2016). Beginning the journey: What motivates therapists to join the profession? In S. Sriram (Ed.), *Counselling in India: Reflections on the process* (pp. 75–90). Springer.

Farber, B. A., Manevich, I., Metzger, J., & Saypol, E. (2005). Choosing psychotherapy as a career: Why did we cross that road? *Journal of Clinical Psychology, 61*(8), 1009–1031.

Gabbard, G. O. (2000). On gratitude and gratification. *Journal of the American Psychoanalytic Association, 48*(3), 697–716.

Hankir, A. (2022). Fighting mental health stigma. *Bulletin of the World Health Organization, 100*(8), 472–473.

Hammer, D. E. (2020). The lived experience of a psychologist activist. *Psychotherapy & Politics International, 202018*, e1536. https://doi.org/10.1002/ppi.1536

Hill, C. E., Lystrup, A., Kline, K., Gebru, N. M., Birchler, J., Palmer, G., Robinson, J., Um, M., Griffin, S., Lipsky, E., Knox, S., & Pinto-Coelho, K. (2013). Aspiring to become a therapist: Personal strengths and challenges, influences, motivations, and expectations of future psychotherapists. *Counselling Psychology Quarterly, 26*(3–4), 267–293.

Hoyt, M. F. (2005). Why I became a (brief) psychotherapist. *Journal of Clinical Psychology, in Session, 61*(8), 983–989.

Ishiguro, K. (1986). *An artist of the floating world.* Faber & Faber.

Ivey, G., & Partington, T. (2014). Psychological woundedness and its evaluation in applications for clinical psychology training. *Clinical Psychology and Psychotherapy, 21*(2), 166–177.

Jung, C. G. (1963). *Memories, dreams, reflections.* Pantheon Books.

Luks, A. (1988). Helper's high: Volunteering makes people feel good, physically and emotionally. *Psychology Today, 22*(10), 34–42.

MacFarquhar, L. (2015). *Strangers drowning: Grappling with impossible idealism, drastic choices, and the overpowering urge to help.* Penguin Press.

McBeath, A. (2019). The motivations of psychotherapists: An in-depth survey. *Counselling and Psychotherapy Research, 19*, 377–387.

Mahoney, M. J., & Eiseman, S. C. (2014). The object of the dance. In W. Dryden & L. Spurling (Eds.), *On becoming a psychotherapist* (2nd ed., pp. 14–29). Routledge.

McAdams, D. P. (2001). The psychology of life stories. *Review of General Psychology, 5*(2), 100–122.

McCullough, L. (2005). Doing something. *Journal of Clinical Psychology, 61*, 991–997.

Neki, J. S. (1973). Guru-chela relationship: The possibility of a therapeutic paradigm. *The American Journal of Orthopsychiatry, 43*, 755–766.

Orlinsky, D. E. (2005). Becoming and being a psychotherapist: A psychodynamic memoir and meditation. *Journal of Clinical Psychology, 61*, 999–1007.

Orlinsky, D. E., & Rønnestad, M. H. (2005). *How psychotherapists develop: A study of therapeutic work and professional growth.* American Psychological Association.

Rober, P., & Seltzer, M. (2010). Avoiding colonizer positions in the therapy room: Some ideas about the challenges of dealing with the dialectic of misery and resources in families. *Family Process, 49*(1), 123–137.

Rumi. (1997). A great wagon. In *The essential Rumi* (C. Barks, J. Moyne, A. J. Arberry & R. Nicholson, Trans.). Castle Books.

Sommers, T. (2012). Shame cultures, collectivist societies, original sin, and pharaoh's hardened heart. In T. Sommers (Ed.), *Relative justice: Cultural diversity, free will, and moral responsibility.* https://doi.org/10.23943/princeton/9780691139937.003.0004

Street, E. (2014). Challenging the 'white knight.' In W. Dryden & L. Spurling (Eds.), *On becoming a psychotherapist* (2nd ed., pp. 130–143). Routledge.

Stirling, F. J. (2020). Journeying to visibility: An autoethnography of self-harm scars in the therapy room. *Psychotherapy and Politics International, 18*, e1537. https://doi.org/10.1002/ppi.1537

Sussman, M. (2007). *A curious calling: Unconscious motivations for practising psychotherapy.* Jason Aronson.

Wheeler, S. (2007). What shall we do with the wounded healer? The supervisor's dilemma. *Psychodynamic Practice, 13*, 245–256.

Victor, S. E., Lewis, S. P., & Muehlenkamp, J. J. (2022). Psychologists with lived experience of non-suicidal self-injury: Priorities, obstacles, and recommendations for inclusion. *Psychological Services, 19*(1), 21–28.

Victor, S. E., Schleider, J. L., Ammerman, B. A., Bradford, D. E., Devendorf, A. R., Gruber, J., Gunaydin, L. A., Hallion, L. S., Kaufman, E. A., Lewis, S. P., & Stage, D. L. (2022). Leveraging the strengths of psychologists with lived experience of psychopathology. *Perspectives on Psychological Science, 17*(6), 1624–1632.

Zerubavel, N., & Wright, M. O. D. (2012). The dilemma of the wounded healer. *Psychotherapy, 49*(4), 482–491.

Chapter 3
Discovering the Self-Of-The-Therapist

As the story goes, Theseus, the mythical founder and hero of Athens, returned from Crete on a ship which was preserved to mark his glorious victory over the minotaur. Over time, the decaying planks were gradually replaced by newer and stronger parts, until none of the original parts remained. The Greek historian Plutarch presented two philosophical perspectives: one which held that the ship had ceased to be the original Ship of Theseus, while the other declared that the restored ship fundamentally remained the same despite the changes. If we think of the ship as a metaphor for the human self, the story raises many questions about identity. What are the parts that make up our self? Are we the same today as we were a few months ago? As things change, are there some intrinsic parts that stay the same? Are we our strongest emotion in the moment or are we our most consistent habits of thought and action? Are we most ourselves when alone or does our range of being emerge in our interactions with the world? What does self really mean and what we are referring to when we talk about the self of the therapist. How do we as therapists stay in touch with our self, and also use this awareness meaningfully in our therapeutic encounters?

The self or personhood of the therapist enters therapy, regardless of the theoretical orientation or approach that is followed. As Satir (2013, pp. 20–21) pointed out, "Techniques and approaches are tools. They come out differently in different hands". The concepts of the self of the therapist, person of the therapist or self as instrument represent a range of actions and experiences, including how therapists relate to clients, get emotionally triggered and use self-disclosure, humour or presence in the therapy room to further therapeutic goals. These concepts also encompass a reflexive awareness of the thoughts, values, experiences, roles and social identities that have developed within the context of relationships, experiences, training and sociopolitical environment (Sude & Baima, 2021).

The self of the therapist has been positioned in varied ways; sometimes as an unwanted entrant in sessions which might interfere with the therapy process. Initially, self-awareness was positioned as a route to keep the therapist's subjectivities and personal issues from spilling into their work. In contrast, Carl Rogers believed that

P. Bhola et al., *Reflective Practice in Psychotherapy and Counselling*,
https://doi.org/10.1007/978-981-96-9732-8_3

it is therapist transparency and authenticity that are powerful facilitators of change for the client (Baldwin, 2013). All of us have quirks and idiosyncrasies that make us who we are—in terms of the language we use, our demeanour, our life experiences and ways of responding to ambiguous situations. We use our emotions, personality, belief systems and relational dynamics as tools for change—it is therefore who we are with our clients. Psychotherapists are now exploring the intentional use of self to influence the client and change process, and this works in tandem with self-acceptance. The maxim 'Love yourself as a person, doubt yourself as a therapist' captures the balance we seek—and it is this combination that is linked with better client outcomes (Nissen-Lie et al., 2017).

In this chapter, we examine the relationship between the personal and professional selves of the therapist and explore two key questions that therapists can answer through reflective practice. How do I become more aware of myself? And how do I understand how to use my self in therapy?

Meeting Our Personal and Professional Selves

While the *personal self* exists in all situations both inside and outside the therapy room, the *professional self* plays the therapist role and is heavily influenced by training and skills (Rønnestad & Skovholt, 2003). Aspects of professional and personal selves percolate into each other. For instance, we may incorporate the communication skills learnt as therapists into our personal repertoire. Similarly, we may apply personality traits like agreeableness or extraversion in forming relationships with clients. An increased awareness of the linkages, interactions and tensions between the personal and professional self can enhance use of self in therapy.

Pause and reflect...

Use words, images, metaphors, songs, or any material or medium (clay, collage, paints), to depict how you see your personal self and therapist self.

As you see what gets created through this creative exercise, reflect on how you experience your personal and therapist selves and think about how they have evolved through your professional journey.

Diverse ways of seeing personal and therapist selves have emerged during several reflective practice workshops that we have conducted with trainees and practitioners. For several participants, the two identities were intertwined in complex ways with personalized meanings. One participant made a creative representation of her personal self as a coiled rope, which gradually untwisted as her professional self was strengthened. Another participant depicted parts of his personal and professional self both hidden and revealed in origami folds, while others drew a Venn diagram with overlapping circles. Some participants related to the image of a railroad track, where both selves moved together in the same direction, sometimes merging and sometimes separating. Others saw a clear wall dividing and separating their two selves. This reflective exercise gave participants a tangible way to represent the relationship between their personal and professional selves. The different levels of overlap and permeability of boundaries between the two selves suggests that this is a very individualized experience.

The *self-schema*, which develops through personal life experiences, is active before a person starts training. The *self-as-therapist schema* gradually becomes more dominant through the process of professional training, and promotes the learning of conceptual, technical and relational skills (Bennett-Levy, 2006). As therapists gather professional experience and confidence and build their therapist identity, there is more comfort in bringing in personal qualities and learnings from life experiences. The self-schema starts to find more expression in therapeutic work. Finding an effective balance between the professional and the personal is considered a hallmark of therapists' development. The two might never balance completely and no matter how congruent we are, we are likely to forefront different parts of ourselves in our personal and professional worlds. The way we are in sessions is influenced as much by the dictates of therapist's role as it is by our personal style of relating and attaching. For instance, we may be calmer, more patient or more accepting inside the therapy room than we are outside.

The post-modern perspective proposes that the bifurcation of the self as personal and professional is an arbitrary and false one. There are, in fact, multiple selves that exist and at each given point in time, the self is being constructed through interactions with the context/co-constructed through interactions with the other. So, there is only the self in the moment and different aspects are activated in different relational contexts with clients. This implies that we may be kind and patient with one client, while we are intolerant of another. Or that we can be very emotionally sensitive to the same client at one point in time, while not being moved at other times. We may have days when we feel like extroverts, enjoying our engagement with everyone we encounter, whether as therapists or as people, and other days when we want the whole world to remain outside. How then can we find a consistent sense of who we are? And do we really need to? These questions open up an important perspective for therapists, because while we may never know ourselves fully, we can know ourselves in the moment with our client.

Discovering the Self

While working with clients, therapists embark on a parallel and ongoing journey of self-discovery. This could include noticing aspects of our personhood that are a consistent professional asset or observing how each client brings our inner world alive in different ways. Sometimes what happens in a session triggers a past memory or brings to the surface an emotion which highlights a bias or reflects a preference.

A client discussing their closeness with their parent may bring feelings of warmth about our own parents, or a client sharing an incident of a conflict with their partner might trigger memories of painful conflicts with our partners. At times, we might miss how certain ways of being (e.g., our tendency to experience anxiety in the face of interpersonal challenges) enter our work. The self is not static but keeps evolving, and each time we look inside, we may find something new. Just as we need to catch up with our friends, regular self-reflection enables us to catch up with ourselves and stay in touch with our strengths and the ways in which we are evolving.

Notions of the self often begin with the *individual self* in terms of the unique constellation of attributes, beliefs, experiences and aspirations. Self-representations also encompass the *relational self*—the aspect of the self that both evolves and operates in relationship with others. The *collective self* represents parts that are shared with members of groups we belong to and also differentiate us from relevant outgroups (Sedikides et al., 2011). The *spiritual self* is often considered the deepest level of self or the core of our being and refers both to what is universal and transcendent within us. All these facets of the self contribute to our overall sense of identity, and interact to determine particular actions and preferences. The process of self-discovery includes building an integrated sense of self that enhances our repertoire of available resources and creates added layers of meaning and experience that can be used to help clients.

Taking self-reflections deeper guides therapists to notice inner and outer layers, parts that are more accessible and visible and those that are not. Delving into the unknown parts of the self is useful for anyone who wishes to understand themselves better and not just for therapists. The construct of the *Johari window* provides a way to conceptualize the known and unknown parts of the self (Luft, 1982). A reflective interaction with others can reduce blind spots (parts of us that are known to others but not to ourselves), as we get feedback on our behaviours. As we open up and share more parts of ourselves, we can also chip away at our façade, revealing parts of us that are known to ourselves, but not to others. Both these moves shift us towards the open quadrant, where inner and outer selves are more congruent. This enables consistency in relationships and open communication, both of which are crucial for the self of the therapist.

Satir (2013) proposed the *personal iceberg metaphor* to gain awareness of our inner world and become more authentic in the therapeutic relationship. Beginning with the behaviours which are at the tip of the iceberg, the model explores what lies below the waterline or what may not be immediately accessible—these could be bodily sensations, feelings, feelings about feelings, perceptions, beliefs, expectations from self and others, yearnings (e.g., for love, acceptance, connection and freedom) and the core self—the sense of who I am (Banmen, 2002). These layers of the self can be accessed through the senses and monitored during sessions through observing and wondering about different layers of experience and how they affect each other. As awareness increases, therapists can work towards building congruence within themselves, thereby attuning better with clients and increasing their sense of professional competence (Lum, 2002). Metaphors like the Johari window or the personal iceberg can give a shape and form to our reflections, as each metaphor offers a different perspective on what lies within.

Pause and reflect...
Imagine a set of matryoshka dolls of different sizes, one nested within the other, as parts of your self.

These could represent your beliefs, emotions, values, traits, desires, roles, memories—those that make you who you are.

You can place each doll, representing a part of your self, in relation to the other dolls (parts) in any way you like.

If you had to put something that represents the core of your self inside the smallest doll, what would that be? This could be an object, an image, a word, a phrase, or a metaphor....

This nesting dolls exercise has been an evocative and powerful reflective tool during our workshops with therapists. Several participants spoke of the innermost doll as signifying something hidden, with the larger dolls creating safe boundaries around the more tender or personal parts of their self. It was interesting to see how some participants responded to the different colours of the dolls while others related more to sizes, with the smaller ones being the parts that they were surer of and the larger ones signifying ambiguity. As a contribution to this dialogue, some of the therapists emphasized the need to meet all parts of the self—even those that might be contradictory or do not fit neatly one inside the other like the nesting dolls. This exercise can open different doors within us, stimulated by reflective questions to interrogate a range of experiences. We can extend the exercise to explore how the self manifests in interactions with our clients. This might involve asking which parts of the self enter the therapeutic space, whether these are immediately visible, gradually revealed or remain hidden from the client.

Self-Of-The-Therapist Work

Self-of-the-therapist work helps us recognize characteristic ways of thinking, feeling, and relating, as well as their potential impact on therapeutic practice. We explore and understand our personal histories, psychological, relational, and spiritual challenges, and struggles—both in terms of how they developed and how they manifest in therapeutic interactions. This awareness helps in crystallizing how we can use our self more consciously and meaningfully in our work. Acknowledging and accepting our own history of struggles and challenges can help us connect more deeply with the vulnerabilities clients experience. It creates room to hold compassion for the current situation and commitment to well-being and growth, both for clients and ourselves. While it may seem that there is an undue focus on the less functional parts of the therapist, it is equally important to be aware of strengths and skills as well. All personal experiences are relevant, and even those that might be considered barriers or constraints can be a strength or resource to draw on (Timm & Blow, 1999). Seeing one side of ourselves in the context of the other side can bring us closer to a more integrated picture of our complete self…opening the door for us to do the same with our clients.

The primary pathway to developing self-awareness is through reflection on experiences in therapy. In critical moments, asking questions that focus on the self of the therapist is helpful—and this is something we typically do, whether alone or in supervision. Pausing at significant moments in role-plays to deep dive into the experiential world helps therapists understand what was going on within them and how it impacted the interaction. For instance, noticing discomfort in our bodies, perhaps a tightness in the stomach when stuck during a session, can prompt reflection on what underlies the experience. This might reveal frustration with the client or ourselves, or a sense of not having anything useful to say. We may interpret this feeling as indicating that we are not being good therapists or that our clients are not being good clients. In the presence of supervisors or peers, we can empathically enter this experience and connect with our need to feel and appear competent. This may lead us to a new understanding of ourselves and perhaps even our clients. Drawing inspiration from triad work proposed by Satir, we recommend role-plays where therapists can play three different roles in turn—that of the client, therapist and observer, operating from different vantage points. When playing the client's role, there is an opportunity to present and explore personal issues and relate more closely to the client's position. In the therapist's role, one can experiment with different ways of being with clients and reflect on the insights of the observer. From the relative distance of the observer's role, therapists can cultivate sensitivity to the therapy process, witnessing the client–therapist interaction and noting the impact of micro and macro processes (Lum, 2002).

As we sit with our clients we often conduct a parallel inner conversation with ourselves, this includes our observations of the client as well as the personal experiences they evoke. Rober (1999) conceptualized this *inner conversation as* the dialogue between the self of the therapist and the role of the therapist. Paying attention to this inner conversation privileges our intuitive and reflective capacities, offering another route to encountering what has not been articulated by the client. For instance, if a client describes preferring to listen to music with his headphones on when his wife is at home, the self of the therapist observes and responds to this. As we picture our client with his headphones on, we may ask ourselves if he fears intruding in his partner's space with his music or if he prefers to keep his experience separate. The experience could also evoke images from our personal lives, perhaps of feeling shut out by a loved one or even wanting to shut them out. Although such connections to our own inner worlds can bring difficult emotions or images, attending to them gives us access to experiences that are yet unspoken. While the role of the therapist brings in theoretical knowledge and hypothesis, it is the self of the therapist that observes the goings-on, evoking a range of images, feelings, intuitions and so on. The act of reflecting on what is observed is a crucial first step, but it is also important to bring this reflection to professional interactions. Discussions with supervisors and colleagues enable therapists to engage with an outsider gaze to externalize and examine inner process. This helps in sifting through and identifying experiences that are more related to our personal histories and need a separate space to be spoken and processed. When therapists share relevant aspects of their personal self with clients, it is important to closely observe the client's response, as it is through these reactions that we discern whether new possibilities have emerged within the therapeutic relationship.

Formal training frameworks that explore the self-of-the-therapist offer a more structured framework to guide reflections. They are often spread over a longer period and require serious commitment to the self-reflective process. The tangible and long-term benefits of learning to work effectively with ourselves can make the investment truly worthwhile. The *Person-of-the-Therapist (POTT)* model (Aponte, 2016) introduces the concept of a signature theme (e.g., need for control, fear of rejection, lack of self- worth and fear of being vulnerable) that often reflects ongoing struggles with the self. A series of reflective questions can bring one closer to understanding their signature theme—asking about sources and areas of anxiety, fear or frustration; recognizing typical responses in stressful situations or difficult patterns in relationships; and contemplating what aspects of themselves they would rather conceal from others (Aponte & Kissil, 2014). No matter where we are on the road to the acceptance or resolution of our signature theme, it shapes our journeys and influences how we think, feel and relate. For instance, a therapist may no longer feel as overwhelmed by their fear of rejection now as at the start of their career. However, the ways in which they overcame that fear and the social skills or self-affirming habits they learnt are likely to remain a significant part of who they now are. Awareness of these themes is beneficial for therapists, as they could enhance recognition of similar themes in clients, separate therapist issues from client issues and use this awareness as an asset or strength. Less aware therapists may feel more easily triggered in sessions, without fully comprehending why and therefore misinterpreting their emotional signals.

A Therapist Speaks: Using the POTT-Er's Wheel to Shape the Self of the Therapist

Maliha Ibrahim

The Person of the Therapist (POTT) model has been a part of my professional life for about a decade, beginning with an immersive exposure to the training modality by working directly with Dr Harry Aponte. As teacher and faculty lead for the practicum in the Master's in Counseling Psychology program, Yorkville University, Canada, I have introduced this training framework to strengthen the clinical competencies of our students, along with increasing their comfort with using self-themes in therapy. The intensive course spans two semesters and is interwoven across the stages of the program, accompanying students through the 30 weeks of their practicum.

As practicum instructor, I meet with students on a weekly basis in group consultation and supervision format meetings, each of 2–3 hours in duration. We begin with exploring underlying core signature themes which impact our relationships with self and others, both inside and outside the therapy room. Each 'wounded healer' becomes more familiar with their signature theme, reflecting-in-action as it plays out in the group. This prepares them for the next stage of learning to assess the link (identification) or distinction (differentiation) from client themes or presenting concerns as they emerge in therapy sessions. Finally, we reflect on how interventions in the therapy room can be more aligned with awareness and analysis of self.

My focus is on moving from more general reflections to more specific ones examining how signature themes play out in each of their experiences and relationships with clients and colleagues as well as during supervision. My role is to scaffold by providing safety and containment, while allowing discomfort to be felt. It is this visceral and emotional discomfort that transforms to deep understanding of self and a growing comfort around vulnerability and the human experience. The transformative potential of reflective practice emerges through the range of the course activities, including journal entries, a case conceptualization paper, reflective narratives and video case presentations. As an instructor, I find that the journals and video case presentations are particularly powerful.

One student reflected on how their signature theme of "a fear of rejection" led to people pleasing behavior with the client and the loss of a sense of self during sessions. The process of consistent journaling helped them recognise how their subjugated parts emerged while getting stuck in a power struggle with the client.

Through the video recordings, I emphasize to students to "invite the self of the therapist" into the conversation. I ask specific questions around; "What are you seeing as you watch the recording?", "What questions do you have about the therapeutic process?", "How does the alliance seem to be?" and finally, "How does this connect to or diverge from your own sense of self?". We spend time deliberating on these aspects, while group members respond to the presenter, and reflect on possible common overlaps and the differences. We discuss how client utterances, reported behaviors and emotional experiences impact 'me' the counselor, asking, "What am I noticing in myself? How am I altering/changing my reactions in the session as a result"? I spend time with students to analyze if self-responses are stemming purely from client concerns or personal issues.

One of the video-recordings brought an awareness about ethical boundary crossings in therapy. The student connected this with her signature theme of personal inadequacy and its derivatives of over-functioning towards burnout, reluctance to access support from supervisors and extending self by being very directive/prescriptive with clients. This process of reflection brought an understanding of how her personal investment pressurized her clients, to the point that it reduced their autonomy.

I have noticed the growth and development of themes over the course of training. For example, one student identified perfectionism as a signature theme early in the practicum course. After a few months, her understanding of self and her signature theme deepened. This opened an understanding of vulnerability when things were beyond her control in her own life, thus leading to perfectionism as an attempt to gain control. Through identifying these aspects, she was able to join relationally with clients at her practicum site, who were survivors of abuse and domestic violence. She dropped the 'expert' and performative aspects of therapy to engage in very raw and real encounters where she connected with their deep feelings of helplessness as well as the life force towards survival and resilience.

Drawing from my experiences as instructor and supervisor, I would advocate the integration of reflective practice in the training curriculum for budding counselors and therapists. While it can be introduced at any stage of training, it is ideal if it is introduced early. For me, it has been a wonderful experience teaching and co-learning in this way, as students develop into self-aware and self-reflective colleagues.

Dr. Maliha Ibrahim *is a counseling psychology faculty instructor and clinical researcher who lives and works in Canada. As a psychotherapist, she uses a relational, systemic, intrapsychic and interpersonal approach to therapy and supervision.*

Therapists may be more inclined to focus on difficulties or pathology, both within clients and themselves. However, this perspective presents only part of the picture, and not necessarily the most useful part. Though it may be necessary to contend with dysfunctional patterns, it is often one's strengths that are drawn upon most consistently in therapeutic work. A positive psychology framework can help tune into the unique combination of character strengths that make a person who they are (Peterson & Seligman, 2004). Discovering our character strengths, perhaps through completing the Values in Action (VIA) Survey of Character Strengths, can bring an intentional focus to their use in therapeutic work. Tools such as this can be used to identify which character strength(s) (e.g., kindness, forgiveness, perseverance, teamwork, self-regulation and spirituality) manifest most strongly in both personal life and therapeutic work. This understanding enhances the use of personal strengths. For instance, if you identify curiosity as a key strength, you can develop it by committing to exploring and learning something new—maybe that pottery class you have been postponing or taking a new route on your morning walk. Spending some time reflecting on how you interact with your strengths can throw up some interesting insights. You may find that you express a strength in interactions with your clients (e.g., kindness) but neglect to apply this to yourself in the same measure. Therapists can also err on the side of overusing some strengths, perhaps extending perseverance into inflexibility or kindness into conflict avoidance. Too much focus on a particular strong suit can lead to neglect of other potential strengths, as we stay within our safe zone. For instance, an overuse of empathy can come at the cost of judgement or perception. Too often though, we are reluctant to take a healthy pride or pleasure in our strengths, whether as therapists or individuals; and this restricts us from a complete experience of ourselves.

Pause and reflect...
In what ways do your key strengths manifest in your therapeutic work?

Which are the strengths that you would want to use more intentionally in your therapy practice?

We can explore ourselves through many possible pathways, arriving at various insights about how we operate. Staying with and reflecting on these insights over a period of time can help us crystallize and integrate an understanding of self. This sets the stage for using our selves more effectively in the therapy room. It seems that it is not the self that matters for our effectiveness as therapists, as much as the *use* we put that self to.

The Relational Self

Building an awareness of the thoughts, emotions and behaviours that are evoked during interpersonal interactions is crucial for the relational enterprise of therapy. This can be understood as the self-in-relationships or the aspects of the self that gets activated during interactions. It can also be extended to the idea of the relational self, a concept that implies that a part of the self gets created through interactions with others. While family members are often the primary crucible for this shaping of self, a typical relational world is made of many more people. Extended family, neighbours, teachers, coaches, best friends...and later, colleagues, partners and even children can shape the way we interact and the way we see ourselves in interactions. This creates a "repertoire of relational selves" (Andersen & Chen, 2002; p. 619) as different parts of the self are elicited in different relationships. These relational selves show up in attachment patterns, relational schema and relational vs independent self-construal (Chen et al., 2011). The relational self is responsive to context and evolves with each new relational experience. A person may choose to spend time with those who bring out the best in them with individuals who create space for the parts they most wish to nurture. In contrast, difficult relationships can leave one feeling unworthy and cautious about the world. In this complex way, it is possible to shape one's relational landscape deliberately, influencing how aspects of personality unfold over time. A sense of cohesion begins to emerge when different parts of the self are linked to past and present experiences across various relationships.

All in the Family?

Revisiting childhood interaction patterns creates new perspectives on individual and relational selves. As adults, there is an opportunity to integrate an appreciation for our strengths with a more compassionate understanding of our vulnerabilities.

Pause and reflect...
Draw a three-generational relational genogram for your own family. Using the relevant symbols to depict close, distant, conflictual, cut-off or fused relationships can help you recognize key interaction patterns in your family.

Think about whom you felt close to or distant from during your growing years. How did your family members express and resolve differences of opinion? How was care expressed? How was anger expressed? Were relationships more hierarchical or more equitable?

Note any multigenerational patterns that seem to reflect in your current interactions and relationships.

Working on a genogram can be both illuminating and emotionally demanding, often bringing up unexpected memories and interactions. This exploration can be more fruitful when conducted in a safe and comfortable space, allowing yourself the time to let your memories unfold. Connecting with specific experiences or memories and noting your age and life cycle stage provides important context for your reflections (McGoldrick & Gerson, 1985). Reflecting on specific adjectives you would use to describe your family members at various ages can be an evocative experience. You might also consider how easy or difficult it was to choose those words. Did you find it challenging to be critical, or was it easier than you expected? What emotions arise as you recall these memories? These reflections can deepen your understanding of your attachment experiences (Rovers, 2004). As you revisit your family patterns, you can appreciate their dynamic nature, observing how certain styles of interaction ebb and flow over time. For instance, you may notice fluctuations in your closeness to your siblings at different life cycle stages. To enhance this experience, consider discussing your genogram with a trusted family member or drawing it together, sharing and comparing memories. Following the exercise, you can engage in focused reflections on any recurring patterns and unexpected findings as you seek to understand your relational self.

Gaining insight into the origins of certain behaviours can provide the freedom to make new choices, allowing for fresh ways of relating to oneself, family and the world. For example, examining how beliefs about marriage from family of origin influence current relationships can lead to a desire to change specific patterns related to gender roles or problem-solving methods that no longer serve a purpose. Of course, the family is by no means the only context in which relational selves are shaped, and we encourage reflection on other key relationships with friends, mentors and partners.

Therapists' Relational Scripts

Each of us respond differently to the relational crucible of therapy, being more or less nurturant, needing more or less power, or more or less autonomy. We have beliefs about what constitutes a healthy interaction as well as a sense of what we need from others and both these shape our choices. Our response can also come from our experiences and roles in other relationships in our lives, so perhaps a therapist who has not experienced assertiveness in relation to their parents or partners will find it more difficult to be assertive in the therapy room. Similarly, if we have learnt to be nurturant and empathetic in our roles as child, partner, parent or sibling that can continue in our role as therapist. The therapist-client relationship is a special one which draws shades from all relationships but does not exactly simulate them. This is a purposeful and intentional alliance in which the therapist is responsible for the client's well-being, while the client does not share that obligation. The therapist role forms the filter through which relational styles are expressed in the therapy room.

By becoming aware of how we typically function in relationships—both comfortable and challenging—we can intentionally shape the therapy relationship into something the client can benefit from. This goes beyond offering empathy or positive regard to meeting the client's (sometimes unstated) relational needs. Clients who remind the therapist of someone they like or admire may evoke a strong desire for connection. This can lead to a wish to protect the relationship, prompting more accommodating behaviour. As a result, the therapist may remain receptive and affirming, while overlooking signs that the client may actually need a different kind of relational stance. Conversely, when the client cues a significant other with whom the therapist had a difficult relationship, this could elicit a self-protective mechanism. The therapist may withdraw emotionally, fearing or expecting a negative interaction, without even realizing what is going on (Andersen & Chen, 2002). When we instinctively move towards or away from a client, we can ask ourselves if they are activating a particular relational self, giving us the chance to choose our response.

Our relational selves may operate within distinct relational schemas which provide information about what to expect from others and can have a strong impact on the response to a client presentation (Tufekcioglu & Muran, 2015). For instance, if a therapist's relational schema suggests that people do not like them easily, they will expect the same from their client. In response they may withhold from the client, waiting for signs of warmth or approval. This withholding can cause the client to be slower in offering positive regard, in turn reinforcing the therapist's schema. Aspects of the therapist's relational self can play out in interactions with clients as they seek closeness or distance and enact their own interpersonal patterns. Similarly, clients may also bring their own expectations to the relationship, anticipating distance, hostility or care from therapists. When the therapist responds as they expect, for instance distancing from a withdrawn client, it reinforces the client's belief that others are undependable and emotionally unavailable, leaving them feeling unworthy of care. If these interaction patterns become rigid and fixed, with both the therapist and client getting stuck in their roles it limits therapeutic progress (Wiseman & Atzil-Slonim, 2018). When therapist fears and blocks are unknowingly communicated to the client, this also constrains therapeutic possibilities. For instance, a therapist who struggles with challenging authority may feel uneasy when a client expresses a desire to confront their boss or leave their marriage. Clients who pick up on this discomfort can unintentionally internalize it, leading them to make decisions influenced by the therapist's relational preferences.

Forming a healthy therapeutic alliance requires the therapist to be aware of, and able to manage their own emotional needs so that they can mentalize, reflect and theorize about what might be happening in the relationship. It is no wonder then that therapists with secure attachment styles are generally found to be effective with clients. The findings regarding anxious and avoidant attachment styles are more varied, with some studies suggesting challenges in forming and maintaining alliances, while others report no significant impact (Heinonen & Nisen-Lie, 2020; Steel et al., 2018). A process based understanding of the interaction between therapist and client attachment styles as well as how therapists experience and express their own attachment will help us be more intentional in how we manage the relationship. There are some indications that clients with an anxious attachment style do better with therapists who are more avoidant in their attachment style, and vice versa (Steel et al., 2018). Going deeper into how attachment styles play out, research also suggests that therapists with a dismissing attachment style may be less empathetic or deep in their interventions and prefer clients who are more intact and less dependent. Therapists who are anxiously attached initially work very hard to create the alliance but later feel exhausted by these efforts. Anxiety can also drive them towards micro-managing the process and can leave them upset at clients who wish to make more independent choices (Talia et al., 2020).

How can we understand such conflicting results? Perhaps the answer lies in seeing attachment as a dimensional construct, with different attachment systems being activated in different relational contexts. Therapists come with many layers to their being—we are not all secure or all insecure, and this may serve us well, as it offers flexibility in response. Combinations of traits can balance each other out; with reflective abilities compensating for attachment vulnerabilities, and secure attachment buffering against lower reflective functioning (Cologon et al., 2017). As we self-reflect and expand our awareness of our relational selves, new ways of being can open for us and our clients.

I to We: Our Collective Self

The collective self not only defines who we are, but also who we are not. The collective self can become visible to others through external markers of group membership, like a particular form of clothing or a preference for a kind of language or lens through which experiences are interpreted. This group identity is not dependent on closeness with other group members, but rather on a shared set of values and behaviours. Some group memberships are ascribed at birth, while others are acquired through interests and activities. Group identities that are valued and bring a strong feeling of emotional connection are more salient to the self-concept. As we navigate through life, we may find ourselves distancing from groups that once held meaning for us while aspiring to join new ones. New groups are constantly being created (e.g., those who were pro-vaccination and those who were anti-vaccination during the COVID-19 pandemic) and some of them can become very central quite quickly. As group memberships evolve and we become familiar with new ways of functioning and being, our collective self also evolves. An important source of our sense of collective self comes from the profession we belong to. Doctor, drummer, dancer…each profession evokes a picture of a particular kind of person—as does psychotherapist.

The memberships we identify with, such as "I am a feminist", can shape our interactions in the therapeutic setting. This influence can occur both when clients are perceived as part of the ingroup and when they are seen as belonging to the outgroup. What will be spoken and what will be withheld, what will be seen or not seen, and who feels more comfortable in contradicting or challenging the other… all of this is shaped by the interactions of our collective identities. Gender, race, geography and the intersections of all our social locations determine the advantages, privileges and power we have access to; and the oppression, internalized stigma and discrimination we might have lived through. This awareness can sensitize us to exploring the meaning and implication of our client's group memberships and also provides another perspective through which we can understand the therapeutic relationship.

The Spiritual Self

The spiritual self refers to the aspect of an individual that seeks meaning, purpose and connection beyond the physical or material world. It is often associated with one's sense of identity in relation to something greater than oneself, such as the universe, a higher power or the collective consciousness. This is a part of ourself that lies within, shaping our ethics and values, and influencing our actions and choices. It can take time and searching to uncover what holds this deeper meaning within. This, in itself, is a spiritual journey that calls for patience and commitment. This personal exploration can take many forms, with some preferring solitary meditation, and others finding connection through community or an immersion in rituals. A therapist's spiritual self can enrich the therapeutic process in diverse ways. It can offer perspectives or approaches that support clients facing existential dilemmas, providing space to express their beliefs and explore their sense of purpose. By embracing this dimension, therapists can create a strong connection with some of their clients, helping them tap into their own spiritual resources as part of the healing process. Not all clients are comfortable with a spiritual language or perspective and spiritually inclined therapists should be careful not to impose this part of themselves onto the client. Outside the therapy room, a therapist can use spiritual practices that they personally value as part of their repertoire for self-care and resilience. While spiritual practices are easier to define and operationalize in research, the inner experience of the transcendent is far more intangible and difficult to capture. Yet, with so much of therapeutic work centred around growth, the search for peace and making meaning of suffering, it becomes important to understand how therapists engage with these processes in their own lives.

For many, engaging with spiritual beliefs and teachings fosters personal growth while cultivating a sense of grounding and connection to oneself and the world. Indian philosophical traditions are among numerous spiritual traditions across the world that offer a metaphysical perspective to guide the process of self-discovery.

A Therapist Speaks: Meditations on the Self

Jyotsna Agrawal

In the Indian psycho-spiritual tradition, the self is differentiated between outer (*ahamkara*) and inner (*antaratman/purusha*). The outer self is constructed by our experiences, memories and actions and tied to our bodies. The inner self is considered transcendental, a spark of divine infinity and a source of sublime knowledge. While the outer self may be helpful initially in individuating from others, going beyond it to discover one's inner self is the aim of these traditions. Connecting with one's inner self is transformative, but it is a hero's journey - effortful and full of adventure - so only a few commit to it. Those who go till the end may find their outer self dissolving like a 'salt doll' when it meets the ocean water (metaphor by the mystic Sri Ramakrishna Paramahamsa) and experience the 'oceanic feeling'.

One way to get closer to one's inner self is to attenuate the outer self, which is made up of our thoughts, feelings and actions. Four psychological components of the outer self have been acknowledged and studied, that is, agency (*kartatva*), identification or our relationship with objects or people (*abhimana*), separation from others (*dwait bhava*) and individuality (*vaishisthya*). Becoming more aware of these four components and their dynamic interplay, and then growing beyond them, can come naturally as people mature, but doing it intentionally is the essence of the yogic path. For example, we may grow to accept that we cannot control our lives. However, we can also deliberately develop flexibility and a healthy separation from the outcomes of our action. Doing things for their inherent meaningfulness and offering one's efforts to something larger than oneself (*karma yoga*) may help us progress on this.

A sense of separation from others and a strong focus on our own unique individuality are two other components of the outer self. While some individuation is healthy, rigid boundaries between self and others may strengthen the outer self, making these boundaries look like walls with shards of broken glasses. The natural way may be to see these boundaries as seashores, where the separation between the earth and water consists of a beautiful back-and-forth dance. We may have our uniqueness and differences, but we also have many commonalities with others in our joys and sufferings. So, balancing our uniqueness with a sense of the collective would bring us closer to the truth and our inner self.

These components have their play both within us and in our therapy room. Our personal growth can bring more healing in our therapy work, as we become open and flexible with our clients, in their uniqueness and differences. We may find it easier to develop genuine warmth and positive regard for clients, especially the ones who challenge us. As we let go of our attachments or fixed agendas, we create a therapeutic space that fosters deeper growth. In growing closer to our inner self, we can convincingly show our clients how far they can go themselves.

Dr. Jyotsna Agrawal *is a clinical psychologist and faculty member in India and is deeply committed to exploring the applications of Yoga and Indian psychology in clinical and community settings, as well as for personal growth. She strives towards an integrative and inclusive approach and also has a strong interest in expressive arts.*

The Revealing and Concealing Self

As therapists, we are guided to be genuine and authentic in our encounters with clients. We are also expected to maintain a professional demeanour and only show parts of us that will be therapeutic for the client. How are we to be both real and therapeutic at the same time? If our personal self is very timid and non-assertive, should we mask this to seem more confident and competent? If we feel moved to tears hearing a client's story, or if our funny bone is tickled at an inappropriate time, how much of this do we reveal to our clients? As therapists, we need to understand how we can reconcile these contradictory but important professional imperatives. Perhaps what is required is a committed search for what can be both real within us *and* helpful to our clients.

Pause and reflect...

Think about the therapy room you usually practice in. What does it look like? Does it have a desk or a low table? Are the chairs formal or comfortable? Do you have any certificates, family photos or art on your wall? What is the colour scheme and the amount of light and air available?

How much of your setting is deliberate and planned with your clients in mind?

What do you think your client might surmise about you from your setting?

As you visualize your space and what it says about you, do you want to change anything about your therapy room?

Based on theoretical orientations as well as personality, therapists may choose to allow more or less of their personal selves into the therapy room. Over time, they often learn to incorporate their personal style into their professional style, leading to an amalgamation that feels both natural and therapeutically effective. Allowing our human side into the room is essential if we are to form a genuine connection with clients. Sometimes when a client asks us a question or their story resonates with our own experiences, we respond spontaneously without much prior thought, perhaps blurting out that we too hate doing household chores or smiling at a political comment. At these times, clients have perhaps reached our personal selves and drawn us out into the session. Such unplanned disclosures can be discussed with clients, and they often bring life into the therapy session and further therapeutic work. We do not need to only show what is healthy about us, and we do not need to get it right each time. In fact, it is this comfort with imperfection and the willingness to acknowledge the messiness of both life and therapy that can resonate with clients who are themselves trying to come to terms with what is messy in their own lives.

There are also occasions where therapists cannot help but reveal themselves—life events like pregnancy, illness or bereavement have a way of intruding into the client's awareness. The choice here is whether to speak about it openly and how much to say. Intentional use of self, on the other hand, involves choosing to disclose either immediate responses or personal stories as a way of addressing therapeutic goals. Therapists might share immediate responses, with the intention of encouraging clients to state their unstated feelings (e.g., "That would make me really sad. I'm wondering if you feel the same way?"), attempting to negotiate (e.g., "It seems that we are both feeling stuck. I know I am feeling frustrated by it. I would like to know what you are feeling?"), enhance the bond (e.g., "I feel particularly worried for you today. What can I do to help?") or repair the relationship (e.g., "I am so sorry that what I said hurt you.") (Hill, 2014).

Current views on therapist disclosures about themselves or their experiences have shifted away from perspectives that this is inherently and universally harmful to clients. Now self-disclosure is seen as another tool in the kitbag, albeit one that is used thoughtfully and selectively. Most often therapists choose to self-disclose as a way of strengthening the relationship or creating change within the client. Disclosures can be soothing for the client to hear (e.g., "Yes, fatherhood can be hard."). Or they can be used to stimulate new thoughts or actions (e.g., "I needed to stick with the exercise program for weeks before I started to enjoy it."). Sharing a similar personal experience with a client can build an emotional connection in ways that merely telling them that their experience is 'normal' may not. When therapists speak about life experiences or their own mental health journeys, this encourages client openness and can leave clients more hopeful and motivated to work on themselves. Importantly, such revelations can also be a means of equalizing power and building solidarity. However, over sharing or unsolicited sharing can be problematic, particularly for vulnerable clients or those with boundary issues. They may feel obliged to respond to the therapist's need and put their own aside, or they may feel overwhelmed and unprepared to be the recipients of a disclosure. When the therapist speaks out of a countertransferential need to share their story, they can disregard client cues or responses indicating discomfort. To disclose or not to disclose is not a single decision but a series of decisions—based on the therapist, client and the moment in therapy.

Being asked a direct question by a client can be an unsettling experience. The way the therapist responds can demonstrate respect and empathy for the client's need to know. Even when therapists do not directly answer the question, it is important to deal with it in an open way, rather than hiding behind rules. As professionals, we owe our clients information about our training, background and approach to therapy. Therapists do sometimes choose to disclose personal experiences—to do so effectively includes being tentative and brief, perhaps starting with non-verbal indications (e.g., nodding) or a simple statement identifying a shared experience. This leaves the door open for clients to ask about the experience (if they are interested). Having shared their story, therapists need to turn the focus back to the client, to see how it might be meaningful for them (D'Aniello & Nguyen, 2017). More caution is recommended in the early stages of therapy, or when the client is already emotionally overwhelmed. At any stage in therapy, therapists need to carefully weigh the potential costs and benefits of self-disclosure and evaluate whether the transparency, respect and trust the disclosure conveys, outweighs any burden the client might feel. It can be helpful for therapists to consult nuanced frameworks to guide their decisions, particularly around revealing lived experiences of mental health vulnerabilities (Dunlop et al., 2022). Our reflections on our self-disclosures (e.g., Why did I that to that particular client at that specific moment in therapy?) continue long after the therapy session is over. As we mull over possibilities and options, we discover other routes we could have taken and things we could have said differently or left unsaid.

Malaika, a young therapist, is going to have a baby and take a break from therapy sessions later in the year. There are six months until the due date and it's still a new and exciting feeling for her. Of course, she needs to inform and plan with all her clients; but it seems harder when she thinks of Lina, a particularly sensitive client who took six months to even begin to speak about the painful feelings around her "forgotten childhood" and "difficult mother".

In the next session Lina says, "I wonder if I can be a good mother? Should I even try to get pregnant? This is what I want to talk about now." Malaika realises that she needs to share the news about her own pregnancy....

Malaika is aware that self-disclosure is inevitable but knows that sensitivity and timing are critical elements of the decision-making process. One route could be to jump straight in with her news and then keep the rest of the session to process it. Or she might choose to first hear Lina out, get a sense of her level of readiness and disclose when the time feels right. Malaika is apprehensive about how her disclosure might affect her client's sense of self. Would Lina feel more inadequate and isolated in her experience of doubts about motherhood? She was also concerned about the possible impact on the therapeutic alliance. Might Lina feel that her therapist would be focused on her own pregnancy and have less energy or interest in Lina's emotions? Deeper reflections on all these possibilities can help Malaika decide when to speak and also how to minimize the potential negative impact on Lina. Disclosures like these are most likely to be well received when the client is feeling attended to and cared for, and is also adequately regulated. Planning ahead is crucial to establish a supportive framework for the client. Emotions can fluctuate over time, and it could take several sessions before the client feels comfortable again. Considering all these factors, Malaika chooses to keep her news to herself in that moment, and address Lina's emotions and emergent dilemma first. She recognizes that remaining silent about something so significant for too long could ultimately be perceived as a betrayal or at the very least a lack of honesty. Malaika resolves to disclose this information within the next few sessions. Finding the right words and timing to initiate the discussion is only the knock on the door. The creation of a safe space for processing Lina's response is much more crucial.

Self-disclosure can go wrong even if we follow all the rules. Our internal or bodily reactions, feelings of stiffness or uneasiness can indicate that we have opened a door which should have remained closed. We may each have a personalized perspective on what it means to be authentic in sessions. This can be influenced by textbook ideas, as well as cultural norms, personal comfort and values. As we tune into what feels real and reflect on how we can be ourselves while remaining professional with our clients, we may discover a truer blend of the personal and professional.

Creative and Experiential Pathways to Self-Discovery

The self is both intangible and unknowable in its entirety. Sometimes we need to feel our way towards the self, rather than think our way towards it. Creative approaches, both verbal and non-verbal, offer meaningful pathways of bringing it all together—discovering aspects of the self, connecting this with therapy and using this knowledge more effectively and meaningfully. Art, drama, storytelling, music, movement and other experiential methods harness the power of imagination. For therapists who are so often anchored to words, this immersion in visual, tactile, symbolic and embodied modes can add a fresh dimension to the understanding of self.

Artmaking and Self-reflection

Artmaking is a powerful tool for self-expression and self-discovery, where the evolving process of creation holds more significance than the final product. Artists like Frida Kahlo used self-portraits as a means of self-expression, embedding deep emotional truths and personal experiences into her work. Surrealist artists sought to depict the hidden, often fragmented layers of the psyche, unveiling the complexities of inner psychological landscapes. Creative expression taps into the unconscious, with symbols and images acting as gateways to deeper self-awareness, as emphasized in the theories of Carl Jung.

Artmaking can be done through a variety of mediums—painting, clay, photography or even digital tools and mixed media—each offering a unique dialogue with the self. For example, one might create collages to represent the layered inner landscape, make masks that embody different aspects of the self or select everyday objects that evoke salient memories, powerful emotions or strongly held values. These forms of artistic expression provide therapists with opportunities for personal exploration, helping them gain deeper insight into their own emotions, beliefs and unconscious processes. What part of yourself would you like to explore through art?

***A Therapist Speaks*: My Strength Tree**

Deepti Guruprasad

Materials: A large sheet of paper, pastels or markers.

Instructions: Lay your hand on the large sheet of paper such that a part of your arm is also on the paper and your fingers remain around the middle of the paper. Spread your fingers open and trace your hand including your arm, leaving the back of the arm and fingertips open. Your arm becomes the trunk of the tree, and the fingertips are the beginnings of your branches. Divide the base of your tree trunk into sections to indicate roots and divide each fingertip into smaller branches. Add leaves to the end of the branches. The leaves should be big enough to write words inside them. There is no right or wrong way to draw the tree. List your core strengths or pillars of support in your journey as a therapist on your roots. On each leaf, list one special skill, unique resource, coping strategy or a contribution to your profession. Your relatively newer skills could be depicted on the smaller leaves, along with any skills you wish to add to your repertoire. You can complete this activity at one go or leave it open for additions and changes. As you grow as a therapist, you may deepen your roots or sprout more leaves.

Reflection questions: How did you experience this activity? Was it easy for you to list your strengths? How active is your inner critic? How often do you reflect on your strengths and spend time appreciating yourself? You could keep this image as a reminder of your growth journey and use it at times when you feel less motivated or perhaps underappreciated in your environment.

Deepti Guruprasad *is a clinical psychologist and registered art therapist with a decade of clinical experience across diverse racial and socioeconomic settings in the*

United States. She has recently moved back to India and follows a strengths-based integrative approach in therapy while emphasising the mind-body relationship in healing.

Self-Discovery Through Reflective Journaling

Journaling is the art of making stories about what is happening to us, and through these stories, making sense of who we are. In the pages of our journals lie possibilities and preferences, not just our pasts but also our potential futures. Hubbs and Brand (2005, p. 60) evocatively refer to a journal as a paper mirror, one that enables us to gaze at our minds and hearts. By its very nature, the process of writing forces one to slow down, mull over ideas, organize our thoughts and express them in a somewhat focused manner. It provides a safe space to explore and express feelings, objectively examine prejudices or set patterns of thought, and even transform as new perspectives are integrated within the self (Mudgal et al., 2025). Because a journal is typically confidential and private, it fosters the freedom to express our complete selves. Journals are usually written in the first person, so the connection with the inner being is inescapable. Unlike other writing that trainees or therapists need to do, the journal does not have to showcase knowledge or achieve an immediate goal. These conditions may be ideal for a free-flowing reflection that takes one to new places while also allowing for the revisiting of old experiences (Wright & Bolton, 2012).

It can be helpful to create a ritual around writing, with some targets for frequency or time spent. Fixing a time, a day or a medium of writing can make it a regular and potentially more useful part of life. Attaching it to other activities (e.g., soon after yoga, before each supervision session) can also anchor the practice. For those who do not like routine, keeping a journal handy to make notes on the go is also useful. To begin with, we recommend keeping aside an hour's time, settling into a space, clearing the mind, looking around and imbibing the surroundings. We can ask ourselves what experience we wish to write about. We may let different thoughts swirl around until something calls on our attention—a block in therapy, a great session, a challenging moment or a typical interaction seen through new eyes. As we open the door into our experiences, a stepwise process of journaling, helps create a reflective loop.

Entering into the experience: A detailed description of the session content and process is a good place to start. Write down what you might be thinking and feeling about it in retrospect. Express yourself as you feel comfortable without being limited by language. If you are multilingual, choose the language you think in, the one closest to your heart.

Reflecting on the experience: Step back and think about what has come up for you and what it means for you. How are your thoughts and feelings about your experience linked to your values, identity and contexts? Are they influenced by theory or what your supervisor might say? Think about what you would hope to do if you had the experience again.

Applying it back to ourselves: Try to crystallize what you might have learnt about yourself as a person or as a therapist, and what you might like to strengthen or change. When we engage in a reflective journaling exercise, it can sometimes bring up painful feelings. Reflection may be deepest when we engage with repeated patterns or strong emotions from the past. We therefore need to be prepared with a safe space and emotional support before embarking on this exercise.

Movement as a Reflective Practice

Our bodies are containers and mirrors for our thoughts and experiences and can be valuable paths to self-awareness. Embodied experiences such as feelings of lightness, heaviness, pain and sleepiness can be markers for understanding deep emotional and mental states. Body-based practices can help tune into unspoken messages in the therapeutic encounter, as our bodies resonate with our mental states and those of our clients.

***A Therapist Speaks*: To Move and Be Moved**

Brinda Jacob-Janvrin

One of my favourite body-based practices is Authentic Movement. In this simple but profound movement discipline, the mover moves with her eyes closed in front of a witness. The mover is not 'performing' for the witness, but waiting to see what the body suggests, thus experiencing the sense of 'being moved' as opposed to 'moving'. During this process, she also tracks her movement, refining her own inner witness. This is accentuated by the presence of the external witness, who not only tracks the mover but also her own responses to the mover. Compassionate witnessing creates a safe and sacred space within which we can encounter both our wounding and our potential—that part of ourselves that is greater than our wounding, the Self with a capital S as defined by Jung.

In my movement exploration at a retreat, I found myself trying to separate from a large mound of earth, which felt like my father who had passed away in 2000. As I struggled to separate myself, I saw (in my mind's eye) images of important men in my life (my husband, past boyfriends) escape from between us. This act of separation was heartbreaking, and I was crying for over 20 minutes. The compassionate witnessing provided by my two teachers allowed me to continue and witness myself experiencing the most devastating pain and grief. I was finally mourning my father, something I hadn't done in 17 years. In doing so, I began peeling away the projections of my father from these various men. The experience also revealed to me my own inner strength that allowed me to stay with this pain. In learning to hold this pain, I learnt to love in deeper ways.

As a trainer, I always begin with a short movement visualization to bring trainees into the space with a heightened sense of presence. They learn to listen to their body signals in the here and now—a tightening of a muscle, the quickening of the heartbeat, sweat on the palms, etc. Interestingly, one part may feel quite different from another—with the lower body feeling heavy and the upper body light, or the right side of the body feeling stiff, while the left part is fluid. When we consciously move our body, we are moving layers of suppressed memory and releasing unexpressed emotion and energy. The body holds incredible wisdom and is always moving towards healing and balance. Our body is our most intimate home and being at home in our body is one of the greatest indicators of positive mental health.

Ms. Brinda Jacob-Janvrin *is a dancer, a movement-based expressive arts therapist, an Authentic Movement practitioner and trainer, and a Natural Dreamwork practitioner. She is the founder of the Studio for Movement Arts and Therapies (SMART) Trust, which provides training in expressive and creative art therapies and offers mental health services to individuals and communities in India.*

Perspectives on Training and Development

Training Frameworks for the Use of Self in Therapy

Use of self training frameworks such as the Person-of-the-Therapist model (POTT; Aponte et al., 2016) and the Self-Practice /Self-Reflection model (SP/SR; Bennett-Levy, 2019) fuse reflection to build a bridge between the self of the therapist and the conceptual and procedural skills of therapy. Such training is time-, knowledge- and resource-intensive and requires commitment from institutions, trainers and participants. If trainees struggle for time in a packed academic and clinical schedule, both engagement and attrition are likely to be problematic. Programmes that are integrated into the curriculum are likely to be more sustainable.

Any sustained focus on the use of self requires a deep emotional investment in accessing and revealing aspects of the inner self. Trainers need to ensure that trainees are prepared for this exploration and feel empowered to decide when, to whom and how much they wish to disclose. Close attention to confidentiality and safety is paramount, and boundaries between self-work and therapy need to be delineated. In the POTT model, personal stories and sharing are invited only when directly relevant to therapy work and therapist development. While certain aspects could be individual reflective exercises, for example, personal histories and genogram, others such as signature themes could be brought to the group. Trainers also require preparation to connect with the language and philosophy of the training model as well as ways to process the emotional impact of this work, which will inevitably evoke aspects of their own selves. This is an area that needs to be addressed more strongly in any training methodology used to facilitate self-exploration.

If training programmes do not have the space to implement intensive modules, we recommend integrating conversations and exercises aimed at self-awareness and use of self into academic teaching, classroom discussions, and most importantly, supervision sessions. Trainers and supervisors could select methods that promote active self-reflection as well as the use of reflective blogs and therapy simulations. Training focused on embodied awareness could add another pathway to the understanding of therapeutic processes such as attunement, relational depth and countertransference. We also anticipate an increased focus on assessment and training of therapist mentalizing ability. When a therapist's ability to explore their own emotions and experiences through a not-knowing stance is strengthened, this can help them understand what might be happening within the client's mind (Barreto & Matos, 2018). There is some evidence that brief experiential training can increase mentalizing abilities among novice therapists, but there is scope for further conceptual elaboration and empirical support (Ensink et al., 2013). Working with experienced practitioners or those in supervisory roles would require tweaking of the content, process and aims of programmes developed for trainees or novice therapists. Therapists may also seek personal therapy or follow paths of self-discovery in ways that feel personally meaningful.

Use of Self-Work Within Supervision

Supervisors play a critical role in helping supervisees translate their therapy experiences into personal and professional growth. Supervisees can be encouraged to bring process notes of therapy sessions along with reflective observations about their emotions, reactions and observations to facilitate this reflective process. Techniques grounded within specific theoretical frameworks can provide a language and method that supervisees can relate to. Depending on the theoretical orientation/s within the training context, supervisees could be encouraged to explore their own life scripts, understand and manage the activation of their underlying schemas and modes, or engage in a value-clarification process. Reflective supervisors can adapt and incorporate methods and perspectives that are consonant with the evolving needs of their supervisee.

Even supervisors who value the use of self in therapy and find it meaningful could hesitate to open conversations on the use of self with their trainees. Supervisors can encounter roadblocks that stem from inadequate theoretical grounding, less experience with self-work or struggles to integrate this along with other competing demands on the limited supervision time. Supervisors need to assess supervisee readiness, use gentle and indirect feedback when needed, and circumvent issues that are too sensitive while trying to build a collaborative space. Reaching out to their own supervision and consultation networks can support the expansion of skills in addressing use-of-self issues.

Conclusion

The self encapsulates not just who we have been and who we are, but also our hopes, goals and aspirations—what Markus and Nurius (1986) refer to as *possible selves*. As new ideas and perceptions come in and the old are discarded, the self continuously changes. These questions about change and persistence can also be extended to understanding our self and identity, thereby making the reflexive process of self-awareness an ongoing endeavour.

References

Andersen, S. M., & Chen, S. (2002). The relational self: An interpersonal social-cognitive theory. *Psychological Review, 109*(4), 619–645.

Aponte, H. J. (2016). The person-of-the-therapist model on the use of self in therapy. In H. J. Aponte & K. Kissil (Eds.), *The person of the therapist training model* (1st ed., pp. 1–13). Routledge.

Aponte, H. J., & Kissil, K. (2014). "If I can grapple with this I can truly be of use in the therapy room": Using the therapist's own emotional struggles to facilitate effective therapy. *Journal of Marital and Family Therapy, 40*(2), 152–164.

Baldwin, M. (2013). Interview with Carl Rogers on the use of the self in therapy. In M. Baldwin (Ed.), *The use of self in therapy* (3rd ed., pp. 28–35). Routledge.

Banmen, J. (2002). The Satir model: Yesterday and today. *Contemporary Family Therapy, 24*(1), 7–22.

Barreto, J., & Matos, P. (2018). Mentalizing countertransference? A model for research on the elaboration of countertransference experience in psychotherapy. *Clinical Psychology & Psychotherapy, 25*(3), 427–439.

Bennett-Levy, J. (2006). Therapist skills: A cognitive model of their acquisition and refinement. *Behavioural and Cognitive Psychotherapy, 34*, 57–78.

Bennett-Levy, J. (2019). Why therapists should walk the talk: The theoretical and empirical case for personal practice in therapist training and professional development. *Journal of Behavior Therapy and Experimental Psychiatry, 62*, 133–145.

Bruck, E., Winston, A., Aderholt, S., & Muran, J. C. (2006). Predictive validity of patient and therapist attachment and introject styles. *American Journal of Psychotherapy, 60*, 393–406.

Bucci, S., Seymour-Hyde, A., Harris, A., & Berry, K. (2015). Client and therapist attachment styles and working alliance. *Clinical Psychology & Psychotherapy, 23*(2), 155–165.

Chen, S., Boucher, H., & Kraus, M. W. (2011). The relational self. In S. J. Schwartz, K. Luyckx, & V. L. Vignoles (Eds.), *Handbook of identity theory and research* (pp. 149–175). Springer.

Cologon, J., Schweitzer, R. D., King, R., & Nolte, T. (2017). Therapist reflective functioning, therapist attachment style and therapist effectiveness. *Administration and Policy in Mental Health and Mental Health Services Research, 44*, 614–625.

D'Aniello, C., & Nguyen, H. N. (2017). Considerations for intentional use of self-disclosure for family therapists. *Journal of Family Psychotherapy, 28*(1), 23–37.

Dunlop, B. J., Woods, B., Lovell, J., O'Connell, A., Rawcliffe-Foo, S., & Hinsby, K. (2022). Sharing lived experiences framework (SLEF): A framework for mental health practitioners when making disclosure decisions. *Journal of Social Work Practice, 36*(1), 25–39.

Ensink, K., Maheux, J., Normandin, L., Sabourin, S., Diguer, L., Berthelot, N., & Parent, K. (2013). The impact of mentalization training on the reflective function of novice therapists: A randomized controlled trial. *Psychotherapy Research, 23*(5), 526–538.

Heinonen, E., & Nissen-Lie, H. A. (2020). The professional and personal characteristics of effective psychotherapists: A systematic review. *Psychotherapy Research, 30*(4), 417–432.

Hill, C. E. (2014). *Helping skills: Facilitating exploration, insight, and action* (4th ed.). American Psychological Association.

Hubbs, D. L., & Brand, C. F. (2005). The paper mirror: Understanding reflective journaling. *Journal of Experiential Education, 28*(1), 60–71.

Luft, J. (1982). The Johari window: A graphic model of awareness in interpersonal relations. *NHL Human Relation Training News, 5*(1), 6–7.

Lum, W. (2002). The use of self of the therapist. *Contemporary Family Therapy, 24*, 181–197.

Markus, H., & Nurius, P. (1986). Possible selves. *American Psychologist, 41*, 954–969.

McGoldrick, M., & Gerson, R. (1985). *Genograms in family assessment*. W.W. Norton.

Mehlomakulu, C. (2017). *Tree of strength art directive*. http://creativityintherapy.com/2017/04/tree-strength-art-directive/

Mudgal, R., Bharadwaj, I. U., & Bhatia, H. (2025). Role of reflective writing: A first person inquiry into the therapist self. *Journal of Constructivist Psychology*, 1–21. https://doi.org/10.1080/10720537.2025.2555437

Nissen-Lie, H. A., Rønnestad, M. H., Høglend, P. A., Havik, O. E., Solbakken, O. A., Stiles, T. C., & Monsen, J. T. (2017). Love yourself as a person, doubt yourself as a therapist? *Clinical Psychology & Psychotherapy, 24*(1), 48–60.

Peterson, C., & Seligman, M. E. P. (2004). *Character strengths and virtues: A handbook and classification*. Oxford University Press.

Rober, P. (1999). The therapist's inner conversation in family therapy practice: Some ideas about the self of the therapist, therapeutic impasse, and the process of reflection. *Family Process, 38*(2), 209–228.

Rønnestad, M. H., & Skovholt, T. M. (2003). The journey of the counselor and therapist: Research findings and perspectives on professional development. *Journal of Career Development, 30*, 5–44.

Rovers, M. (2004). Family of origin theory, attachment theory and the genogram. *Journal of Couple & Relationship Therapy, 3*(4), 43–63.

Satir, V. (2013). The therapist story. In M. Baldwin (Ed.), *The use of self in therapy* (3rd ed., pp. 19–27). Routledge.

Sedikides, C., Gaertner, L., & O'Mara, E. M. (2011). Individual self, relational self, collective self: Hierarchical ordering of the tripartite self. *Psychological Studies, 56*, 98–107.

Steel, C., Macdonald, J., & Schroder, T. (2018). A systematic review of the effect of therapists' internalized models of relationships on the quality of the therapeutic relationship. *Journal of Clinical Psychology, 74*(1), 5–42.

Sude, M. E., & Baima, T. (2021). Training the self of the therapist through marriage and family therapy role-plays. *International Journal of Systemic Therapy, 32*(1), 23–40.

Talia, A., Muzi, L., Lingiardi, V., & Taubner, S. (2020). How to be a secure base: Therapist's attachment representations and their link to attunement in psychotherapy. *Attachment and Human Development, 22*(2), 189–206.

Timm, T. M., & Blow, A. J. (1999). Self-of-the-therapist work: A balance between removing restraints and identifying resources. *Contemporary Family Therapy, 21*, 331–350.

Tufekcioglu, S., & Muran, J. C. (2015). Case formulation and the therapeutic relationship: The role of therapist self-reflection and self-revelation. *Journal of Clinical Psychology, 71*(5), 469–477.

Wiseman, H., & Atzil-Slonim, D. (2018). Closeness and distance dynamics in the therapeutic relationship. In O. Tishby & H. Wiseman (Eds.), *Developing the therapeutic relationship: Integrating case studies, research, and practice* (pp. 81–103). American Psychological Association.

Wright, J., & Bolton, G. (2012). *Preparing for the journey. Reflective writing in counselling and psychotherapy* (2nd ed.). Sage.

Chapter 4
Adopting a Theoretical Lens

What is a good life? How do people live, strive, grieve and connect? How much free will do people have? What is knowable and unknowable about human experience? How can we understand and respond to inevitable problems and struggles? What are the ways in which meaningful change, growth and healing can occur? In its essence, psychotherapy is a response to such philosophical questions about the human condition. At the heart of the therapeutic endeavour lies the effort to alleviate emotional distress and suffering, and theoretical frameworks represent ways of understanding and responding to this experience. Rather than techniques and strategies, it is the deeply embedded philosophical assumptions about human nature that both unite and differentiate the theoretical paradigms which guide the therapeutic process. Each theoretical model of psychotherapy proposes a route to facilitating emotional and behavioural change for better mental health and well-being. It offers a language to communicate with clients, shows ways to listen, observe and do, and becomes a guide as we travel together on the journey of change. Theoretical frameworks help to make meaning of clients' stories and shape therapeutic relationships. In this process, both therapist and client find newer ways of understanding and responding to the self, others and the world.

Our first encounters with these theories and their applications are often during psychotherapy training, where we are introduced to one or several theoretical models. Theory provides a lens through which to view the world and helps in exploring situations, emotions or relationships that are often complex and challenging. As we progress as therapists, many of us identify a framework with which we feel more connected and prefer to work. The traditional schools of therapy: psychodynamic, cognitive behavioural, humanistic–existential and systemic, have been joined by approaches which are situated within newer post-modern and social constructivist frameworks. Therapies which have emerged from feminist theory, critical psychology and social justice have firmly placed the individual back in their social context, highlighting how structural inequities, systemic oppression and experiences of marginalization shape people's identities and contribute to emotional distress. This evolution

P. Bhola et al., *Reflective Practice in Psychotherapy and Counselling*,
https://doi.org/10.1007/978-981-96-9732-8_4

of theoretical models parallels the larger paradigm shift from modernist approaches that focus on objective truths and empirical validation to post-modern frameworks which value subjective knowledge and shared meaning-making.

Increasingly, theoretical orientations are seen as representing different doors through which to enter the therapeutic arena. The choices are multitudinous, and each theoretical orientation uses a different set of metaphors to enter the psychological world. Theories tend to merge and divide, reminding us of the familiar dodo bird verdict which suggested that all forms of therapy are equally effective (Rosenzweig, 1936). This landmark finding marked a shift away from polarized or competitive approaches to a growing recognition of the contribution of common factors like the therapeutic alliance, therapist characteristics and skills, and influences that originate outside the therapy room (Wampold, 2015).

The emergence of integrative and transtheoretical models has opened new arenas for reflection on the many ways of seeing and doing in our therapy practice (Fleuridas & Krafcik, 2019). The field is not static, and in the spirit of continued reflecting and questioning there have been calls to move away from fixed orientations. Instead, therapists are urged to adopt a pluralistic approach and engage in a dynamic process of choosing methods drawn across orientations. The choice of method is responsive to an individual client's needs and preferences and also rooted in the therapist's knowledge and experience (Cooper & McLeod, 2012). More recently, we note the emergence of a plethora of 'newer' theoretical models that are integrative in their conceptualization. For instance, mentalization-based therapy which draws from psychodynamic, cognitive-behavioural, systemic and ecological approaches and emotion-focused therapy that draws from experiential, systemic and attachment-based approaches. There are continued developments both within and outside these frameworks, and if one is curious, there is always more to learn. With this profusion of information and perspective to navigate, it is useful to remember that "Models are words on paper, and as such are not 'effective' in and of themselves; rather, models help *therapists* be effective" (Blow et al., 2007, p. 308). The professional journey of a therapist often begins with translating theory into practice. Over time, reflections on practice inform and deepen the understanding of theory, creating a continuous cycle of learning and growth.

In this chapter, we explore the ways in which therapists can intentionally position themselves vis-à-vis theory. We reflect on the numerous factors and experiences that influence the choice of theoretical orientation or model, as well as the evolution of that choice, acknowledging the dynamic relationship with one's orientation. Each therapist evolves a unique personal connection with theoretical orientation and its practice, and we also explore this process. Throughout the chapter we have used the words model, orientation or approach interchangeably, recognizing that theories offer a framework as well as a lens to shape our therapeutic work.

Positioning Ourselves

The ways in which the therapeutic role is imagined stimulates a deeper exploration of what each theoretical framework means for a therapist. While some of us carry a clear image of who a therapist is and what they do and feel certain about our model of choice, others may still be on the journey of discovery.

Pause and reflect...
We invite you to picture each of these images as possible reflections of who a therapist is and what a therapist does. Do you see a therapist as a mother, an architect, a scientist, an angel, an archaeologist, a magician, an explorer, a guru, a detective, a puppeteer, a healer, a gardener, or perhaps a co-traveller...?

Which images resonate with how you see your role as a therapist?

Do any of these possible ways of seeing a therapist make you feel uncomfortable?

Do you imagine a therapist in any other way?

Think about what you associate with each image.

If you connect with several images, consider how these different ways of being a therapist fit together for you.

In our experience during workshops on reflective practice, this activity invariably evokes a wide range of responses from participants. Some view themselves as an archaeologist excavating into the past and meticulously joining lost pieces; or as a detective, possibly in disguise engaged in sifting through clues and searching for evidence. Others relate more closely to the metaphor of a gardener who clears weeds and cultivates growth, or a mother who offers unconditional care and support. What is striking is how the same image can be perceived differently by different people. For instance, the image of mother can be perceived as being more supportive or more cloying, depending on the therapist's personal history. This highlights how past experiences shape the ways in which therapists approach therapy and relate to clients. Equally important is listening carefully to how other therapists respond to the images and engaging in discussions with them. This dual process of introspection and dialogue enriches the reflective activity, promoting growth, awareness and a more nuanced understanding of therapeutic processes. We also encourage spending some time reflecting on the images that evoke some discomfort. Often, these are the images of a magician or puppeteer and sometimes the angel or guru. This can deepen insights into how you relate to concepts of agency and power in therapeutic interactions, how these are embedded across different theoretical orientations, and how they are experienced within you. Each therapist's choice of images conveys something about the techniques they prefer to use in the therapy room. For instance, how much you hold the client and how much you encourage them to hold themselves can relate to whether you see yourself more as a parent or more as a teacher. Through a reflective exercise like this, therapists can also engage with therapeutic goals that they are yet to realize (e.g., "I should be more of a scientist in my sessions"), or parts of therapy they dislike (e.g., "Was I being too manipulative in trying to help that client?").

These images can serve as prompts for reflecting on the methods and perspectives one tends to prioritise, as well as one's positioning vis-à-vis various theoretical frameworks. Therapists may identify with one of the major traditions, or feel like outliers, being drawn to perspectives that are less familiar to many of their contemporaries. Many alignments are possible, and in fact, it may be quite rare for a therapist to be very exclusive in their preferences. It is more fruitful to understand how each theoretical orientation can influence therapeutic work and contribute to professional identity, rather than ranking or choosing between them.

Opening Gambit: What We Listen for and What We Do

Naisha came into the session looking distraught. She shared how her husband "really cares" for her, but sometimes this got too much. Just as her mother used to do, he did everything for her, including carrying her bags and doing her bank work. When he did this, Naisha expressed how it felt like he did not respect her or think of her as competent. She spoke of her fears trying things out on her own, feeling sure that she would make a mistake. With her husband, she was often withdrawn, irritable or silent. In response, her husband was more affectionate and constantly checked on her. Her mother did not like her husband at all, and Naisha felt pressured to change him or leave him. She was not sure if she had the strength to do either.

Our theoretical lens can influence what we observe, attend to and encourage our client to share during a therapy session. It can manifest in the choice of questioning style, the specific techniques used, our relational approach or the goals we are working towards. If you were Naisha's therapist, what would you observe, listen and ask for? What are the focal problem areas that you would identify as needing more exploration and attention in therapy? How might your theoretical lens impact this process?

While there are definite overlaps between orientations, particularly in terms of attention to client experience and building the therapeutic relationship, each orientation also has some unique foci. Practitioners from the cognitive-behavioural tradition might first focus on identifying Naisha's beliefs about herself and her abilities, understanding the cognitive filters through which she makes sense of her experiences. After assessing the interpersonal and emotion regulation skills she needs to navigate her life, the focus shifts to helping her think more logically and realistically about herself and her environment. This process also involves making concrete plans to bring about the changes she desires. Skills are usually taught during the session and reinforced through homework assignments. The dynamically oriented therapist might listen for what she is not saying, as they attend closely to her emotions. At the appropriate time, the therapist may draw attention to possible parallels between her emotional experiences with her husband and her mother, and patterns in her interactions with them. Exploration of her dreams and fantasies as well as her interpersonal experience in the therapy room is used to illuminate the deeper layers of her consciousness. The humanistic therapist is likely to explore all levels of her experience (her thoughts, feelings, behaviours, bodily reactions, meanings, values, etc.) and try to draw connections between them, helping her become more aware of herself. The therapist might ask how she feels in her body when her husband takes her bag from her or urge self-reflection as Naisha gives her bag to him (again)? The intervention process is aimed at helping her to get in touch with who she wants to be in the world, contrasting this with who she thinks she is and trying to arrive at a realistic and compassionate picture of who she actually is. A systemic therapist will delve into interaction patterns with her husband, eliciting the thoughts, behaviours, feelings and meanings associated with each interaction. The focus would be on helping her understand how she influences her family and how they influence her, perhaps seeing how very responsive she and her husband are to each other's slightest communication and how this leaves both of them feeling stuck. A narrative practitioner will seek to unpack her story of herself, looking at where she might have picked up a script of herself as an ineffective woman through examining her personal experiences as well as cultural messages and strictures. Therapy would work though looking for exceptions to this story and expanding on experiences where she was able to take decisions or control. The goal would be to help her build a new and constructive story for herself.

Each theoretical orientation raises distinct questions, depending on which aspect of human experience is viewed as most fundamental to psychological development and distress. For instance, all orientations ask the therapist to observe non-verbal behaviour, the emotion being conveyed, and to note verbal and non-verbal discrepancies. Therapists aligned with the psychodynamic approach use this data to build awareness of their own and client's emotions as they are being experienced and to identify processes like projective identification. Therapists from the cognitive-behavioural tradition use the same data to identify the dysfunctional assumptions that bias how the client views the world. Reflecting on how we listen to clients, engage with their narratives and choose which experiences to emphasize can reveal how theoretical models inform our work, and how we, in turn, shape the application of those models.

Pause and reflect...

Take a moment to consider how you would respond if a new client asked about the theoretical model which informs your work.

Is this a question that is easy for you to answer, or does it leave you feeling uncertain? What does your response say about your relationship with psychological theory?

Is there any one (or two) theoretical orientation(s) that emerges as a dominant influence on your practice? Or is it a combination that is difficult to articulate?

While thinking about your theoretical lens, keep in mind that actions do not always align with intentions. The overlap in foci and methods across orientations indicates that they are not watertight categories, with techniques neatly divided into boxes. Further, the adherence to stated protocols is influenced by the knowledge, comfort and experience with diverse techniques. Most of us tend to use the techniques we feel surer of rather than venturing into new territory. In the evolving process of therapy, some interventions are executed according to plan, while others might emerge more spontaneously. Good therapists are responsive to the unfolding interactions and circumstances in sessions and can stray from their theory to meet their client's needs. So, neither theory nor therapists are fixed and immutable; and our choices, both deliberate and accidental, allow for a flexible and responsive process of weaving between orientations. Bringing session transcripts or detailed notes into supervision, along with annotations and reflections, is an invaluable aid for identifying the processes and techniques used in work with clients. Through this process, therapists can gain insight into how they engage with and respond to clients, monitor their level of activity in sessions, and determine whether their focus leans more towards the past, present or future. Reflecting on the similarities and differences across clients and sessions helps crystallize a clearer understanding of what therapists actually do in practice.

Watching experienced therapists in action can make theoretical orientations come alive. Utilizing video resources, such as those from the American Psychological Association, is a valuable practice. These videos showcase how master therapists from cognitive therapy, emotion-focused therapy and psychodynamic therapy orientations translate these different concepts into practice with the same client. Videos allow for the careful tracking and gradual understanding of how model-specific interventions can be applied and how clients respond to them. The goal is not to unthinkingly emulate the therapists in the video demonstrations, but to link these observations to our own experiences as therapists. While watching, we recommend placing yourself in the therapist's chair and realizing what you might have done in the same situation. This represents another layer of learning about the varied ways that theoretical frameworks translate into practice. A close observation of how interactions unfold brings a more nuanced understanding of how techniques can be delivered in different ways. For instance, a client's response might illustrate that the effectiveness of a transference interpretation depends not only on its content, but also on the timing and the manner in which it is introduced by the therapist.

There is a flood of information from each therapy session, about emotions, ideas, processes and moments, and it is not always easy to look back and identify particular techniques used. A more structured approach can support reflection-on-action after the session. We have used the Multitheoretical List of Therapeutic Interventions (MULTI; McCarthy & Barber, 2009; Solomonov et al., 2019) in psychotherapy training contexts, asking trainees to reflect on their most recent therapy session and identify how typical their use of the various interventions was. This scale can be used to understand the frequency and patterns of interventions used across a wide range of psychotherapy orientations—psychodynamic, process-experiential, person-centred, cognitive, behavioural, dialectical-behavioural, with the recent addition of mentalization-based therapy. The use of common factors across orientations, such as attentive listening or expressions of empathy and support, can also be tracked. Trainees who engaged in this process spoke of an increased awareness of their actions within the session. In retrospect, they recognized how some of the listed interventions might have been beneficial in the session but were not used by them. They also raised questions and shared their thoughts about the focus on certain theoretical orientations and the exclusion of others—such as narrative and feminist therapies. Some trainees were struck by the realization that their responses reflected only the therapist's perspective—their client might have experienced the approaches and activities in the same session quite differently. Our discussions also revealed that the use of techniques outside of their planned theoretical approach was certainly not uncommon.

As therapists deepen their understanding of different theoretical orientations and their own practice, they can reflect on why they remain within the frame of their self-identified orientation/s and when they borrow from other perspectives. These shifts may be part of the initial plan or emerge spontaneously in response to what unfolds moment to moment with a client during a session. These explorations can bring therapists closer to understanding the amalgamation of change processes and the ways therapeutic techniques can be tailored to the unique needs of each client. The process of finding or choosing a theoretical orientation could probably be better seen as a journey rather than a single decision point, with a range of factors that influence choices along the career path.

Influences on the Choice of Theoretical Orientation

It seems obvious that who we are as people has a role to play in determining the orientations that resonate with us. Early research focused on identifying potential differences in *personality traits* between the adherents of different orientations, though the findings remain inconclusive. In a review of studies on determinants of the choice of orientation, Arthur (2001) paints a picture of the active, rational, assertive cognitive therapist, and contrasts it with the more intuitive, thoughtful dynamic therapist who is comfortable with ambiguity. Comparative trends have been reported in more recent research, where trainees with different theoretical preferences varied in the description of their own interpersonal style. For instance, trainees with a psychodynamic orientation perceived themselves as more intuitive, introspective and accepting in their close personal relationships than did trainees from cognitive-behavioural and systemic approaches (Messina et al., 2018). The search for distinctive personality traits that predict choice of orientation has waned, and the expanded focus on the personal now encompasses therapists' learning approaches, value systems and interpersonal styles (Tartakovsky, 2016) . For instance, students who preferred a *feel and watch* learning style were drawn to the slower-paced, emotional and relational foci of the psychodynamic orientation while those who gravitated towards a *think and do* style preferred the structure of CBT with its stepwise description of interventions and strategies (Heffler & Sandell, 2009). There is a suggestion that when the prescriptions and philosophies of therapeutic orientations do not match with personalities and value systems, this cognitive dissonance leads to increased dissatisfaction with work life (Topolinski & Hertel, 2007). Exploring a niggling sense of dissatisfaction or a mental block against certain interventions and connecting this with personality or belief systems can help therapists understand what draws them towards or pushes them away from certain styles of working. While creating this picture can be an interesting exercise, relying on such patterns may also risk reinforcing limiting stereotypes. We also need to remember that no two therapists are the same and individuals with diverse personalities and beliefs might find themselves drawn to the same orientation. Orientations are not narrow boxes, and there can be room for different personalities to express themselves within the framework of each theory.

Personal life experiences also influence the choice of orientation. As therapists, we can recognize bits of ourselves in different theories, and approaches that have proven effective or meaningful in our personal lives may be the ones we most believe in. Some of these connections seem obvious, for instance, growing up in a family that emphasizes gender equality could create an affinity for feminist therapies. Our life experiences also influence us in implicit and complex ways, and we may not even be aware that we are searching for answers to personal questions as we encounter different theoretical orientations. Sometimes, it is only during the process of training that a therapist joins the dots, realizing for instance how childhood experiences have influenced their current relationships.

The initial choice of orientation is often influenced by *training and professional contexts*. Therapists may naturally align with the dominant model of their training centre, as they are often immersed in its principles and practices, learning both how it works and how to apply it effectively. Admired theorists, influential ideas and compelling books can all influence the preferred therapeutic orientation, drawing practitioners into new intellectual worlds. Teachers or mentors often become professional role models, and trainees might find it easier to trust orientations that come from authority figures or sources they look up to. When this resonance continues with practice experiences, the allegiance to a particular theory is reinforced. Training in a single model can sometimes feel limiting as it restricts the possibility of encountering other orientations. Therapists need not be confined by this, as the rise of online training opportunities has expanded access and exposure to various theoretical orientations and their offshoots. For those who are inclined, this allows for explorations of different orientations without being constrained by what their training context has to offer.

Client needs and preferences can exert a strong influence on the orientation one works with. Clients may come in with their own notions of what therapy is, what they want to talk about and how they wish to approach themselves. So sometimes, the therapist adapts a therapeutic approach to fit the needs and realities of the client. For instance, dynamic therapy can become briefer to fit the needs of clients who do not have the resources for long-term therapy. Or a therapist might notice that her clients are more accepting of the cognitive-behavioural therapy format when there is less emphasis on homework. Therapists also have to be mindful of how much they direct the course of therapy. Some clients may resist being pushed, preferring a more collaborative, hands-off approach, while others feel lost without adequate leadership and structure.

Our *clinical experience* and reflections on what seems to be needed and effective with clients or what does not seem to be working can draw us towards certain orientations. For example, a therapist who works with many individuals from marginalized communities during their training might realize that traditional therapeutic models do not always fully address the complex realities and systemic barriers their clients face. This experience could draw the therapist towards frameworks that incorporate a social justice perspective, enabling them to address broader societal issues and offer interventions that align with their clients' lived experiences. Choices are also made based on an understanding of the *cultural fit* and acceptability of dominant counselling and psychotherapy theories. The therapy session is a microcosm of the world outside the room and *global events*, such as the COVID-19 pandemic, armed conflicts, refugee crises and terrorism, all impact which theoretical frameworks feel most relevant. As a result, there has been an increased focus on crisis interventions, trauma-informed and trauma-focused interventions, reflecting the evolving needs and perspectives of both clients and mental health practitioners.

When it comes to exploring the determinants of our preferred model, it helps to understand the complex interactions of multiple factors rather than focusing on a single pathway. Clearly, the personal and the professional are intertwined, even in the choice of theoretical orientation. Our awareness of these myriad influences can make us active participants in our professional journey and help shape our work lives to the benefit of ourselves and our clients. In this process of exploration, we may find that there are both an element of choice (what is the kind of practitioner I want to be?) and an element of discovery (what is the kind of practitioner I am inside?).

Pause and reflect…

Reflect on the possible determinants of your theoretical lens(es) and depict them in a pie chart. The size of each slice of the pie chart can indicate the relative strength and significance of each of the influences.

Dwell on how each of these influences played a role in your initial choices or experiences.

Has the impact of these influences waxed and waned through your ongoing journey as a therapist?

Me and My Orientation: An Evolving Relationship

Choosing or discovering the theoretical framework(s) we believe in is certainly not a linear process. Not all of us are clear about which orientation resonates the best with us or even which one we use the most. When training is limited to a single orientation, we may not know enough about other orientations to make a genuine choice. On the other hand, when training covers multiple orientations, there is less time and space to reflect on which one we actually prefer. Some therapists prefer not to think too much about theory, finding it intimidating or preferring to trust their instincts. There are of course therapists who find their theoretical home quite easily. They are the true believers or purists and have a strong adherence to one theory, often in combination with active rejection of others. Such ideological purity allows for a deepening of mastery and competence and a clear therapeutic focus, emphasizing depth over breadth. The clarity and simplicity that comes from following just one framework can feel both attractive and limiting. It is good to remember that a deep commitment to one model need not preclude being open to other ways of thinking and practising.

Therapists may also find themselves transitioning from one framework to another, or combining different approaches over their years of practice, based on what they have found helpful or effective. Some therapists try two or three orientations before settling on one that fits. Personal preferences and philosophies can influence this process of exploration. As individuals, we have differing needs for certainty, and differing comfort levels with change. Some therapists may move from model to model because they do not wish to commit and prefer flirting with possibilities and looking for the next good thing. Therapists who are attracted to more integrated or eclectic approaches may be uncomfortable with absolutes and wish to be more contextual in their approach. Adherence to a single model can meet a need for belongingness as much as it meets a need for clarity. Understanding the why beneath our what can help us think more intentionally about our choice of theoretical orientation.

Therapeutic frameworks and techniques continually evolve over time, adapting in response to new research, shifts in societal values and advances in understanding human behaviour and mental health. Theories that were mainstream during one time period have later been seen as outdated and even oppressive. In 2019, the American Psychological Association Division 39, Society for Psychoanalysis and Psychoanalytic Psychology, tendered a public apology for their past alignment with theories that viewed homosexuality as a disorder (LeRoy & Tummala-Narra, 2019). In this letter, they acknowledged that both psychoanalytic theories and several psychoanalysts had stigmatized, pathologized and excluded members of the queer community, and emphasized the need to move towards a new way of thinking and theorizing. In the shifting landscape of theoretical approaches, therapists can choose to stay loyal to early allegiances or to reassess both the theories and their own perspectives when necessary. At any time, there will be some orientations that are more prominent, garner more research funding and appear to offer better professional prospects. These trends can influence the direction of practice, pushing some therapists to align with popular approaches. There are also variations in the salience of specific orientations across contexts and countries. The analytic psychodynamic tradition is almost synonymous with the term psychotherapy in the popular imagination, and nearly 60 per cent of therapists surveyed in a large international study indicated that this orientation was a prominent influence on their therapeutic work (Orlinsky & Rønnestad, 2005). However, while the psychodynamic orientation remains popular in some countries like Poland (Suszek et al., 2017), it is rarely endorsed by trainees and practitioners in other countries, for instance in India (Bhola et al., 2017; Kumaria et al., 2018). Cognitive-behavioural therapy (CBT) is increasingly favoured by psychotherapists and has been widely integrated into mental health systems worldwide. The evolution of CBT can be traced through its various waves, progressing from traditional behaviourism to cognitive-behavioural approaches, and finally to mindfulness and acceptance-based techniques that emphasize psychological flexibility and holistic well-being, incorporating social and contextual factors. Additionally, there has been a resurgence of psychodynamic therapies, characterized by briefer formats and heightened attention to cultural and contextual influences. Each therapist can choose to align with current trends or swim against the tide, depending on their evaluation of what is clinically effective and personally resonant.

Even after therapists have worked successfully using one theoretical orientation, there can come a time when it no longer feels satisfactory, prompting them to consider other options. At times like this, it can be useful to remember that as a system of helping people, therapy is not perfect. Being aware of where it falls short or contradicts its own ideals can help therapists accept themselves and therefore their clients a little better. The process involves questioning orientations, reflecting on what feels comfortable and uncomfortable, and whether there is enough space to explore other orientations. Whatever we choose, this search involves a process of immersion in theory, efforts to understand ourselves and our clients and reflections about issues relevant to training, practice and research in psychotherapy.

Finding a Theoretical Home

At some point in your career, there comes a moment when your identity, what you do in session and what works with your client align. You may feel a click—a thrill that brings a release of a breath you did not know you were holding. When that moment happens, you can catch it and cherish it as one of the most remarkable experiences in your professional journey. Keep in mind though that this journey does not end in a single orientation, and you may find yourself exploring new paths again.

A Therapist Speaks: What Feels True

Malika Verma

The modality of psychotherapy that we choose to practise is very much about what is the best fit with our own personality, what feels true to us. Psychoanalytic psychotherapy suits me best. My thoughts here are not about the nature of the various therapies but rather about how I have experienced them. I initially trained as a CBT therapist and enjoyed my work very much. It made me feel very competent. I always had the right words, the right answers, a solution. I wore them like an armour suit. The avoidance of pain and reality is an aspect of my personality. I feel that being a clinical psychologist allowed me to be an expert, someone who will never be in the position the patient was in. I saw my patient's struggle as an illness and a pathology of which I could cure them. I worked mainly with severe, chronic and complex mental health conditions but I never felt ruffled or frustrated. The truth was perhaps closer to the fact that I felt omnipotent and had no real understanding of the patient's pain or their reality.

One must wonder what made me leave this for psychoanalytic psychotherapy. I think it was starting my own therapy. For the first time, I really knew what my patient's experience was, because I was one too. I knew now what it felt like when I said I was going on a break, or that we don't need to meet weekly anymore, or that we must now end. For the first time, I could allow myself to be real instead of competent. I didn't want the body armour anymore. I trained in interpersonal therapy alongside psychoanalytic training and never felt attached to it. Both CBT and IPT now felt constraining and rigid. I felt that neither allowed me a real relationship with my patients. I enjoyed the rigour and demand of psychoanalytic training at Tavistock Clinic, UK. My own analysis, 5 days a week for 5 years, was invaluable to me both personally and professionally. Now I only practice psychoanalytic psychotherapy and psychoanalysis. I am often lost for words, but I can share with my patients the silence to convey that for which there are no words. I don't have solutions, but I have the capacity to bear with my patients that which feels unbearable and intolerable. I work with aspects of my patients and with patients that others would not wish to work with. I fail often, and the patient is not the only one in the room who has failed and is floundering, and so we continue. Not all psychotherapists will want this. Not all patients will want this. Whatever feels true to you.

Ms. Malika Verma *is a clinical psychologist and psychoanalytic psychotherapist who currently has a private practice in Melbourne, Australia. Her initial training was in India, after which she worked in National Health Service (NHS) in the UK for 7 years, and later trained and worked at the Tavistock Clinic, UK.*

The search for a shoe that fits is a process of self-exploration, as much as an exploration of theoretical orientations. Congruence between the self of the therapist and the theoretical orientation can create a powerful synergy for change in therapy. When therapists have a deep sense of conviction in a theory of change and experience a sense of easy attunement, this resonance increases their sense of hope, tenacity and allegiance with the theory (Blow et al., 2007). A therapist's genuine commitment to their theoretical orientation is also conveyed to clients. The stronger the therapeutic relationship, the more clients are likely to trust and be motivated by the therapist's beliefs. This, in turn, enhances the credibility of the theory in the eyes of the client, leading to greater engagement and lower dropout rates (Bartle-Haring et al., 2022).

Pause and reflect...

Have you found your theoretical home?

What guided you to this place?

Looking Through the Integrative Prism

Integrative thinkers have the capacity to hold opposing and sometimes paradoxical ideas in their mind. Instead of resolving these tensions by picking one over the other, they are able to create something new that weaves select elements together in a creative synthesis. There is no single integrative model but many ways of integrating, with each therapist charting their own path and integrating theories to varying degrees. Norcross and Alexander (2019) recognize four routes to integration: *common factors* (i.e., focusing on effective therapeutic practices which are common to all approaches), *technical eclecticism* (i.e., using effective ingredients or techniques from different approaches), *theoretical integration* (i.e., synergizing two or more models at a theoretical level) and *assimilative integration* (i.e., working primarily from within one model but integrating aspects of others when needed). Reflecting on integration includes considering where it is useful to combine theories to arrive at a more complete understanding of the client, or where a technique from one orientation can enhance the effectiveness of another orientation. Therapists need to be intentional in their experimentation, always keeping an eye on what can create the most therapeutic change. By taking the best of what each orientation has to offer, therapists can tailor their interventions to meet the needs of the client sitting in front of them.

A Therapist Speaks: My Integrative Journey

Shigeru Iwakabe

Psychotherapy integration has been an integral part of my professional life both as a practitioner and a researcher. To me being 'integrative' involves openness and flexibility. As psychotherapists, we need to be flexible and open to new and different ideas so that we can be responsive to *each* individual whose uniqueness needs to be understood and appreciated if psychotherapy is to be of help to them.

In my journey toward becoming an integrative psychotherapist, my interest in psychotherapy process research and emotion played two central roles. In my graduate school days at McGill University, I joined a research group where members listened to and watched renowned psychotherapists' sessions and rated each client and therapist utterance, using process scales such as the Experiencing Scale and therapist response modes. This was not an easy task. We had to listen to short segments, pause, and discuss our ratings, and when we disagreed, rewind and listen over and over until we resolved our rating discrepancies. This seemingly tedious and laborious task sensitized me to observe subtle changes in vocal and nonverbal cues and moment-to-moment change processes (e.g., facilitating emotional awareness, insight, corrective emotional experience, etc.). It also helped me go beyond looking at psychotherapy from a macro level in terms of overall theoretical orientations and develop a process-oriented view of change that can cut across different models of psychotherapy.

As I listened to these psychotherapy session tapes, I became very interested in the role of emotion in psychotherapy. When clients experienced emotions in therapy, time flew differently. The air in the room changed. I was convinced that emotion was central to understanding effective psychotherapy. This led me to learn affect-focused integrative approaches such as emotion-focused therapy and accelerated experiential dynamic psychotherapy in depth, as well as those new cognitive behavioural approaches that focus on emotion. I studied basic emotions such as shame, sadness, and anger: how different psychological problems are related to different shame experiences and expressions. I started to get interested in positive emotions too as they are essential ingredients of effective therapy from the very beginning of therapy: we need to feel trust and feeling of safety to disclose about ourselves, and we need to feel hope to continue to work on difficult issues.

My interest in integration may also be driven by many personal factors including my past and recent life experiences - some of which I might not be completely aware of. One of such personal factors is my exposure to different cultures. I grew up in Japan at the time when economic prosperity and security was so prized, which I questioned and could not buy into. My personal search for the meaning of life started. I first studied economics in a university in Japan. Then I decided to go to Canada to study psychology. I craved to know different ways of life and I enjoyed learning diverse values and life philosophies. I certainly needed to learn about myself. I cannot help but think that I am always 'integrating' and 'synthesizing' all these things that I learn into a coherent whole.

My most recent interest is the relationship between therapist's own experience of emotional injuries and corrective emotional experiences that they provide to their patients in psychotherapy. We as humans can never be free from getting hurt emotionally and we are all wounded healers. These painful experiences can teach us important lessons in life and also become our embodied wisdom to help others. This is an integration of a therapist's personal life and their interventions. I am still excited about new integrations that I might be trying out in the future.

***Dr. Shigeru Iwakabe** is a clinical psychologist and Professor at Ritsumeikan University, Japan. He is the President-elect, Society for Psychotherapy Research and former President, The Society for Exploration of Psychotherapy Integration.*

Developing a Personal Theory of Change

During training, it often seems as though there is a theory "out there" (Rogers, 1986, p. 9), a guiding map that already exists that we merely need to follow. The truth is that even before we begin any formal training, we have a theory within us (Fall et al., 2017). This personal theory of change relates to our beliefs about what drives psychological change and which interventions will lead to particular outcomes. Beliefs about what causes personal and interpersonal problems as well as beliefs about what are desired outcomes are also implicit in this understanding. These convictions evolve through reflections on the intersections between self, ideology and therapy practice. As we move between experiencing ourselves and experiencing our clients, some aspects of theoretical frameworks may start to resonate more strongly as others lose ground. Together, these elements shape our personal theoretical orientation, one that resonates with us as human beings and allows us to stay authentic as we go about the tasks of therapy. As Carl Rogers famously said, perhaps the best school of therapy is the one we have developed ourselves (Rogers, 1986).

We do not always interrogate underlying beliefs or consider framing them into a clearly articulated position. When left unarticulated, these beliefs can influence our choices in therapy without our awareness. Many of us begin our careers believing that human beings can transform their personal selves completely, and that this is the purpose of therapy and the ideal outcome of personal growth efforts. This understanding becomes more nuanced when we observe change journeys within ourselves and within clients. As we encounter what changes easily and quickly, and what changes more slowly; we can also grow to accept, value and embrace parts of ourselves rather than looking for a complete overhaul. Our understanding of the scope of therapy can then shift from listing everything that should change to discerning what are the things that need to and can change.

Because a psychotherapist's personal theory of change is as an extension of the self, parts of different theories may ring true to us. We can resonate with the narrative approach to therapy that views feelings like depression or worry as a natural response to difficult life circumstances; with the psychodynamic notion that anxiety emerges from internal threats to the ego; and the cognitive therapy based perspective that the way we process information affects our experience of reality. We form impressions about human nature, such as seeing people as inherently altruistic or selfish, motivated by a desire for self-actualization or peace. These beliefs draw us towards theories that echo our deeply held convictions. Reflecting on our beliefs about human nature, psychological vulnerabilities and change agents, provides insights into how they shape our overarching narrative of how therapy works and what a psychotherapist needs to do.

We have an internal picture of what it means to be mentally healthy as well as a philosophical or value-based picture of what it means to live a good life. Both can interact to influence the goals we pursue for our clients. Therapists who define mental health in terms of self-awareness or authenticity are likely to prioritize achieving this inner experience. Similarly, therapists who value being well adjusted with the context, being able to carry out roles and tasks or being aligned and connected with members of the community, are likely to encourage clients to look in these directions. Similarly, beliefs about what creates change within a human being (whether a corrective emotional experience, an acceptance of self or the learning of a needed skill) determine the tasks of therapy.

Embracing the ways in which context shapes perceptions and experiences can enhance and redefine our theory of change. It has become increasingly difficult for therapists to work from within their ivory towers, separated from what is happening outside the safe space of the therapy room. Issues such as systemic racism, economic inequality and the impacts of climate change have highlighted the interconnectedness of individual mental health and broader societal factors. An awareness of social suffering can lead us to question the scope and purpose of psychotherapy, refiguring our ideas about what an effective mental health system needs to provide.

Finally, our beliefs about the relative roles of the therapist and client impact the way we conduct therapy and the nature of the therapeutic relationship. We can see the therapist as holding an objective truth or deeper understanding of human nature that they use to guide clients, or we can see therapy as a more mutual process of arriving at truths or stories of self that the client can live with. Of course, we may also notice ourselves moving between positions based on the need of the moment. Our personal beliefs and understanding of theory really come together in interactions with clients. For instance, we can question the value of digging up old wounds when we see a client continuing to express intense distress or when we continue to experience pain from our old wounds. But we can feel differently if a client says that confronting their past trauma has freed up their emotional energy in the present, and they find themselves laughing more and loving easily. In this process we also encounter the client's theory of change and start to notice where it agrees with or differs from ours. Through negotiating a shared understanding with the client, we can find our own theories evolving as well.

The development of a sense of connection and flow as we grow into a theoretical orientation has been described as a process of metabolizing theory, a personal endeavour that happens inside the therapist, and in the interactions between the therapist and client (Betan & Binder, 2010). As psychotherapists we actively make meaning of the models taught to us, and select ideas, techniques and stances, often drawn from a range of theories. These learnings amalgamate values, life experiences and accumulated wisdom to create a personalized and idiosyncratic model of being a psychotherapist and doing psychotherapy. As Carere-Comes (2001, p. 107) put it, "We have almost as many psychotherapies as psychotherapists"... and we feel that this is as it should be.

Pause and reflect...

Reflect on varied representations of a *Personal Theory of Change*. Do you find a resonance with any of them?

Does your personal theory feel like an edifice that is neat and organised, with specific pathways to get from floor to floor?

Does it feel more like a tree, growing organically as it responds to its environment, and adapts to unexpected circumstances?

Would you describe your theory of change as a messy desk, with some important objects and a lot of stuff that needs to be sifted through.

A search for an embedded orientation, one that fits with our personality, values and world views, may not happen during the training phase itself. As trainees, we may not know enough about our selves or theory to speculate on the possibilities of resonance or incompatibility with diverse theoretical orientations. However, this is where we begin to create spaces for reflection on our own ideas about helping and change, as well as our experiences with clients. Starting early facilitates the eventual emergence of a personal theory of change (Spruill & Benshoff, 2000). Coming up with a personal theory is never an easy task, and nor is it a one-time exercise. At times, the ideas may seem disjointed and incomplete, and it can be hard to pull the theory together. Starting with an existing theory, small adjustments can be made to incorporate ideas and techniques from other models that resonate personally, gradually extending through individual reflections and experiences. This process resembles learning a new language; as knowledge is synthesized, assimilated and transformed, spontaneous moments may begin to emerge in therapy sessions. This journey also involves learning to tolerate ambiguity when theory does not provide immediate answers. A receptive stance towards learning from therapeutic encounters fosters a thoughtful exploration, rather than a hasty application of theory to explain a client's experiences.

Over time, an awareness of the alignments or misalignments between theory and our personal style, beliefs and values may lead to a closer integration between our self and our orientation. We also have moments of learning in our own lives; when we become parents, lose a parent, overcome a challenge or experience an adverse event.

These developmental transitions constantly feed into our understanding of ourselves and the world—we keep growing and so does our personal theory of change.

Over the years of professional development, accumulated wisdom integrates into theory, resulting in an increasingly sophisticated process of integration. Looking back, experienced therapists can recognize the gradual shift from a detached understanding of theoretical ideas and techniques to a feeling of belongingness and integration. A rigid adherence to theory can limit the space for the client's experiences, the development of therapists' relational skills, and our capacities to accept and accommodate limitations, vulnerabilities and uncertainties within the encounter (Råbu & McLeod, 2018). Therapeutic wisdom then lies in a nondogmatic appreciation of theory, allowing for diverse truths and uncomfortable questions. This approach reduces the pressure to completely emulate a particular model and allows for a better fit between the person and the emergent model of practice. With a more in-depth understanding of theory and practice, it becomes easier to allow our personalities and world views to enter the room. If we look at theoretical orientation as a "framework and not a strait-jacket" (Casement, 1985, p. 4), this leaves room for clinical intuition, flexibility and our personal styles to emerge in the therapeutic process. This adds another layer to our theoretical orientation, as each of us develop a personal style that feels authentic and effective in our work with clients. This can include the language we use, our sense of humour, our affability, dependability or any other trait that we value. Fernández-Álvarez et al. (2003) proposed five dimensions that can capture the distinctive ways in which each therapist does therapy: whether there is a relatively *broad or narrow focus* in therapy and how receptive we are to what our clients share; how *flexible or rigid* the regulation of the therapy setting is (e.g., schedule, fees and tasks); the *distance or closeness* in terms of the emotional communication and engagement with clients; the *level of engagement* reflected in the involvement and commitment to clients in relation to other aspects of our lives; and the degree to which interventions are *spontaneous or planned*. As therapists develop their own style, it becomes clearer that the theoretical orientation does not entirely define the kind of therapists they are. The practice of therapy involves more than dipping into a compendium of skills. Intuitive, flexible and nuanced responses and actions during sessions can feel akin to painting or composing a symphony, and it is these creative and artistic elements of our work that allow for a deeper connection with human experience.

Pause and reflect...

How would you describe your personal style as a therapist?

Where would you place yourself on the five dimensions outlined by Fernández-Álvarez et al. (2003)?

Perspectives on Training and Development

Exposure to Diverse Theoretical Models During Training

There is evidence that early exposure to multiple theoretical orientations has a positive impact on professional growth trajectories (Orlinsky & Rønnestad, 2005). Trainees can benefit from learning the language of diverse theoretical models through formulating clients' stories from multiple perspectives. Case conceptualizations and discussions using different theoretical models can provide an initial exposure to the links between theory and therapy, even if therapy training is not as broad-based. Where possible, we recommend opportunities for critical engagement with more than one orientation during clinical rotations and internships. Some training institutes are defined by their allegiance to a specific theoretical orientation, and this allows for an immersion into its philosophy and methods. Even when training is focused in this way, it is important to create a space where other perspectives are valued and discussed. Supervisors need to build time and space for reflections about theoretical orientations where trainees can be encouraged to articulate their philosophies about human suffering and change, and their experiences with theories and interventions. Even as supervisors make their own orientation/stance known, they can leave room for trainees to question and debate about diverse theories and techniques.

Training in Integrative, Eclectic and Pluralistic Approaches

With many therapists shifting towards eclectic-integrative positions as they move along their career trajectories, there are proponents for an early initiation into integrative approaches. However, Castonguay (2005) argues that integrative practice should be preceded by a deep understanding of the theoretical, clinical, empirical and epistemological bases of different orientations. Trainees may struggle to grasp the nuances and complexities of diverse orientations, and their common threads and possible combinations, all at once. Additionally, all training sites may not have the resources to provide the theoretical knowledge and therapeutic skills reflected in each orientation.

We believe that training contexts need to provide some theoretical anchors and help trainees build a foundation from which to explore and integrate. It is through exposure to different models, using a range of methods, that trainee therapists can experiment and understand how to put them together (Aafjes-van Doorn et al., 2018). Didactic methods have their place in exposing trainees to the concepts underlying integrative, eclectic and pluralistic approaches. In our experience, trainees respond well to additional learning opportunities such as viewing videotapes of varied theoretical models and demonstrations of integrative approaches, building case formulations using different models and through using supervision as a space to hold different, even contradictory, perspectives at the same time. Trainees also need explicit support in articulating the theories that resonate with them as well as how they wish to approach the integrative process.

Training in Change Processes and Pathways

While psychotherapy training in most centres is model-driven, there is value in including training in change processes and pathways that cut across these distinctions. This approach enables trainees to move beyond merely following the steps of a model or adopting it in a fragmented manner. Gaines et al. (2021) recommend the development of specific modules to train therapists in the identification of key moments during sessions, and in the use of transtheoretical change strategies that are flexible and personalized. Close observations of the oscillations in the therapeutic process can help trainees be more attuned to their experiences of relational depth as well as recognize any signs of ruptures in the alliance. Therapists could be trained in ways to build a strong therapeutic alliance and also to mark implicit and explicit indicators of feedback from clients so that they can make responsive changes (Westra, 2023). The rapid advancements in neuroscience, coupled with a growing interest in more holistic approaches, suggest an increased focus on embodied processes in future. Experiential methods are particularly effective in helping trainees attune to internal experiences during sessions and draw on these signals to inform the therapy process.

Theoretical Orientations and Contextual Sensitivity and Relevance

All theoretical orientations are drawn from human experience—thoughts, feelings, behaviours, memories, needs and motivations—and some aspects of these are universal. However, theoretical orientations have been developed largely from Eurocentric or Anglo-American perspectives and we cannot assume that their applications are always equally relevant and responsive to needs and expectations across cultures and contexts. It is important for training centres to examine their curricula, learning resources and pedagogies and consider the need for adaptations or the inclusion of locally rooted epistemologies and approaches. In this process, we caution against the use of simplified categories such as West vs East or West vs the Rest, as this can lead to an essentialized understanding of culture. A critical engagement with context can guide the choice, translation and adaptation of theoretical orientations, so that they can be used more intentionally and flexibly in therapeutic work. Trainers and supervisors can help trainees reflect on the times when the infusion of cultural idioms, metaphors and practices can enhance the applicability and impact of theoretical models. Adaptations of interpersonal therapy in some Asian countries have included goals and processes consonant with cultural beliefs and values (e.g., family cohesion, relational hierarchies and spirituality) and involved family members in therapy when needed (Stuart et al., 2021). A more flexible approach to cognitive-behaviour therapy, with adaptations in the relational stance, therapy length and the application of select techniques, has been documented across several countries in Latin America (Neufield et al., 2021). In order to ensure that psychotherapy remains contextually relevant, we look for more documentation and research examining the relationship between theoretical orientations and culture. Most of the adaptations made as part of research studies are not translated into training contexts or into practice and even when practitioners make adaptations, these are not documented or disseminated. As we reflect on why this is so, we can also generate ways of overcoming these barriers.

Engagement with Key Questions and Debates About Theoretical Orientations

As therapists, we are not just recipients of theoretical orientations but active partners on how they are conceptualized and practised. The movement towards cost-effective short interventions continues to influence what research is funded, what therapy services receive insurance coverage, what types of training are available and eventually where the field moves. There are ongoing tensions between low-intensity standardized evidence based interventions, such as the *NHS* Talking Therapies for anxiety and depression programme in the UK, and other interventions that involve deeper and longer engagement. As practitioners, we do need to stay updated about the evidence for the effectiveness of various therapeutic approaches. However, there are attendant concerns about the over-dependence on empirically supported treatments and the narrowing of theoretical orientations at training sites. These interventions are often validated through randomized controlled trials which use carefully controlled participants, processes and treatments that may not accurately reflect real-world conditions. Contemporary trends in research methodology now involve recruiting participants with complex and comorbid presentations, alongside adopting a dimensional lens that better represents conditions in naturalistic settings. This approach shifts the focus from merely statistical significance to clinical significance, expanding the range of outcomes to include factors beyond symptomatic improvement and tracking these outcomes over extended periods. Additionally, explorations of the mechanisms of change enhance our understanding of how different theoretical orientations function (Lilliengren, 2023). There are increasing calls to incorporate qualitative research on therapeutic processes and outcomes to strengthen the evidence base for clinical practice guidelines in psychotherapy (Levitt et al., 2024).

The growing popularity of treatment manuals, mobile applications and online web-based programmes is other trend that does not easily encompass all theoretical orientations. New waves of research are also exploring how various therapies and techniques can be adapted for delivery through technology. While short-term interventions, especially cognitive-behavioural approaches, offer clear benefits in public mental health initiatives, they also present challenges for therapists. Therapists may struggle to balance the demand for efficiency with the complex needs of their individual clients. As trainees and practitioners explore the world of theoretical orientations, their training options may be constrained by the dominance of time-limited and empirically supported therapies. We are concerned that this growing reliance on select theoretical orientations and frameworks could edge out longer and more intensive psychotherapy formats which have their own place.

It can be an unsettling experience to realize that a particular theoretical lens might not be adequately responsive to the inequities in clients' lives and experiences. The figure and ground varies across different theoretical models, and this can influence whether you see your client as depressed or oppressed. We recommend that practitioners continue expanding their theoretical frames to incorporate social justice and human rights paradigms and hope that pedagogies and practices in counselling and psychotherapy will include these perspectives more uniformly.

Building Practice–Research Networks and Access to Collective Resources

Partnerships between practitioners and researchers can inform more meaningful and practice-friendly research on theoretical orientations. In some ways, therapists are constantly building hypotheses in their work with clients and there is so much potential for using their experiences to inform research questions which can then feedback into improving practice. Therapists and researchers need to find a common language and spaces to engage with each other. The gatekeeping of knowledge means that many therapists have limited access to published research, and this is coupled with the significant economic barriers and global inequities in most of the open access pathways. The emergence of alternative ways to make research findings more accessible and user-friendly, for instance through the inclusion of practice-focused summaries in journals, helps in bridging the research-practice gap. While both quantitative and qualitative research methods have value, there is an underrepresentation of psychotherapy case studies in both journals and professional forums. Case studies can help us engage deeply with the therapeutic process and the complexities of the decision-making process. We welcome the development of shared resources and archives, such as the Single Case Archive (www.singlecasearchive.com), to share this wisdom within the professional community. There is much potential for therapists and researchers to collaborate and work together to respond to their separate and combined questions about the processes and outcomes associated with various theoretical models. It is these learnings that can percolate into psychotherapy training processes and support the development of therapists from the initiation of their journeys.

Conclusion

As psychotherapists, it is imperative that we locate ourselves on the complex map of theoretical orientations. As we move along our professional trajectories, we build our toolbox, explore and understand diverse theories, and engage in the process of reshuffling or strengthening alignments. A reflective and flexible stance leaves room to continue our search within one orientation or explore divergent models and practices. In this ever-evolving journey, we not only expand our professional repertoire but also deepen our empathy and understanding of the human condition.

References

Aafjes-van Doorn, K., Klinar Alfaro, D., Fialová, M., & Kamsteeg, C. (2018). Psychotherapy integration training around the globe: A personal and empirical perspective. *Journal of Psychotherapy Integration, 28*(4), 505–520.

Arthur, A. R. (2001). Personality, epistemology and psychotherapists' choice of theoretical model: A review and analysis. *European Journal of Psychotherapy & Counselling, 4*, 45–64.

Bartle-Haring, S., Bryant, A., & Whiting, R. (2022). Therapists' confidence in their theory of change and outcomes. *Journal of Marital and Family Therapy, 48*, 1190–1205.

Betan, E., & Binder, J. (2010). Clinical expertise in psychotherapy: How expert therapists use theory in generating case conceptualizations and interventions. *Journal of Contemporary Psychotherapy, 40*(3), 141–152.

Bhola, P., Raguram, A., Dugyala, M., & Ravishankar, A. (2017). Learning in the crucible of supervision: Experiences of trainee psychotherapists in India. *The Clinical Supervisor, 36*, 182–202.

Blow, A. J., Sprenkle, D. H., & Davis, S. D. (2007). Is who delivers the treatment more important than the treatment itself? The role of the therapist in common factors. *Journal of Marital and Family Therapy, 33*, 298–317.

Carere-Comes, T. (2001). Assimilative and accommodative integration: The basic dialectics. *Journal of Psychotherapy Integration, 11*(1), 105–115.

Casement, P. (1985). *On learning from the patient*. Tavistock/Routledge.

Castonguay, L. G. (2005). Training issues in psychotherapy integration: A commentary. *Journal of Psychotherapy Integration, 15*(4), 384–391.

Cooper, M., & McLeod, J. (2012). From either/or to both/and: Developing a pluralistic approach to counselling and psychotherapy. *European Journal of Psychotherapy & Counselling, 14*(1), 5–17.

Fall, K., Holden, J. M., & Marquis, A. (2017). *Theoretical models of counseling and psychotherapy* (3rd ed.). Routledge.

Fernández-Álvarez, H., García, F., Lo Bianco, J., & Corbella Santomá, S. (2003). Assessment questionnaire on the personal style of the therapist PST-Q. *Clinical Psychology & Psychotherapy, 10*(2), 116–125.

Fleuridas, C., & Krafcik, D. (2019). Beyond four forces: The evolution of psychotherapy. *SAGE Open*. https://doi.org/10.1177/2158244018824492

Gaines, A. N., Goldfried, M. R., & Constantino, M. J. (2021). Revived call for consensus in the future of psychotherapy. *Evidence-Based Mental Health, 24*(1), 2–4.

Heffler, B., & Sandell, R. (2009). The role of learning style in choosing one's therapeutic orientation. *Psychotherapy Research, 19*(3), 283–292.

Kumaria, S., Bhola, P., & Orlinsky, D. E. (2018). *Influences that count*: Professional development of psychotherapists and counsellors in India. *Asia Pacific Journal of Counselling and Psychotherapy, 9*(1), 86–106.

LeRoy, M., & Tummala-Narra, U. (2019). Letter of Apology to LGBTQ+ Communities and APA Division 39 Members (past and present) On Behalf of the Board of Directors, APA Division 39 - Society for Psychoanalysis and Psychoanalytic Psychology. https://div39members.wildapricot.org/LGBTQ-Apology/

Levitt, H. M., Hamburger, A., Hill, C. E., McLeod, J., Pascual-Leone, A., Timulak, L., Buchholz, M. B., Frommer, J., Fuertes, J., Iwakabe, S., Martínez, C., Morrill, Z., Knox, S., Langer, P., Muran, J. C., Weie Oddli, H., Řiháček, T., Tomicic, A., & Tuval-Mashiach, R. (2024). Broadening the evidentiary basis for clinical practice guidelines: Recommendations from qualitative psychotherapy researchers. *American Psychologist*. https://doi.org/10.1037/amp0001363

Lilliengren, P. (2023). A comprehensive overview of randomized controlled trials of psychodynamic psychotherapies. *Psychoanalytic Psychotherapy, 37*(2), 117–140.

McCarthy, K. S., & Barber, J. P. (2009). The multitheoretical list of therapeutic interventions (MULTI): Initial report. *Psychotherapy Research, 19*(1), 96–113.

Messina, I., Gelo, O. C., Gullo, S., Sambin, M., Mosconi, A., Fenelli, A., Curto, M., & Orlinsky, D. E. (2018). Personal background, motivation and interpersonal style of psychotherapy trainees having different theoretical orientations: An Italian contribution to an international collaborative study on psychotherapy training. *Counselling and Psychotherapy Research, 18*, 299–307.

Neufeld, C. B., Szupszynski, K. P. D. R., Barletta, J. B., Romero, F. A., Rutsztein, G., Airaldi, M. C., Ruiz, P., & Keegan, E. (2021). The development of cognitive behavioral therapy: Practice, research, and future directions in Latin America. *International Journal of Cognitive Therapy, 14*(1), 235–246.

Norcross, J. C., & Alexander, E. F. (2019). A primer on psychotherapy integration. In J. C. Norcross & M. R. Goldfried (Eds.), *Handbook of psychotherapy integration* (3rd ed., pp. 3–27). Oxford University Press.

Orlinsky, D. E., & Rønnestad, M. H. (2005). *How psychotherapists develop: A study of therapeutic work and professional growth.* American Psychological Association.

Råbu, M., & McLeod, J. (2018). Wisdom in professional knowledge: Why it can be valuable to listen to the voices of senior psychotherapists. *Psychotherapy Research, 28*(5), 776–792.

Rogers, C. R. (1986). Rogers, Kohut and Erickson: A personal perspective on some similarities and differences. *Person-Centered Review, 1*(2), 125–140.

Rosenzweig, S. (1936). Some implicit common factors in diverse methods of psychotherapy: "At last the Dodo said, 'Everybody has won and all must have prizes.'" *American Journal of Orthopsychiatry, 6*, 412–415.

Solomonov, N., McCarthy, K. S., Gorman, B. S., & Barber, J. P. (2019). The multitheoretical list of therapeutic interventions - 30 items (MULTI-30). *Psychotherapy Research, 29*(5), 565–580.

Spruill, D. A., & Benshoff, J. M. (2000). Helping beginning counselors develop a personal theory of counseling. *Counselor Education and Supervision, 40*(1), 70–80.

Stuart, S., Pereira, X. V., & Chung, J. P. (2021). Transcultural adaptation of interpersonal psychotherapy in Asia. *Asia-Pacific Psychiatry, 13*(1), e12439. https://doi.org/10.1111/appy.12439

Suszek, H., Grzesiuk, L., Styła, R., & Karwczyk, K. (2017). General overview of psychotherapeutic practice in Poland. Results from a nationwide survey. *Psychiatric Quarterly, 88*, 571–584.

Tartakovsky, E. (2016). The motivational foundations of different therapeutic orientations as indicated by therapists' value preferences. *Psychotherapy Research, 26*(3), 352–364.

Topolinski, S., & Hertel, G. (2007). The role of personality in psychotherapists' careers: Relationships between personality traits, therapeutic schools, and job satisfaction. *Psychotherapy Research, 17*(378), 390.

Wampold, B. E. (2015). How important are the common factors in psychotherapy? An update. *World Psychiatry, 14*(3), 270–277.

Westra, H. A. (2023). The implications of the Dodo bird verdict for training in psychotherapy: Prioritizing process observation. *Psychotherapy Research, 33*(4), 527–529.

Chapter 5
Connecting with Clients and Building a Therapeutic Alliance

Moments where we truly feel connected with the other are precious—whether it is whirling dervishes dancing in oneness with the universe, a musician reaching the flow state, or a mother who tunes out the world to be with her child. Seeking attunement and connection is also what lies at the heart of the client–therapist relationship. The therapeutic alliance (also referred to as working alliance or helping relationship) has been recognized as key to facilitating therapeutic growth. The relationship between therapist and client is often both the context and the impetus for therapeutic change. Acceptance by the therapist is what helps clients accept themselves and gain the confidence to make changes in their lives. Psychological interventions are thus deeply embedded within the relationship—marking the difference between advice from a self-help book and care from another human being. The intimate and continued interactions between therapist and client create a shared microcosm that enables the work of therapy to be carried out. The relationship between the quality of the therapeutic alliance and therapy outcomes is robust and enduring, holding true across client characteristics, varied alliance and outcome measures, theoretical orientations and both in-person and online modes of therapy (Flückiger et al., 2018). Of course, clients and therapists may perceive the depth of the alliance in different ways. It is our *clients'* perception of the alliance that often has the most powerful impact on the progress and changes achieved in therapy (Castonguay et al., 2006). This underscores the importance of continually attuning to their experience and ensuring that the therapeutic relationship feels collaborative, safe and empowering.

Connecting with our clients is not a one-time event but a process which is replayed and strengthened session after session. In this chapter, practitioner narratives have been used to capture the almost intangible essence of what it is to be with a client and reflect on some of the ways to deepen this experience. We start by focusing on how therapist presence can build attunement with clients and then move to examining how to repair that connection when the inevitable ruptures occur. We then highlight the role of reflective practice in managing countertransference and balancing power between a therapist and a client. Finally, we turn to the joys and sorrows of therapy termination.

P. Bhola et al., *Reflective Practice in Psychotherapy and Counselling*,
https://doi.org/10.1007/978-981-96-9732-8_5

I'll Be There for You: Presence and Attunement in the Therapeutic Relationship

Implicit in the therapeutic contract is the idea that we will be there for our clients. This is built into the frame of therapy, through having regular sessions, seeking to understand what the client needs from therapy, working hard to help them get there and above all being a caring presence in their lives. As therapists, we are not just there for the client, we are also present with the client. We tune into their moment-to-moment feelings and experiences, sensing them not just with our minds but also through our embodied responses. When we do this, we can connect with their internal world, experiencing (for instance) the tension in their shoulders, their frantic thoughts and even the tearing feeling of an inner conflict. As we articulate these fragments, images and insights to our client, they may truly feel seen and begin to experience themselves through our eyes. As we hold the client in our minds, the client is able to hold themselves in their mind.

In order to be so present with the client, we also need to be present with ourselves. Our awareness of our embodied experience, non-verbal reactions and feelings; our personal histories and sensitivities; our knowledge, professional skill and wisdom—all contribute towards our awareness of our therapist self in that moment with the client. We can use this awareness to separate ourselves from the client, seeing more clearly how we are impacting each other in each interaction cycle. In this manner, our presence helps us to be more attuned with our clients, and it is in these moments of connection that clients are able to transform. Therapeutic presence then is "a way of *being* with the client that optimises the *doing* of therapy" (Geller, 2018, p. 108; italics in original).

A Therapist Speaks: The Girl in a Locked Room

Poornima Bhola

Some of our deepest learnings emerge from experiences of our struggles to connect with our clients. I remember a young woman Maya, a reluctant client, angry with her family, herself and with me. Sitting with arms crossed, she would talk about being detached from everyone and everything and being attracted to darkness and the imagined possibility of death. Often quoting from the Japanese novelist Haruki Murakami, she spoke of the futility of human attachment and was clearly angry when she realized that I had read his books too. Maya reminded me of the girl in a locked room, from Murakami's book *Norwegian Wood.* Most often I was outside the door, tentative and uncertain or trying to knock and get her to open. There were fleeting moments of connection and progress during sessions, but at other times she looked out of the window or laughed at my "weird" facial expressions. She kept coming for sessions, always five minutes early, but the therapeutic alliance certainly did not seem on firm ground.

During one session, I spontaneously shared how I experienced her internal struggles and our time together. It was a visual metaphor about a bird, something that seemed to have just popped into my mind – my inner thoughts making themselves heard as I began to speak. Maya narrowed her eyes and asked angrily, "Did you read my diary" Reaching into her bag, she opened a page in a journal and showed me the same metaphor—a line in a poem she had written about herself. We sat in silence for some time. This shared experience opened a space for us to work together in the next few sessions.

This brief but powerful encounter helped me learn many things about connecting with clients. Clients will often tell us how they have experienced relationships-what they yearn for and what they fear. This may need to be understood through the way we relate with each other. We may be too eager to close the distance and open closed doors—we may be ready (even anxious)—but our client may not. This therapeutic experience has stayed with me and reminds me that empathic attunement between the client and therapist can occur silently and slowly. It is also interesting for me that the two of us could connect and resonate in this way only when I stepped back from struggling with her and entered a more reflective space.

Dr Poornima Bhola *is a clinical psychologist from India who is deeply engaged with the training, supervision, 'research and practice of psychotherapy. She hopes to strengthen connections among psychotherapy researchers and practitioners in Asia in her role as Vice-President, Society for Psychotherapy Research – Asian Area Affiliate,*

Both presence and attunement are pantheoretical constructs central to the therapeutic relationship and prerequisites for the work of therapy. They demonstrate a fascinating interplay between neurobiology and interpersonal phenomena. This kind of attunement can help a client to experience interpersonal safety which, in turn, allows them to regulate their affect and enter their window of tolerance, to access and process their thoughts and feelings in a constructive way (Siegel, 2020). Over time, such encounters can build the client's capacity to self-regulate, as their neural systems entrain with those of the therapist (Geller & Porges, 2014).

As therapists, we can build our capacity to be present by developing an awareness of ourselves, developing an awareness of our client and learning how to communicate this in sessions. Long-term practices like mindfulness mediation, yoga or even chanting or music can help us to tune into our embodied state. We can prepare for each session by using a centring or grounding ritual to access a state of calm receptiveness, even bringing an image of the next client into our minds and setting an intention for the session.

Pause and reflect...
As therapists, we often have busy days, where we rush from session to session.

On a typical day, is there anything specific you do to enhance your presence and center yourself?

Are there any practices that you would like to integrate into your routine?

Therapeutic attunement implies letting clients know that we have the capacity to receive their communication and the complexity of their experience. Therapists who are preoccupied with their own worries have less room to fully embrace and hold the client's distress. While therapists usually strive to bring their best self to the therapy room, keeping their personal concerns contained, this can build pressure in the long term. A more sustainable solution lies in taking care of the self. Paying attention to one's own well-being, building long-term relationships and finding meaning in life can go a long way in sustaining the capacity to be present with clients.

Presence can be demonstrated through the quality of listening (without interruptions), maintaining eye contact and matching the rhythm of breathing, tone and prosody with that of the client (Geller, 2018). This can help us sense when we want to explore client's distress and when we may need to prioritize soothing or regulation. Being present is not just about mirroring the client but also responding to both where they are in the moment and what they may need from us through the course of therapy. When we note a particular experience, we often respond with reciprocal affect. So, when a client shows anger, the therapist responds with attentiveness or concern rather than mirroring their anger. Or when a client shows fear, the therapist responds with protectiveness and support (Erskine, 1998). As we put these observations together, larger emotional and interpersonal patterns like attachment styles or relational schemas emerge.

Attuning to Attachment Needs

As therapists, we need to reflect on the sense of connection and the patterns of the closeness and distance we experience with clients at different moments over the course of therapy. Attunement can be more challenging with clients who are primed for dysregulation and heightened threat perception because of their attachment histories or trauma experiences. They may perceive themselves to be in constant danger and respond defensively or aggressively even when there is no risk. This can make it harder to forge a meaningful connection (Geller & Porges, 2014). Clients with anxious or ambivalent attachment styles often exhibit a hyperactive need for proximity, looking to their therapist for consistent reassurance and emotional support. In contrast, those with avoidant or dismissive attachment styles tend to have a deactivated need for proximity and may find it easier to regulate their emotions when on their own (Mallinckrodt, 2010). Each client can have quite differing needs from their relationship with their therapist. Our awareness of our own attachment needs, whether for closeness or distance, can help us be aware of when we are feeling pushed or pulled, and also enable us respond appropriately to the client's need.

Clients who seem to need more than we can give often leave us feeling overwhelmed and inclined to protect ourselves by drawing stronger boundaries. With clients who are anxiously attached, we need to initially offer some of the comfort and care that they need, while keeping a firm eye on the frame of therapy. As they grow to trust that our care is consistent, their ambivalence and anxiety in relationships reduce. As they start to feel safer, we experiment with changing our stance, occasionally refraining from offering comfort or soothing and gently encouraging them to search for their own solutions. While the client may initially feel frustrated that their needs are not being met, over time they can learn to tolerate these feelings and develop their ability to understand and regulate themselves.

On the other hand, clients who seem not to need us at all can raise our anxieties. This can cause us to try moving closer, almost insisting on a connection. These experiences can be particularly hard for therapists who are anxiously looking for that sense of connection from their clients. We need to be able to hold that anxiety and offer our clients the safety of distance, letting them know that we are willing to meet them within their comfort zone. Without necessarily asking them to share or pressurizing them to change we gradually build a connection by consistently tuning into their feelings. We can then push for more emotional exploration, discussion of distressing material or of the therapeutic relationship itself. The client may initially feel discomfited, but then gradually feel more comfortable with intimacy in a relationship. In this way, the therapist can initially sense and match the client's style and slowly expand their interpersonal repertoire (Mallinckrodt et al., 2015).

The task of the therapist here is not just to find the correct attachment box to put their clients in, but to be sensitive and flexibly responsive to the client's interpersonal patterns and expectancies. Each client is likely to have a unique goal of how much connectedness or distance they wish for in their relationships, and this could be based on their cultural value system as much as their childhood experiences. As therapists, we also tune into clients' cultural locations, interpreting their behaviours through this lens. For instance, in India, the therapist may be referred to as akka,[1] indicating that we have been given the position of a respected but approachable family member. While this can feel inappropriately close in some cultures, it is the appropriate amount of distance in others. Our reflections can help us stay present and attuned, enabling us to forge the therapeutic connection while still working within the realm of therapeutic boundaries.

Tuning into the client helps us contextualize what we do, when and how we do it, as well as what we do not do in the session. As we reflect on the pushes and

---

[1] Elder sister in several Indian languages.

pulls in the therapeutic interaction, we come closer to understanding how we create the safety and trust that are prerequisites of therapeutic change.

Can We Fix This? Responding to Ruptures in the Therapeutic Alliance

Rafoogari, the traditional art of darning from India and the subcontinent, involves the repair and preservation of torn, frayed and fragile heritage textiles. This can be a powerful metaphor about healing, which "honour(s) the place, significance and act of visible and invisible 'darning' in the fabric of any life" (Mehra, 2018). Rafoogars are like artists, who mindfully suture, strengthen and restore the injure' fabric, often using threads extracted from the original cloth. In the warp and weft of our relationships in life and in psychotherapy, there are frictions, injuries and ruptures…and they hold within them the potential for repair and transformation.

Pause and reflect…

Think about a disruption in one of your personal relationships - perhaps a misunderstanding with a friend or a conflict with a partner.

How did you feel and respond during that time?

What might have helped to resolve the strain?

A threat to any significant relationship (including the therapy relationship) evokes a very personal response in each of us. Minor gaps in understanding or communication in the therapeutic relationship are often easily resolved and tided over. But there are also times when there is a significant push or pull between the client and the therapist. When the client appears tentative, reluctant, withdrawn or hostile at the beginning of therapy, these signs are easier to recognize. When the early alliance is positive and strong, therapists might expect the relational trajectory to remain smooth, possibly overlooking shifts in the level of connection. Therefore, therapists must remain sensitive to fluctuations, both in the emotional atmosphere of the session and within themselves.

These strains in the therapeutic alliance can arise out of disagreement on one or more dimension of working alliance (Bordin, 1979)—the goals of therapy (e.g., the therapist wants to focus on understanding deeper emotions, while the client wants to improve their organizational skills), the tasks of therapy (e.g., the therapist recommends mindfulness to become more aware of thoughts and emotions, while the client prefers a more structured approach) or the nature of the therapeutic bond (e.g., the client experiences the therapist as unavailable or too demanding). Over the past two decades or so, the seminal work of Safran and colleagues on the cycles of alliance ruptures and responsive processes of repair has provided a clinically sensitive and research-based model to help therapists think relationally (Muran et al., 2021).

Ruptures can have varied manifestations and underpinnings as they emerge at different times in the therapy process. The tensions might be subtle and transient or much more intense and prolonged. The more obvious manifestations are when a client directly confronts the therapist, expressing anger or dissatisfaction with specific interventions or the pace of therapy. These *confrontation markers* can be directed both against the person of the therapist and the interventions being used, evoking confusion, ambivalence and negative feelings within us. Faced with such direct expression of intense feelings, the therapist can struggle to remain open and empathetic to client experience, obviously impacting the therapeutic alliance and process. Clients also express their relational distress through more indirect *withdrawal markers,* such as long silences, changing the topic, rambling storytelling or apparent unconcern. Here, rather than moving against the therapist, the client moves away. Clients can also withdraw from meaningful engagement by becoming overly deferential or acquiescent when they sense a disturbance in the relationship. Sometimes, the complete absence of strain can reflect a hesitation to enter more challenging aspects of therapeutic work or a reluctance to endanger the relationship. Of course, both types of markers can occur in the same session, with the client initially being more hostile or challenging and later being more withdrawn or quiet, as if they have given up on getting the therapist to hear them (Eubanks, Muran, & Safran, 2015).

Pause and reflect...

Think about the ways in which you typically respond to a client's anger during sessions.

Think about the ways in which you typically respond to a client's disengagement during sessions.

Are you more comfortable with one over the other?

Why do you think this is so?

For the therapist, staying attuned to micro-processes in therapy and recognizing often subtle relational disruptions requires a lot of focus and effort. Even where we do recognize our client's discomfort, we might attribute it to something that belongs only to the client, or even skirt around the conflict or impasse hoping that it is transient. Our assumptions about therapy, therapists and clients or our reticence in recognizing our own errors or misjudgements can all pose barriers to the reflective process. So, while we learn to recognize ruptures, we can also reflect on the reasons why we may not recognize or attend to them.

The art of repair involves the creation of a shared reflective space where the rupture can be named and anchored to what is happening in the present. Clients can express their dissatisfaction in a direct verbal manner or through a more subtle non-verbal shift in emotional tone. When therapists notice a potential or ongoing rupture, they need to pause to explore these experiences together with the client and initiate the process of repair. It is good to begin by ensuring that the client feels safe and validated enough to discuss their difficult feelings. Their attention can then be drawn towards the interruption in connection by asking what they are experiencing in the here and now and exploring their response to what transpired during the interaction. Clients can be reluctant to bring up their negative or conflictual feelings, and therapists need to work a bit harder to invite them in, perhaps by asking, "What is it that you are finding hard to express right now?" The conversation moves between exploring the client's reluctance to express their feelings and exploring the feelings as they emerge. Through this process the client also learns to examine and express their interpersonal needs constructively (Muran et al., 2021).

Once it is clear that the client has examined their experience and brought it to the table, the next step is to respond to their concerns. Acknowledging the client's perspective in a non-defensive manner and taking responsibility for the rupture, is crucial. For example, saying, "Yes, I can see how ignoring your story about your boss was disrespectful of your struggles at work". This is better than saying 'I can see that you *felt* disrespected'—where the more accusatory tone could imply that there is some problem with the client's feelings. Time is then spent exploring the meaning of the experience for the client and gently encouraging them to identify what can help heal the current rift in the relationship. A sensitive invitation to consider their role in the rupture can help construct a more complete interaction cycle. The final step involves using the understanding of this rupture and repair process to assist clients in examining other interaction patterns in their lives (Safran & Muran, 2000).

When a rupture occurs, interjecting our own perspectives, quick-fix solutions or interpretations can risk leaving the client feeling unseen or misunderstood. Taking the time to slow down and reflect on the rupture allows for greater awareness of potential misunderstandings regarding what is important to clients. They might point to misjudgements about the timing of interventions or a lack of discussion regarding the rationale for a therapeutic task. Repair strategies can be chosen in response to the kind of marker clients display, as well as our understanding of their relational style. The dynamics of a rupture often reflect the tension between a client's need for agency and their desire for relatedness (Safran & Kraus, 2014). Clients who value agency may be willing to confront the therapist and risk losing the relationship. Resolving such a rupture involves guiding them towards acknowledging their feelings of hurt or disappointment while accessing their vulnerability and need for nurturance. In contrast, clients who value relatedness may withdraw to protect the relationship rather than expressing their dissatisfaction. By encouraging these clients to voice their needs and feelings, space is created for them to articulate their discontent and assert their needs.

Repair strategies can be executed immediately, as soon as the rupture is noticed, and this responsiveness can have a strong impact on the client. For instance, clarifying a misunderstanding or adjusting the agenda for that session as part of the ongoing conversation challenges the client's negative expectation that others will not notice or attend to their need (Muran et al., 2021). Therapists can also respond to observations of client emotions without bringing them into open discussion. For instance, if a therapist notices a client becoming uncomfortable with a line of exploration and retreating into avoidant storytelling, an immediate response might be to attune to their unspoken needs and slow down the exploration (Eubanks et al., 2015). Alternately, therapists can choose to wait if they feel the timing is not right, sometimes choosing to address many smaller ruptures together. Of course, it can also happen that a rupture is only noticed later while reflecting on a session or writing notes, or when the client brings up an experience from a previous session. It can be helpful to rewind, returning to the experience and reflecting with the client on how it impacted the relationship and how each person experienced what happened. A therapist could bring this up by saying, "The last session felt different from the usual for me. Would it be okay for us to talk about it?" (Safran et al., 2011). Expressive strategies involve therapist metacommunication, being mindful of the interaction as it unfolds and communicating about it. An openness about acknowledging possible therapist contributions and exploring possible reasons and patterns around it, can help the client understand and accept themselves better (Muran et al., 2021). The dance of rupture and repair is spontaneous rather than choreographed, often led by client needs and not something we can anticipate. By reflecting-in-action and matching our client's rhythm we can ensure that the therapeutic relationship is not irrevocably damaged.

Successfully attending to ruptures in the relationship creates a corrective experience that can be very therapeutic. Missteps in the therapeutic interaction create possibilities to recognize what the client is trying to communicate in therapy and to understand their possible reactions to relational conflicts outside therapy. When therapists work towards resolving ruptures, it demonstrates the value of addressing differences in relationships rather than remaining silent or passive. The onus is on the therapist to take the first step to work towards resolution. Therapist readiness to take ownership of their actions and recalibrate therapy tasks and goals can strengthen the therapeutic bond, operate as a powerful mechanism of change, and contribute to better therapy outcomes (Eubanks et al., 2018). The therapeutic relationship is strengthened when clients can feel that the therapist cares about their feelings and is willing to address their needs. As our clients grow more secure with themselves and the relationship, they may become more flexible in their understanding and negotiation of interpersonal difficulties both within and outside the therapy room.

***A Therapist Speaks*: Warp and Weft**

Susan Howard

Sophia came in with difficulties in her relationship with her two- year-old son, Hugo. Our early work in repairing this relationship could not be done without reference to Sophia's own difficult experiences of being mothered and her troubled relationships with others. Sophia's early transference was dominated by idealization - of my ability to help her with Hugo and my knowledge and qualifications. I had gently challenged this idealization to avoid a catastrophic rupture once I (inevitably) did something to upset or disappoint her.

The first major rupture came after Sophia mentioned being pregnant. She had previously spoken of her dissatisfaction with the marriage and had discussed ending it. My surprise was evident, and she immediately accused me of not being pleased for her. I understood this accusation as the projection of her own negative feelings about the pregnancy and realized how desperately she needed my support. As I paused to think carefully about my response, Sophia said, "I knew you didn't approve. I could see it in your face". As her therapist, she felt that it was my job to be pleased for her. It required considerable effort to remain in touch with Sophia's underlying fear and anxiety and refrain from defending myself from such an unfounded and vitriolic attack. I took a direct approach, which both confirmed and challenged her reality: "You were right about seeing something in my face. But what you saw was surprise - I hadn't known that you were thinking of having another child. But surprise isn't the same as disapproval". We did enough work to repair the rupture and continued to discuss this and Sophia's own feelings about the pregnancy over later sessions. She became open to thinking about how difficult my disapproval would have been and what my active support meant to her, given the poor relationship with her mother.

I was better prepared when the next significant rupture occurred a year later, at a time when overseas teaching and illness had kept me away from my practice more than usual. When we met after some trouble rescheduling a therapy session, Sophia averted her eyes. I recognized this as a sign of both her anger and a potential rupture. She began by saying that this would be her last session; I was too unreliable, and she was now used to managing without me. I knew that Sophia struggled being dependent on me and with the inherent power differential in therapy—illustrated by my ability to change sessions when she could not. My reflections showed me that she had a legitimate complaint—I had not given her enough opportunity to complain about my recent absences. I began by addressing her feelings about me as an unreliable object. Initially, this unlocked a torrent of anger, but I did not defend myself. I also shared my hypothesis that she had come to the session wanting to find a way of staying rather than leaving. My apology for not being sufficiently attuned to her feelings and this open acknowledgement of my own contribution to the rupture deepened our therapeutic relationship.

Dr Susan Howard *is a visiting lecturer at the Department of Psychology, University of Surrey, UK, and has a private practice where she sees clients for short and long-term psychoanalytic psychotherapy and for interpersonal psychotherapy.*

The Third Space: Recognizing and Using Countertransference

Psychotherapy is an emotional enterprise, one in which both client and therapist experience and express positive and negative emotions and evoke them in each other. Images of the therapist as the neutral and controlled expert, or as a benevolent, ever-empathic figure are both caricatures. Just like clients, therapists also experience their share of emotional reactions during the therapeutic process. No therapist is immune, and most of us would have experienced countertransferential feelings of deep care and concern, inadequacy and helplessness, boredom or detachment, anger, envy or frustration towards our clients. Misch (2000, p. 192, italics in original) reminds us that "countertransference is *always present,* to a greater or lesser degree, in every psychotherapy and with every psychotherapist". Although the concept of countertransference emerged from the psychoanalytic tradition, it is now considered a pantheoretical idea, encompassing the entire gamut of conscious and unconscious sensory, affective, cognitive and behavioural reactions of therapists in the process of relating with their clients (Gelso & Hayes, 2007).

Reactive countertransference refers to feelings evoked by clients that can help therapists empathize more deeply with the client's inner world. For instance, concordantly feeling the same pain as the client, when the client is sharing a painful memory (Clarkson, 1991; Racker, 1953). Therapists might also react in ways that are similar to another person from the client's life, thus recreating the client's earlier relationship experience. For instance, if the client behaves in ways that are rebellious, a therapist might respond in a critical controlling manner, closely mirroring the client's early relationship with a parent (Kernberg, 1965). Within the object relations framework, transference and countertransference have also been explained through the defence of *projective identification,* where the client unconsciously projects into the therapist a self or object representation and then through subtle interpersonal pressure nudges the therapist to take on the feelings and behaviours characteristic of the representation (Gabbard, 2004). In this way, our emotional reactions to our clients present another way to listen to and understand their stories.

As therapists, we also bring something to the relational table in the form of *proactive countertransference*, reactions that have roots in our own histories (Clarkson, 1991). For instance, a therapist who experiences the need to do more than usual to help an older client might recognize the roots of their behaviour and feelings in their own unresolved grief around the loss of a grandparent. Another therapist's intense feeling of powerlessness in response to a challenging client might stem from difficulties with authority figures in their own life. There is a curious alchemy in this encounter between client and therapist. As our feelings, thoughts and ideas come together as unique co-created patterns of countertransference, they create a bridge of meaning between us and our clients.

In its current avatar, countertransference is not seen as something to be feared, circumvented or eliminated but to be harnessed as a valuable transtheoretical lens and as a reflective tool to help us navigate the therapeutic process. A curious and receptive attitude towards our emergent (and indeed inevitable) feelings is the first step of this journey. Some experiences of countertransference may be intense and easy to identify while other reactions are more subtle, fleeting or disguised, and may elude awareness. Our negative feelings may be reflected in our behaviour during sessions, even when we deny or minimize our feelings. We might have become less responsive to the client, withdrawn or overly task-oriented and directive, ending our sessions early or even wishing for termination of therapy. Our self-protective instincts often arise when emotions are particularly confusing and distressing, and we remain oblivious to our internal turmoil. This need for protection is more likely if we carry an idealized image of a therapist as someone who cannot or should not have negative feelings towards the client. Sometimes we are more focused on the doing in therapy rather than on the being. It is often only in retrospect that we realize how our emotions were hidden in plain sight. Of course, all our emotions cannot be equated with countertransference; a therapist may well be irritated or distracted due to bad traffic, a long and tiring day or a deadline to file tax returns.

We might believe that our positive and protective feelings towards our clients are not really problematic, but that is a comforting myth. Positive feelings that are parental or protective may indeed be less distressing, but they could also cloud our thinking, constrain therapeutic possibilities and result in over-involvement or boundary violations. We may become too effusive and emotionally available and preoccupied with clients' lives and emotions in a way that their actual needs are not addressed. At times, what we want so desperately for our client is what we have missed ourselves. For instance, a young therapist may feel overly invested in pushing adolescent clients to achieve goals or make choices that she was unable to exercise in her own life. A therapist's needs for special closeness, intense maternal or sexual feelings could be enacted in the relationship with a client, if they are not recognized, contained and constructively processed (Little, 2018). Often, both positive *and* negative feelings towards our clients are intertwined, and it is particularly important that we recognize and accept this within ourselves. This can open possibilities for our clients to accept how feelings of love and hate can coexist within ourselves and in our relationships—including of course the therapeutic relationship.

Pause and reflect...

At the end of the day, after you wrap up your sessions and gather your thoughts, focus on any client who evoked a strong emotional response from you. It could be someone you really looked forward to meeting or someone you struggled to empathize with.

How did you feel just before your session with this client?

Did you notice any emotions that stayed with you through the day?

Sometimes we need to listen to what our body is telling us and decode any sudden sensations of muscle tightness, pain, cold, heat, numbness or suffocation during sessions. This embodied resonance often emerges when clients are unable to connect with and express their feelings in words. Diamond (2013) describes struggling to stay awake and feeling overwhelmed by boredom and disinterest during sessions with a client who lived alone and was seeking a partner. This was a powerful mirroring of the client's internal experience, stemming from early parental neglect, where the client felt that she meant nothing to anyone. When the therapist was able to tune into this deep sense of nothingness, it deepened their understanding of the client's relational experiences.

The maxim about tuning into our reactions when they are "too much, too little, too positive, too negative" (Gelso & Hayes, 2007, p. 37) is a useful guide to recognizing manifestations of countertransference. We need to look out for exceptional feelings that arise with a specific client or during a particular session or phase of therapy, reactions that stand out because they are unexpected or are difficult to understand. We may also recognize repetitive patterns in our sessions, such as the desire to protect clients or a discomfort with clients' risk-taking behaviours. If we avoid experiencing our feelings, believing that feeling anger towards our clients (for instance) is the same as acting on that anger, they are likely to negatively impact the therapeutic process and outcome. Allowing ourselves to be tangled in the experience for a while brings it closer to our awareness. And reflecting on the meaning of our reactions can protect us from being sucked into the maelstrom of countertransferential feelings.

Countertransference can work as a diagnostic tool or a compass that directs us towards what is important and helps us create a different relational experience for the client. As therapists, it may be helpful to anticipate and tune into our emotional reactions during the therapeutic process with certain clients. Our experiences as therapists and supervisors suggest that more intense and challenging countertransferential reactions may arise in work with clients who have experienced trauma, have certain personality constellations or are at risk for suicide. Reflections on the origins and intensity of our client's emotions and on our own reactions can lead us to a deep understanding of their central vulnerabilities and their relational patterns outside of therapy. However, one of the challenging tasks in understanding countertransference reactions is trying to locate which thoughts and feelings belong to the client and which belong to the therapist's inner world. It may be easier to attribute our emotional reactions to something the client brings. However, our understanding of countertransference is incomplete if we do not turn the reflective lens on our own wounds and vulnerabilities. For instance, a therapist who recognizes their own need for distance is better placed to differentiate between when they are pulling away and when their clients are pushing them away. A therapist who is unaware of their own needs and believes that they are solely responding to their client's concerns can misinterpret their own need for distance as the client's need for space.

Opinions about disclosure of countertransferential feelings to the client are divided, and like all therapist self-disclosures, there are caveats regarding the degree, type and timing of such revelations. It is argued that when therapists share their feelings in the here and now, this could potentially deepen the therapeutic alliance and counterbalance therapist–client power equations (Gelso & Hayes, 2007). However, the client's well-being is always at the forefront. We need to judge whether sharing will be helpful, whether the client has the resources to use this information and whether the alliance is strong enough to sustain the challenge. When emotional reactions stem primarily from our unresolved or unprocessed difficulties, they are best bracketed and explored in the safe space of supervision or personal therapy. Else, we may be taking time and space away from our client and unwittingly making them feel responsible for both our emergent feelings and their resolution. At times, our countertransferential feelings can be so intense and difficult to resolve that we might even consider referring the client to another therapist. Managing countertransference can be complex and challenging but perhaps we may learn to welcome the awareness of our experience as an invitation to be more reflective and responsive in the relational space.

A Therapist Speaks: Do You Want to Switch Seats with Me?

Jyotsna Chandur

Tara, a 23-year-old woman, came into therapy with severe dissociative episodes, an ambivalent attachment pattern and a long, complicated experience with psychotherapy. Through the first year, Tara spoke of her fears about trusting me, explicitly stating that my opinions of her do not count - I was only her therapist, being "paid" to just listen to her. Despite this, she was particular about attending every session and I could see that she felt safe in this space.

Any attempt to provide comfort through validation or interpretation was received with sarcasm or irritation. This was followed by a profuse apology from Tara, accompanied by a palpable fear of abandonment. I was acutely aware of fighting intense anger, resentment and helplessness within myself during sessions. Although supervision helped me recognize how I was being pulled into an enactment, I was unable to find the words to take this forward.

During one session, she expressed feeling completely isolated and angry with everybody over the week. Yet another attempt to connect with her and offer some reflections was met with sarcasm and annoyance. In exasperation, I revealed how useless I felt in our sessions, almost irrelevant. She was able to stay with my comment and not break out into a string of apologies, blaming herself. Perhaps this was because I was genuine in sharing my emotional reaction, and/or we had worked on building a therapeutic alliance that was strong enough to cushion the impact of this intrusion. I shared my feelings of anger and helplessness and how I dared not say that out loud, without feeling like this would crush her. She instantly identified with that feeling and said, "Hey, look at that. You turned into me!" She shared how she always felt like this around her mother, worried about saying something to tip the delicate balance.

This honest exchange helped both of us reflect on our own experiences in the presence of the other in the room. Earlier, supervision and personal reflections had helped to see that my reactions to Tara signalled that there was something she really wished me to know. However, it was only in this interaction that I could fully grasp both the depth of my reactions and their significance for Tara. Prior to exploring my own countertransference, my interpretations were more detached, intellectual and may even have sounded jarring and stilted. This was perhaps my way of protecting myself from the discomfort evoked within me. I am now able to slow down and stay with her, look underneath my immediate responses and find a way for us to connect, instead of forcing her to immediately 'make meaning' of her experiences. This has created space for more authentic and meaningful moments between us.

Dr Jyothsna Chandur *is a clinical psychologist and psychoanalytic psychotherapist with a private practice in India. She works with individual adults in long-term analytically informed psychotherapy.*

Meeting in Difference: Power in Therapeutic Relationships

Many of us are ambivalent about holding power, viewing it as a potentially negative force. Power is often associated with domination or control, but it is important to distinguish between having power over someone and having the power to accomplish something (Göhler, 2009). We would have all experienced feelings of being powerful and powerless, at different points in our lives. The meaning we make of these experience shapes our subsequent responses in unique ways. An experience of powerlessness can leave us hoarding our power fearing another exposure to the (often) intolerable experience of vulnerability. Conversely, it can impel us to be watchful about any power imbalances in our relationships, never wanting anyone else to feel as inadequate and helpless as we once did. Holding power can bring a range of mixed feelings—safety and a certain satisfaction but also guilt and feelings of heightened responsibility. The way we feel about power also plays out in the therapeutic space, where there is an undeniable power differential between therapist and client. Expressions of power emerge in overt and covert ways, even as we imagine being an egalitarian relationship—in the seating arrangements in the therapy room, in the way in which therapist and client greet each other and how they reach an understanding about the client's story. What we pay attention to, what we ignore, where we choose to interrupt and where we stay silent are all subtle indicators of the balance of power in the therapeutic encounter. The unequal sharing within the relationship—where we know all about the client, but the client knows very little about us—is just one of the ways in which therapists retain control over the frame of therapy. The power difference can be more palpable in certain contexts. For instance, it is not uncommon for clients from rural India to remove their footwear before entering the therapy room or to touch the therapist's feet as an expression of gratitude and deference. Clients can put therapists so much at the centre of their emotional worlds, whether they are expressing their needs, gratitude or even hostility, that it can be difficult to resist the temptation to see ourselves as special or our words as inherently powerful (McWilliams, 2004). Even with benevolent intentions, such as withholding certain information because we believe the client isn't ready, therapists still retain power over the therapeutic process. As we open some doors and close others, we direct the process of therapy in specific ways.

Of course, clients are not entirely powerless and most of us can remember clients who challenged our authority and the status quo in subtle or direct ways. Consider a client who slams the money down on the table after a particularly challenging session or an adolescent client who saunters into the therapy room, puts his sunglasses on and sits back with a nod to the therapist. The power play can be much more subtle and expressed even in the way in which clients ask about their therapist's age or professional qualifications. When clients hold a more privileged social location vis-à-vis their therapists, this can give rise to unarticulated power imbalances. For instance, an older man may automatically expect a degree of deference from their younger woman therapist, and the therapist can find themselves automatically responding according to this script. Expressions of power can have distinct meanings for each client, whether a need to protect against internal feelings of powerlessness, an assertive stab at reclaiming power or even a thoughtless expression of privilege. By paying close attention to the interactions surrounding these power shifts, therapists can gain valuable insights into the client's internal experience. Engaging in an active process of reflection on possible power plays and strengthening the reflexive awareness of our own feelings about power are both critical.

Pause and reflect...

Can you recall a time when you felt powerless in your own life?

In a therapy session?

In what ways did you experience and respond to these feeling of powerlessness?

Our awareness of the power landscape in the room can help us regulate the relationship: holding, shifting or sharing power as the need arises. This enables us to stay connected with the client through the course of therapy, regardless of who holds the power in a particular moment. In the early stages of therapy, the therapist is seen to hold more power as the holder of knowledge, and this is often true. This relational asymmetry is not inherently problematic and can be liberating for a client, who may benefit from receiving the therapist's knowledge and skills without the pressure to reciprocate (Altimir et al., 2017). Some clients are more sensitive to interpersonal imbalances and wish to retain a sense of power, even as they are being helped and supported. Regardless of the client's initial need, empowering clients and supporting their inherent capacity to make decisions, change and grow remains one of the basic goals of psychotherapy.

There are times in therapy when we are more likely to walk alongside our clients rather than leading them. This levelling of the relationship can have great meaning for the client. Clients can and do have preferences and every disagreement with the therapist does not indicate resistance. It is also possible that they are just expressing their rights. We can respond by encouraging them to become aware of their preferences and making explicit space for the same in therapy. We may also need to examine our own stance and actions to understand what the client is not getting from therapy and why. Sometimes our attempts to help and support clients can serve to undermine them. The desire to play the role of a rescuer and protector is more readily evoked when the client seems particularly vulnerable and disenfranchised, and we see them as a victim of systemic oppression. This can push us to intervene and engage with societal and governmental institutions on their behalf. While this can be helpful to clients on an immediate basis, it also means that they can only exert their power through the therapist, and as such, it keeps them dependent. Though the balance of power often shifts as therapy progresses, there are moments of crises when we may need to take back our power. A client experiencing suicidal ideation, an impulse to harm themselves or a difficulty controlling their craving for a substance can be relieved to have the therapist in the driver's seat, at least temporarily. The therapist still needs to remain on guard not to slip into an unequal relationship. Once we have suggested to the client that ours is the voice of authority in the session, it can be difficult to change that pattern down the line. We may expect the client to accept our suggestions, provide unsolicited advice or otherwise overextend our care in inappropriate ways.

Both therapist and client are impacted by the power plays between them. When we notice a power negotiation in the therapy room, it is helpful to acknowledge it to our clients and wonder aloud about what it might mean. A therapist can say, "I have noticed that often when I offer an idea, it feels like we get caught up in negotiating who has control rather than what can help you feel better. I wonder if you have noticed anything similar. Perhaps we can talk about it?" Naming the struggle can help both become more aware of when there is a felt need to assert power and how this need manifests. This enables therapist and client to directly negotiate their experience of each other and reduces the likelihood of secret or unconscious manipulation (Totton, 2009). As therapists, we need to do more than this; we must also make an effort to understand the vulnerabilities the client might be feeling, which could have led to their need to assert themselves. When we reflect more deeply, we may recognize that some of our client's behaviours or apparent resistance can also signify their own sense of powerlessness and a need to reassert some control. Rather than engaging in a power struggle, it is better for the therapist to hold the client's emotions. By surviving the intensity of their negative feelings, we demonstrate that their power is not necessarily destructive—and it is this response that can be healing for clients. When clients are ambivalent, wanting to be in control and yet asking the therapist to lead the way, Short (2011) suggests that therapists attempt to meet both needs by taking turns with who is in charge. These power plays have their own value; as the therapist and client accommodate each other, the client learns that the world is negotiable and that it is composed of persons with separate subjectivities (Muran & Hungr, 2013). Flexible responsiveness in our power positions can strengthen our ability to create a robust therapeutic alliance with a range of clients.

Pause and reflect…

Think of a time when you shifted the power differential or shared power with a client.

How did you do this?

In what ways did this impact the process of therapy with this client?

Attending to power is a significant way in which we can maintain an authentic and flexible connection with our clients. The canvas of power extends beyond the therapy interaction. Both therapist and client have experiences of power and powerlessness as a part of their lives, stemming from their social locations as well as individual histories. We can grow more nuanced in our understanding of power when we examine, question and redefine power that is embedded in our models of therapy, mental health systems and policies. Post-modern theories have engaged most deeply with issues of power in therapeutic relationships and privilege the client's personal power and vantage point (Sanders, 2011). We see this position reflected in their therapeutic processes and methods. For instance, in Tom Andersen's innovative reflecting team approach in family therapy, families are invited to switch places with therapists and observe and join the reflecting team's discussions about the therapy process. Irrespective of our theoretical orientation, careful consideration of power and control dynamics and how they sway the therapeutic relationship is warranted. Going beyond orientations, we are also aware that mental health systems and policies themselves act as either enabling or constraining frameworks (Andersen, 1990).

***Interview*: Power, Policy and Mental Health Practice**

Soumitra Pathare

This is an excerpt from our conversation with ***Dr Soumitra Pathare****, where he spoke of the role of power in mental health work and care*

Q. How does power play out when a client interfaces with the mental healthcare system?

The therapist–client/doctor–patient relationship is inherently unequal. It's better to acknowledge this inequality, because then you can try and address the power dynamic. We are an extremely hierarchical society where people are culturally attuned to say, "Since you know more than me, you should make the choice". The most common thing therapists say is, "Well … my client prefers it that way, so shouldn't I then do what my client prefers?".

Q. What would your advice be to therapists on negotiating power with clients?

I think you just need to make an effort. You need to put it back to them and tell them that I will give you as much information as you need, in a language that you can understand, and answer your questions, but I want *you* to make the choice. Often people get into healthcare settings because they like to be in a position of power to decide for people's lives. There is no space in our training for clinicians to reflect on that because our role models are all based on this notion of the "benevolent patriarch". Paternalism in healthcare has nothing to do with gender—it is a style, and women in healthcare can be as paternalistic as men. Somehow, our training does not actually challenge that and, in fact, medicine and all of healthcare takes pride in being paternalistic. Young therapists need to reflect, "Am I being paternalistic and is that a good thing for anybody, including me? Am I beginning to enjoy this?"

Q. How could mental healthcare initiatives with communities address the issue of power?

While working with communities, the rule is to try and make it as participatory as possible. This means listening to the community and understanding what they feel is likely to help them, and *then* presenting your point of view. It's a matter of dialogue—not as a tick box to be completed or a focus group discussion.

Q. You were part of the Policy Group appointed by the Ministry of Health and Family Welfare, Government of India, to draft the National Mental Health Policy. How did you handle these issues of power during your mental health policy work?

There are no easy answers to that question. A certain degree of honesty is required from everyone who is engaged in that process - a bureaucrat, an activist or a representative of the professional community. In negotiating policy, you are trying to do the greatest good for the greatest number of people. One's role as an honest broker in that policy process is to try and create a level playing field while ensuring some philosophical, moral and ethical basis to these actions. At the patient level, the notion of a nominated representative reflected the voices and concerns of two disadvantaged groups—women's groups saying, "I don't want the usual system where the husband makes decisions for me", and the LGBTQI groups saying, "I don't want anyone in my family to make decisions for me. I want to choose who should make decisions for me when I can't make decisions for myself". Going down that route was obviously criticized as against our Indian culture, where the family decides and knows what is best for you.

Let us say that in a room full of 10 people, if nine people agreed on everything, that does not necessarily mean that it's the right thing to do. Democratic policy making requires taking care of the needs, wishes and fears of the minorities, as much those of the majority. This requires time and effort, and it ends in a slightly messier solution, but is more inclusive. Everyone leaves the table thinking that I did not get everything I wanted, but I got quite a few things, and I didn't get anything less than what everybody else got.

Dr Soumitra Pathare *is a consultant psychiatrist and the director of the Centre for Mental Health Law & Policy, in India. He has been involved in drafting India's National Mental Health Policy and the Mental Health Care Act, 2017. He is also engaged in suicide prevention policy and strategy development, and in implementation research projects on suicide prevention.*

The End Game: Termination of the Therapeutic Relationship

Termination is an inevitable part of the therapeutic process, sometimes mutual and planned and at other times forced or unilateral. Perhaps a good beginning for our reflections is to think about how we view the termination of therapy. The word termination is derived from *Terminus*, the Roman deity who protected boundaries and borders, ensuring that they remained clearly demarcated and impervious. The phase of termination in therapy often carries a sense of immovability and finality. But this is not always the case—many of us remember our relationships with clients years later, and sometimes, former clients knock on the door again. We may choose to look at this phase as signalling the permanent end of the therapist–client relationship or as a period for processing a relationship that often endures in our memories. The end of therapy can seem like a door that closes, or as a transformative bridge to a new beginning hat is built through the consolidation of gains and changes. Our perspective will impact what we feel at the culmination of this shared journey, the ways in which we understand and respond to our clients' feelings and how we make sense of our experiences.

Session endings can be microcosms of therapy endings, and we need to be finely tuned to how these are experienced. The end of the therapy session can feel abrupt or awkward, and the emotional transition from deep connectedness to "see you next week" can be hard for both therapist and client. As the hour draws to a close, clients may express intense emotions or make an unexpected disclosure, making it harder to say, "Our time is up for today". These endings are not sacrosanct, and the therapeutic frame does not have to be an unyielding fence. Therapists can selectively extend session time if the context calls for it. However, if this happens all too often, our reflections can tell us what we need to work on. Is it about our idea of what therapy is? The role we wish to play in our client's life? Or our discomfort with not being liked? Negotiating session endings provides a practice ground for learning closing words and rituals and prepares both the client and therapist for the eventual termination of therapy (Sher, 2014).

Some termination experiences might be more difficult than others, particularly with vulnerable clients who have a history of previous losses and attachment vulnerabilities. Our understanding of clients' attachment styles can help us anticipate their approaches to termination and tailor our responses accordingly. For instance, clients with an avoidant style may deny the importance of termination or of the relationship and slip back into their comfort zone of detachment. It is important to help them stay connected with their feelings and those of others and encourage them to draw on learnings within the co-created emotional space in therapy. For an anxiously attached client, possible feelings of anger, anxiety, grief and abandonment may be overwhelming, and the therapist would have to step in more actively to structure the process to help them work through their intense cognitive and emotional responses (Zilberstein, 2008). Handling the termination more carefully with clients who have attachment injuries, by preparing early for termination, and allowing time to work through their feelings can mitigate some of the complicated and ambivalent reactions (Juul et al., 2020).

As therapists, we need to reflect on our early relational experiences, how we are in our current relationships, and our feelings about distance and intimacy. Reflections on our personal experiences with losses, transitions and endings; during travel to another country on vacation, a change of school, a breakup or the death of a family member, can increase awareness of our comfort with separations, change and ambiguity. A therapist who is uncomfortable with closeness may stay in the safe zone of positive emotions, without tuning into or processing the messier emotions experienced by the client. Termination of therapy may sometimes be advanced to prevent the development of dependency and to limit the intensity of the relational dynamics between the therapist and client (Holmes, 1997). The therapist who is a bit more anxious about relational separations may experience difficulties during termination, and these feelings may overshadow the client's reactions and needs. As feelings of sadness and guilt arise about abandoning the client, we may hesitate to call an end to the ongoing relationship. To navigate the termination phase effectively, it is essential to address emerging vulnerabilities and ensure that our own needs do not dictate the session process. Therapeutic endings may have different meanings across orientations but deserve attention in both time-limited and long-term therapies. The awareness of the inevitable endpoint makes termination the central issue in time-limited therapies, and possibly accelerates the pace of change. Therapies with a more circumscribed time frame place constraints on the nature and the amount of therapeutic work that can be done. This means that we must assess whether clients have adequate resources and support, as their journey continues without the therapist. Even when termination is expected, it remains essential to explore our clients' emotional responses to this predetermined ending. The challenges differ in long-term psychotherapy, where the client and therapist may not always agree on when their journey together should conclude. At times, it can be difficult to reconcile the complex needs of vulnerable clients with the growing emphasis on short-term therapies that demand predictable and inflexible endings. Speaking of thirteen years of her therapeutic journey with Donna, through periods of hope and despair, moments of insight and repeated cycles of crisis, McWilliams (1986) makes a case for interminable engagement with those of our vulnerable clients who need this.

Pause and reflect...

What do you feel about the idea of seeing a client with no foreseeable plan for termination?

Have a discussion with your peers about how therapeutic systems, funding and policies for mental health care can impact our decisions about termination.

The reasons for ending therapy and the context of termination—whether forced, client-initiated or therapist-initiated, planned and collaborative or unexpected and unilateral—all influence how we understand and process the experience. During our training years, much of the focus is on how to build and sustain our connection with clients, and relatively less is said about the emotional demands and challenges of saying goodbye. As trainees, we often experience interruptions and forced terminations due to the structure of placements and internships. There is no turning back and little opportunity to prepare for these endings, adequately process our emotions, such as sadness, guilt, anger and relief, or critically reflect on these endings. Creating a reflective space to acknowledge and process this end of the relationship is invaluable.

It can be particularly challenging when clients terminate therapy without discussing it with their therapist, leaving unanswered questions and complex emotions in their wake. Such experiences could spill over into our personal lives, impacting both our sense of self and the ways we manage distance and closeness with future clients. We may protect ourselves by focusing on client-related factors, attributing premature departure to their psychopathology. In doing so, we may overlook the potential contribution of therapist-related factors, the dynamics of the evolving therapeutic relationship or contextual influences that also shape the client's decision to disengage. Looking back, we may wonder if we adequately prepared our clients for the work of therapy or if any countertransferential processes had led to the termination. We may also question at our own skills and expertise, wondering if we were responsive enough to client needs or their expectations from the relationship about the alliance. We need to guard against self-criticism or lingering feelings of shame when clients leave therapy prematurely. While such departures can feel personal, they often stem from external factors such as affordability, accessibility of treatment or shifting life circumstances. Processing these endings need not be a solitary journey—peers and supervisors can offer support, perspective and shared learning. Engaging in this reflective and reparative process not only benefits our future clients but also contributes to our own ongoing professional development. While premature terminations are often initiated by clients, we might have experienced moments when a client leaves us feeling so confused, depleted and inadequate that we wish for an end to these interactions. We might also weigh this option of terminating therapy when progress seems blocked, or the relationship seems to have broken down irretrievably. When such strong emotions are fuelling our thoughts and decisions about termination, we should reflect and seek consultation or supervision to find direction and closure.

A good-enough termination allows for the exploration and validation of emotions about ending the relationship and resolving any ruptures, a review of pivotal moments and changes in therapy, and a sense of looking ahead for both the client and therapist (Norcross et al., 2017). In some time-limited therapies such as cognitive analytic therapy, goodbye letters are used to take stock and share feelings, with planned follow-up sessions to monitor and support change (Ryle, 2005). In response to developmental considerations of working with children, therapists may take the extra step of tangible reminders that can be revisited, such as creating an album of the therapy work done together. Discussing what the child would like to remember and how they would like to be remembered by the therapist can also provide a sense of closure and continuity (Zilberstein, 2008). Adults may need similar care as they prepare to separate from the emotional connection formed in the therapy room. When we memorialize the relationship and the learnings from experiences in therapy in tangible ways, these transitional objects accompany our clients as they journey ahead.

Clients can also value the chance to plan their own termination, indicating to the therapist when they wish to slow down and taper sessions and when they feel ready to stop. Discussing what support they would need during this process while expressing trust in their ability to manage their own lives can provide the secure base from which they can continue their life journey on their own.

A Therapist Speaks: On Letting Go

K. Dharani Devi

I began seeing Mira, a single woman in her late thirties with a mood disorder and personality vulnerabilities. Mira grew up feeling unsafe in a chaotic and unstable home, with experiences of sexual abuse, complicated relationships with her mother and brother, and a father who had completed suicide. Since childhood, she had experienced her mother as "pretending" to care for her while simultaneously being hostile and critical and failing to protect her from harm. She was now estranged from all family members and lived alone.

Our relationship evolved over the course of four years. Her previous therapist described Mira as a "difficult patient" and cautioned me about "defending boundaries". Over the course of therapy, I slowly had to relax some of my strict rules and boundaries, and she had to learn to follow some. Through the course of our work together, I alternatively felt proud of her, worried about her and her lack of social support, was frustrated with her and admired her resilience—much like a mother. She had become quite special to me.

The termination of therapy occurred abruptly in the initial stages of what was later identified as a clear psychotic breakdown. Entire sessions were dominated by her insistence that one of her colleagues was sexually harassing her, and I found it difficult to relate to her interpretation of her colleague's actions. After one such session, Mira emailed me stating that she did not want to continue therapy. While I cannot say that this unilateral decision was totally unexpected, it still surprised me. The session seemed to have gone well despite our differing perspectives, and we had agreed to disagree. I tried reaching out to her, but she responded saying that she was okay and did not want to meet me. Accepting what I felt and staying with it opened the door for other thoughts and emotions - worry, anger, frustration, hurt and guilt. Had I let her down in the same way everyone else in her life had? Was it my fault and lack of competence that she felt this way, despite our long alliance? I also felt frustrated that this had happened just as we were making progress, and she had remained stable for an entire year. I felt betrayed and was angry with her for not having trusted me to know better.

In fact, it was an email from my client that brought things into perspective—she understood my concerns but wanted me to let her go. A few months later, I met her while she was recovering from her psychotic episode. She expressed that she had missed me and appreciated the therapeutic journey. It was not that she didn't care, but felt that we had achieved everything we could have together. She spoke of her anger at feeling unsupported at a crucial point in her life but believed that my intentions were good. She wanted to resume therapy, just not with me. This experience uncovered my hidden beliefs regarding successful therapy and therapists, and the role of power and control. Gradually, I appreciated how Mira had come a long way and had exercised her sense of agency in the relationship. Termination is the client's prerogative—this was one of the most important lessons for me.

Dr K. Dharani Devi *is a clinical psychologist and psychotherapist. She uses an attachment and mentalization framework in her individual and group work with persons with borderline personality vulnerabilities.*

Each ending may be different and is a time and opportunity to learn something about ourselves, our clients and the process of therapy. We may also need to accept that things do come to an end, especially therapy relationships. And an ending is not necessarily a bad thing. For the client, it can mean an end to suffering or an end to a bad phase in their life. Therapy endings usually mark the beginning of new possibilities. It could be so for the therapist as well.

Perspectives on Training and Development

Training and Frameworks for Relational Skills

Training programmes need to incorporate frameworks that explicitly focus on developing competencies related to the creation, cultivation and maintenance of the therapeutic relationship. Drawing from our observations as supervisors, as well as feedback from trainees, we suggest several focal areas that merit attention in training.

Working with couples, families and groups requires therapists to develop the ability to build, balance and, when needed, repair multiple alliances—while also attending to shifting alignments between members of these systems. Power dynamics often become central targets of intervention in such work. These dynamics must be addressed both in terms of relationships among family members and between the therapist and the system. In couple therapy, for instance, therapists may aim to strengthen the relationship by supporting the less powerful partner and encouraging the more powerful partner to share their power. Trainees engaged in conjoint therapies will require additional support, both didactic and supervisory, to navigate these complex relational tasks.

In the context of telepsychotherapy, trainees often need support in managing the alliance and finding ways to make meaningful contact across the screen. Early in training, it can be challenging to appropriately challenge clients while preserving the therapeutic relationship. Nuanced training methodologies—such as micro-skill building, experiential exercises and live supervision—can facilitate the development of these subtle but critical competencies.

Trainee therapists have also highlighted the need to strengthen their relational skills when dealing with alliance strains and power struggles. This is particularly evident when working with clients who present with narcissistic personality structures, or when client disclosures contradict the therapist's core values. Additionally, we have observed that some trainees experience difficulty bridging the gap with clients whose lived experiences differ greatly from their own. These differences may stem from age (e.g., younger trainees working with older clients), life experiences (e.g., parenting) or social location (e.g., socioeconomic class). Addressing these gaps requires reflective practice and support to build cultural humility and relational flexibility.

Another area that warrants attention is the emotional and relational impact of premature terminations and case transfers, which occur frequently during clinical rotations and internships. These transitions can be destabilizing for all involved: the trainee may experience a sense of unfinished work, the client is required to separate and form a new therapeutic relationship, the incoming therapist must navigate someone else's ongoing process, and the supervisor needs to hold and support the entire system. Despite their frequency, these transitions are often insufficiently addressed in training. Anticipating such occurrences and integrating protocols for navigating these transitions should be a core component of any clinical programme.

The use of diverse methods to assess and reflect on presence and alliance can enhance trainees' awareness of relational processes. In our training settings, we have encouraged trainees to observe therapy sessions through role-plays or video recordings and use brief alliance measures to evaluate relational dynamics. Transtheoretical training in the identification of key relational markers, as well as in the repair of alliance ruptures, can be an effective way to strengthen relational competencies (Eubanks et al., 2023).

Furthermore, therapist training can benefit from integrating transtheoretical models for recognizing and managing countertransference (Cartwright et al., 2018). Research suggests that therapist qualities such as self-integration, empathy, self-insight and the ability to mentalize one's own feelings, needs, beliefs and intentions play a crucial role in countertransference awareness and in navigating closeness–distance dynamics (Barreto & Matos, 2018; Bhola & Mehrotra, 2021; Sikand & Bhola, 2024). These findings offer clear guidance for incorporating self-reflective and emotionally attuned practices into therapist development frameworks.

Building Relational Skills in Supervision

When trainees experience disruptions in the therapeutic relationship, an exploration of the role of one's own attitudes, biases and assumptions, personal issues or interpersonal skills needs a facilitative supervisory space. Trainees learn not just from the course content but more significantly from the attitudes and stances they see in their trainers. When our supervisor can attune with us, and soothe us with their presence, we experience the power of co-regulation first-hand. Where our supervisors and trainers attend to ruptures in our relationship with each other and do so respectfully and caringly, we experience that those relationships can be rebuilt and strengthened in the process. We can learn how to connect with clients when our teachers connect with us. Effective training in relational skills can only occur in a sensitive and safe training environment in which we learn that all therapists encounter relational challenges, feel comfortable in sharing our experiences and emotions around therapeutic relationship difficulties and strengthen our repertoire of skills.

Conclusion

With every client, a new journey begins—to know and be known. Both the client and therapist discover parts of themselves as they meet another person and encounter their perspectives, values, experiences and feelings. Although the therapeutic contract may end, and the therapy process may be terminated, the therapeutic bond remains as the client and the therapist live on in each other's mind.

References

Altimir, C., Capella, C., Núñez, L., Abarzúa, M., & Krause, M. (2017). Meeting in difference: Revisiting the therapeutic relationship based on patients′ and therapists′ experiences in several clinical contexts. *Journal of Clinical Psychology, 73*(11), 1510–1522.

Andersen, T. (1990). *The Reflecting Team: Dialogues and dialogues and dialogues*. Borgman.

Barreto, J., & Matos, P. (2018). Mentalizing countertransference? A model for research on the elaboration of countertransference experience in psychotherapy. *Clinical Psychology & Psychotherapy, 25*(3), 427–439.

Bhola, P., & Mehrotra, K. (2021). Associations between countertransference reactions towards patients with borderline personality disorder and therapist experience levels and mentalization ability. *Trends in Psychiatry and Psychotherapy., 43*(2), 116–125.

Bordin, E. S. (1979). The generalizability of the psychoanalytic concept of the working alliance. *Psychotherapy: Theory, Research & Practice, 16*(3), 252–260.

Cartwright, C., Barber, C., Cowie, S., & Thompson, N. (2018). A trans-theoretical training designed to promote understanding and management of countertransference for trainee therapists. *Psychotherapy Research, 28*(4), 517–531.

Castonguay, L. G., Constantino, M. J., & Holtforth, M. G. (2006). The working alliance: Where are we and where should we go? *Psychotherapy (Chicago, Ill.), 43*(3), 271–279.

Clarkson, P. (1991). Through the looking glass: Explorations in transference and countertransference. *Transactional Analysis Journal, 21*(2), 99–107.

Diamond, N. (2013). *Between skins: The body in psychoanalysis – contemporary developments*. Wiley.

Erskine, R. G. (1998). Attunement and involvement: Therapeutic responses to relational needs. *International Journal of Psychotherapy, 3*, 235–244.

Eubanks, C. F., Muran, J.C., & Safran, J. D. (2015). *Rupture Resolution rating system (3RS): Manual*. Unpublished manuscript, Mount Sinai-Beth Israel Medical Center, New York.

Eubanks, C. F., Muran, J. C., & Safran, J. D. (2018). Alliance rupture repair: A meta-analysis. *Psychotherapy, 55*, 508–519.

Eubanks, C. F., Muran, J. C., & Samstag, L. W. (2023). Alliance-focused training: Teaching therapists to navigate alliance ruptures. In L. G. Castonguay & C. E. Hill (Eds.), *Becoming better psychotherapists: Advancing training and supervision* (pp. 107–126). American Psychological Association.

Flückiger, C., Del Re, A. C., Wampold, B. E., & Horvath, A. O. (2018). The alliance in adult psychotherapy: A meta-analytic synthesis. *Psychotherapy, 55*(4), 316–340.

Gabbard, G. O. (2004). *Long term psychodynamic psychotherapy: A basic text*. American Psychiatric Publishing Inc.

Geller, S. M. (2018). Therapeutic presence and polyvagal theory: Principles and practises for cultivating effective therapeutic relationships. In S. W. Porges & D. Dana (Eds.), *Clinical applications of polyvagal theory: The emergence of polyvagal informed therapies* (pp. p106-126). Norton.

Geller, S. M., & Porges, S. W. (2014). Therapeutic presence: Neurophysiological mechanisms mediating feeling safe in therapeutic relationships. *Journal of Psychotherapy Integration, 24*(3), 178–192.

Gelso, C. J., & Hayes, J. A. (2007). *Countertransference and the therapist's inner experience: Perils and possibilities*. Lawrence Erlbaum Associates Publishers.

Göhler, G. (2009). Power to' and 'power over. In S. R. Clegg & M. Haugaard (Eds.), *The Sage handbook of power* (pp. 27–39). Sage Publication.

Holmes, J. (1997). 'Too early, too late': Endings in psychotherapy—An attachment perspective. *British Journal of Psychotherapy, 14*, 159–171.

Juul, S., Simonsen, S., & Bateman, A. (2020). The capacity to end: Termination of mentalization-based therapy for borderline personality disorder. *Journal of Contemporary Psychotherapy, 50*, 331–338.

Kernberg, O. (1965). Notes on countertransference. *Journal of the American Psychoanalytic Association, 13*(1), 38–56.

Little, R. (2018). The management of erotic/sexual countertransference reactions: An exploration of the difficulties and opportunities involved. *Transactional Analysis Journal, 48*(3), 224–241.

Mallinckrodt, B. (2010). The psychotherapy relationship as attachment: Evidence and implications. *Journal of Social and Personal Relationships, 27*, 262–270.

Mallinckrodt, B., Choi, G., & Daly, K. D. (2015). Pilot test of a measure to assess therapeutic distance and its association with client attachment and corrective experience in therapy. *Psychotherapy Research, 25*(5), 505–517.

Mehra, P. R. (2018). The *Rafoogar's* yarns crossing time. *Inter-actions, 1*. Retrieved from https://lilainteractions.in/priyas-write/#_ftn1

Misch, D. A. (2000). Great expectations: Mistaken beliefs of beginning psychodynamic psychotherapists. *American Journal of Psychotherapy, 54*(2), 172–203.

Muran, J. C., & Hungr, C. (2013). Powerplays, negotiation, and mutual recognition in the therapeutic alliance: "I never met a client I didn't like…eventually." In A. W. Wolf, M. R. Goldfried, & J. C. Muran (Eds.), *Transforming negative reactions to clients: From frustration to compassion* (pp. 23–44). American Psychological Association Books.

Muran, J. C., Eubanks, C. F., & Samstag, L. W. (2021). One more time with less jargon: An introduction to "rupture-repair in practice." *Journal of Clinical Psychology, 77*(3), 61–368.

McWilliams, N. (1986). Patients for life. *The Psychotherapy Patient, 3*(1), 55–69.

McWilliams, N. (2004). *Psychoanalytic psychotherapy: A practitioner's guide*. Guilford Press.

Norcross, J., Zimmerman, B., Greenberg, R., & Swift, J. (2017). Do all therapists do that when saying goodbye? *Psychotherapy, 54*, 66–75.

Racker, H. (1953). A contribution to the problem of countertransference. *International Journal of Psychoanalysis, 34*, 313–324.

Ryle, A. (2005). Cognitive analytic therapy. In J. C. Norcross & M. R. Goldfried (Eds.), *Handbook of psychotherapy integration* (2nd ed., pp. 196–217). Oxford University Press.

Sanders, C. J. (2011). An exploration of knowledge and power in narrative, collaborative-based, postmodern therapies: A commentary. *The Professional Counselor, 1*(3), 201–207.

Safran, J. D., & Muran, J. C. (2000). Resolving therapeutic alliance ruptures: Diversity and integration. *Journal of Clinical Psychology, 56*(2), 233–243.

Safran, J. D., Muran, J. C., & Eubanks-Carter, C. (2011). Repairing alliance ruptures. *Psychotherapy, 48*(1), 80.

Safran, J. D., & Kraus, J. (2014). Alliance ruptures, impasses, and enactments: A relational perspective. *Psychotherapy, 51*(3), 381–387.

Sher, M. (2014). Words and rituals: The significance of 'smaller' endings. *Reformulation, 43*, 33–36.

Short, D. (2011). I dare you to try and heal me': Alliance formation for cases of complex resistance. *Psychotherapy in Australia, 17*(2), 56–61.

Siegel, D. (2020). *The developing mind: How relationships and the mind interact to shape who we are* (3rd ed.). Guilford Press.

Sikand, M., & Bhola, P. (2024). Push and pull: Role of therapist mentalizing in navigating therapeutic distance. *Indian Journal of Psychological Medicine, 46*(3), 260–263.

Totton, N. (2009). Power in the therapy room. In *Therapy today* (pp. 16 –19). Retrieved from http://homepages.3-c.coop/erthworks/power.pdf

Zilberstein, K. (2008). Au Revoir: An attachment and loss perspective on termination. *Clinical Social Work Journal, 36*, 301–311.

Chapter 6
Understanding Personal and Professional Values

The Empathy Museum is an international travelling participatory art project which allows us to look at the world through another person's eyes. Visitors to the *A Mile in My Shoes* exhibit are invited to literally walk in someone else's shoes, while listening to an audio story about the actual shoe owner's life. These immersive experiences provide an opportunity to understand stories and lives we know less about: a sex worker, war veteran, neurosurgeon, refugee or prisoner turned artist. In the *Human Library* exhibit, we can borrow a person for conversation, someone whose values and experiences may be quite different from our own. These experiential exhibits create spaces for reflexive listening, and for asking questions—even difficult ones. The act of being a therapist and engaging with clients is much like a daily visit to an Empathy Museum. We meet as strangers, but through the process of therapy, we engage with the choices, emotional experiences, beliefs and underlying values of our clients—and in turn our own.

Values lie at the core of who we are and are a central (and sometimes unacknowledged) aspect of our sense of self. They influence our thoughts (e.g., I believe that each human being should be treated with dignity), our feelings (e.g., I feel strongly offended when I see people being rude to a person who may not be as privileged) and our behaviours (e.g., I am always polite to wait staff at a restaurant). Values reflect the understanding of what is good and bad, right and wrong, important and unimportant. When we value something, it acts as an internal standard, and we are impelled to act in ways that are consonant with this belief. When a value is violated, we might experience a visceral aversion that emerges from a deep part of our self. Considering how central values are in our lives, it becomes imperative to ask ourselves what role they play in our psychotherapy practice.

The traditional analytic stance positioned the therapist as a blank screen, fostering an environment where their personal values, attitudes and beliefs remained hidden and were seen as irrelevant or even harmful in the therapeutic space. The aim was to keep the therapeutic space safe for clients to share their thoughts and feelings, choose their goals and make decisions without having to necessarily adopt the therapist's

P. Bhola et al., *Reflective Practice in Psychotherapy and Counselling*,
https://doi.org/10.1007/978-981-96-9732-8_6

value lens. This value-free or value-neutral stance perhaps reflected the pressures on psychotherapy to be a scientific discipline and disregarded the ambiguity, irony and paradox inherent in practice (Holmes, 1996).

Over time, there has been a growing acknowledgement of the inevitable interplay between therapist and client values. Complete value neutrality on the part of the therapist is no longer considered either tenable or desirable. Values are recognized as implicit (and sometimes explicit) in therapeutic work, calling for intentional awareness. Indeed, Tjeltveit (2021) contends that it is an ethical imperative for therapists to be aware of the values guiding their judgements of what is right, virtuous or obligatory in therapy practice. What personal and professional values do we hold? How do values enter our therapeutic space and how do we make choices around them? When do we speak about them and when do we guard against them influencing our clients negatively? In this chapter, we present perspectives to engage with these questions and trace pathways for therapists to negotiate the value conflicts that emerge in therapy.

Unpacking Our Personal Values

A lawyer who pushes for justice, a photographer who is motivated by creativity and passion, a nurse who is dedicated to comforting and caring for the sick, these examples depict the deeply held convictions that people live and work by. It is not always easy to give values a label or define them clearly, and sometimes they only reveal themselves by how we respond or behave in situations. For instance, an awareness of how much we value independence may not surface until a situation challenges our sense of autonomy. Values also become apparent during times of crisis or decision-making and are useful in making meaning of the situation and taking appropriate action. Our awareness deepens as we ask ourselves what we are committed to upholding and what we find very difficult to accept.

Pause and reflect...

List out 10 things you value the most in your life. This could be a person, place, object, significant experience and even a life goal. Organize your list in order of priority, with more important items coming first.

Consider if there is any value you would pick as central to you.

How do you think this value manifests in your beliefs, feelings and behaviours?

Would your friends also realise how much you care about this?

Mapping values on a pre-existing framework is useful as it enables a complex understanding of self. We recommend Schwartz's (2017) circumplex model as it is well researched across several countries and cultures. This model is useful as it does not just provide a list of basic values like benevolence, tolerance, achievement or security; but also organizes them under three levels of super-ordinate themes. A map like this can be used to understand and navigate complex value landscapes which connect with behaviours and life choices. For example, an individual's belief in equal rights for everyone in society may manifest through actions such as volunteering their time or pursuing training in human rights law. While some values seem to go together quite naturally, others feel inherently conflicting. A commitment to promoting the welfare of humanity aligns well with a belief in helping individuals in need. This can sometimes conflict with a value like power, which emphasizes personal success and self-enhancement. Gaps often emerge between stated values and those embodied in one's interactions, decisions and behaviours. Such discrepancies become visible only through an interrogation of actions and choices made, revealing the underlying values and beliefs that lie beneath. A single behavioural choice may be shaped by multiple values, but it is in the subtle nuances of thought and action that the value taking precedence in a given moment becomes apparent. Internal discomfort and difficulty in decision-making often arise when values are in direct conflict. For instance, the pursuit of recognition or promotion for contributions to a team effort may at times conflict with the desire to remain supportive and caring towards colleagues who are struggling.

Most values are learnt and imbibed from family environments, often through interpersonal identification with parents (Podolskiy, 2012). This process can be implicit or explicit, extends across generations and is often reflected in family rituals and maxims or proverbs heard at home. For instance, a grandparent might remind us that "Family comes first", while a parent emphasizes, "As you sow, so shall you reap", and a sibling declares, "Live and let live". A belief like "Family comes first" represents core values of collectivism, loyalty and interdependence. This can lead to actions and decisions that prioritize harmony and the well-being of the family, sometimes above personal or professional needs. It can also lead to a deeper investment in emotional bonds and connection with family members and a commitment to keeping family secrets. Collective observations and experiences regarding what was prioritized and rewarded at home, along with the ways family members responded to challenges and conflicts, come together to shape the values we hold as central even in adulthood. These values are then transmitted to the next generation through both instruction and example.

Each of the groups and communities that we belong to, including educational institutions, sports teams, and religious and professional organizations, has set (if sometimes tacit) standards about the right way to do things. For instance, sportspersons are encouraged to persevere and compete to win—values that they tend to internalize over the years. On a larger scale, values such as individualism which prioritizes independence, and collectivism which emphasizes interdependence are culturally embedded. Generational shifts from Boomers, Gen X, Millennials to Gen Z bring in unique sets of values, which emerge in the context of the social, political and technological landscape around each generation. Generations that experienced scarcity may be more conservative in their approach, preferring to conform or work towards security. On the other hand, generations that experienced economic stability may be drawn towards pleasure, stimulation, change or growth. Values are continually strengthened, recalibrated or transformed through life events such as migration, or in response to global challenges like climate change. Periods of rapid societal change are often accompanied by a recalibration of individual and collective belief systems and norms. Ways of parenting, gender-power structures, sexuality and attitudes towards work and family are all evolving, generating a range of value dilemmas and confusion. Different contexts, such as family, community and sociocultural environments, carry distinct embedded value systems that could conflict with one another. Navigating these influences often involves a process of selectively adopting, questioning or distancing from particular values, shaping a personal sense of what matters and why. Sometimes, values and their possible origins become more discernible only when challenged by an alternate way of viewing the world. Delving deeper into how value systems have evolved can help examine similarities and differences between values learned early in life and those that may have developed later during adolescence or adulthood. Changes in values can be insidious and may go unnoticed unless interrogated every now and then. The process of actively questioning and negotiating values can result in the emergence of newer, more contextual values.

Pause and reflect...
Reflect on a value that was strongly emphasized in your family.

As an adult, what is your relationship with this value?

Values and the Practice of Psychotherapy

Certain values are inherent in a helping profession that seeks to understand and support people in their emotional journeys. Many of these values are embodied in the general principles of ethical guidelines and form the foundation from which the therapeutic endeavour emerges. Choosing to become a therapist can itself be viewed as a value-driven decision. Even when not explicitly acknowledged, the synchrony between personal and professional values may be one factor that draws individuals towards the profession. Additionally, each theoretical orientation is grounded in certain values and ways of looking at the world. The humanistic basis of client-centred therapy is well known, as are its goals of promoting growth and self-actualization while preserving human dignity. Therapists who value tolerance, protection or care above interpersonal effectiveness or dominance are likely to be drawn towards this orientation. Working with theoretical models that align with core value systems tends to strengthen a therapist's belief in their efficacy (Tartakovsky, 2016). Professional values can also be internalized during the process of training and through experiences in therapeutic work. For instance, the value of self-awareness and authenticity may be reinforced as a therapist develops their understanding of client-centred theory and works with individuals who feel uncertain and incongruent within themselves. In such encounters, values are also shaped directly through interactions with clients, whose experiences, struggles and resilience can inspire the therapist to incorporate aspects of their value systems into their own life (Duggal & Sriram, 2021). The values one grew up with, those acquired during training, and those reinforced or challenged during the practice of therapy all interact, often strengthening and supporting each other.

Pause and reflect...

Pause to think about the values that seem central to your preferred theoretical orientation/s.

In what ways do these values resonate with your personal values and beliefs?

These interactive value systems feed back into therapeutic work, guiding a therapist's expectations, their hopes for the client and the overall process of therapy. Value choices are reflected even in the frame and structure of practice, for instance, in how sessions are charged, the typical number of sessions offered, and whether inter-session contact is encouraged. Our values determine how we approach diagnosis (e.g., Do we value the precision and dependability of categories or do we find more meaning in the client's subjective experience of themselves?), how we conceptualize our clients' concerns (e.g., Do we see a client who wants to stay single as someone who values independence or as someone who is avoiding intimacy?) and the nature of the goals we set (e.g., Do we encourage a client to risk an alternative career or value the security of a regular job?). In fact, values lay the template for our entire stance and way of being in the therapy room.

A therapist might seek congruence between key personal values and their work by choosing practice settings aligned with those values. A therapist strongly committed to feminist principles, for example, may establish a community organization that engages in advocacy and provides services for women experiencing intimate partner violence. Another practitioner might explicitly state the affirmative values that inform her therapeutic practice on a professional website, thereby communicating her approach and priorities to potential clients.

As we progress along our professional journey, we hopefully search for and find an increasing resonance between personal and professional values. If we stay connected to core values early in our careers, we could be better positioned to make choices that allow the personal and professional to align.

A Therapist Speaks: No Choice but to Be a Feminist Therapist

Laura S. Brown

I had wanted to be a psychotherapist from around the time I was nine years old. Family dynamics, and the privilege of being in a middle-class public school district that had a school psychologist to whom a troubled child could go for help, convinced me that this was my path in life.

Imagine my horror when, as an undergraduate, I began to encounter the work of radical psychiatrists and the Mental Patients' Liberation Front, both of which exposed the ways in which my chosen profession colluded with oppression. And then, just as I encountered feminism in the fall of 1971, I also became aware of how the so-called "mental health" system in the US was rife with misogyny, informed by the work of such pioneers as Naomi Weisstein and Phyllis Chesler. What I read was reinforced by what I saw, working as a low-level psychology technician/nursing assistant on an inpatient unit, at what was considered the best psychiatric hospital in my home town.

I considered giving up my career dreams. After all, how could I become part of a system that systemically oppressed women, LGBT people, BIPOC[1] people, poor people, that punished those who deviated from a bizarre notion of "normalcy" used to silence those who spoke inconvenient truths. I brought my dilemma to my consciousness-raising group, whose members were older and (I thought wiser) than I was, and who were almost all doctoral professionals in the mental health field or studying to become one.

They convinced me that I had an ethical obligation as a lesbian feminist to go forward with my career plans because, "You have good ideas, but if you're not Dr. Brown you're not going to get listened to". So I applied, for a second time, to graduate school in psychology, was accepted, and arrived on that campus declaring to anyone who would listen that I was a feminist therapist.

Because how could I be anything other than a feminist therapist once I had even an inkling of the truth about the ways in which my discipline had not simply colluded, but had actively promoted and built systemic forms of oppression and devaluation into the treatment of suffering human beings? This was not a choice; it was an absolute political and moral imperative. I began to organize women students in my psychology program to act against particularly egregious examples of sexism and misogyny among peers and faculty. I found comrades, and because of my early involvement in the Association for Women in Psychology, mentors. I discovered that what my consciousness-raising group members had told me was true. Laura Brown was just another crazy radical lesbian feminist in overalls. Dr. Laura Brown, with a growing list of publications, was someone to whom people had to attend, even when they flinched at what I had to say.

There has never been a place where Laura the person and Laura the feminist therapist have not converged in the last 50 years. My personal and professional

[1] Black, Indigenous and People of Color.

values are one and the same. My deepening understanding of intersectionalities expressed itself in my work and in my life. When I found myself, seemingly by accident, working with many trauma survivors, it was clear that feminist analysis had prepared me to be fully present with these individuals, that the feminist attention to power and powerlessness lent added value to my work that no intervention could possibly provide.

Thus, the human I am is a decolonial, liberatory, intersectional feminist who at times finds the world an uncomfortable place. The professional work that I do is decolonial, liberatory, intersectional and feminist. Sometimes this is challenging for me, as my commitments require me to be honest about my privilege and the ways in which I have benefited from the oppression of others. More often, though, this complete synergy between Dr. Brown and Laura the person has given me joy, connection, and a sense of meaning that has made my life better than I could have ever imagined having when, as a troubled child of nine, I walked into the school psychologist's office and, after our first session, asked him, "what do they call what you do?".

***Laura S. Brown**, PhD is a psychotherapy consultant in the USA. She is the author of several important books about feminist therapy and trauma treatment and was a founding member of the Feminist Therapy Institute. She is the past president of the Society for the Psychology of Women (APA Division 35), the Society for the Study of Sexual Orientation and Gender Diversity (APA Division 44), and the Division of Trauma Psychology (APA Division 56).*

The Elephant in the Therapy Room: Recognizing Our Values

Both client and therapist values enter the therapy room in many different guises. At times, their presence is unmistakably clear, such as when clients openly bring concerns related to marriage, divorce, childrearing, birth control, abortion, extramarital relationships, suicide, child abuse and numerous other complex issues. Reflecting on these moments invites therapists to consider not only the client's values but also how their own values interact within the therapeutic encounter. A client could experience an internal conflict between two (or more) of their own values, thinking, "I wish to be there for my new baby, but I do not wish to compromise on my career". They might also wonder how to express their values in their relationship, saying, "I wish to be there for my new baby, but my partner wants me to focus on my career". At times, resolving such conflicts can be the entire work of therapy.

Values are often expressed in subtle ways and may go unnoticed unless the therapist remains alert to their presence. This awareness typically begins early in therapy when identifying the client's goals and the core values these goals reflect. For example, understanding whether a client's desire to improve interpersonal skills is motivated by a need for achievement, a need for affiliation, or both will shape the focus and type of intervention. Therapeutic work with a client who values self-direction can be very different from work with one who values power, even when both share the stated goal of improving their work relationships. A client's values often emerge in their choice of words and the emotional intensity with which they describe their experiences or stance. There are times we make inferences from the appearance, clothing, setting and non-verbal behaviour of our clients, drawing (sometimes incorrect) assumptions about their value positions based on that. While it is true that certain groups of values tend to cluster together, it is not uncommon for values to appear in seemingly surprising combinations. We may imagine that somebody who is very outspoken does not care much for the opinions of others. But it is possible for a person to prioritize being true to themselves and expressing their genuine feelings and thoughts, yet also value conformity to societal norms or group. So, authenticity and conformity can exist side by side. When it feels like a particular value is being drawn on to understand a client, it is important to bring it into open discussion. This not only prevents the therapist's unstated value assumptions from colouring therapy but also creates an opportunity for clients to better understand their own value systems.

Therapists may not become aware that their own values have been activated until experiencing an unexpected emotional reaction. Feelings of disengagement from the client, along with difficulties in establishing a therapeutic relationship or creating a shared goal, can indicate possible value differences. Sometimes we feel an affinity towards a particular client, because of the resonance between their choices or behaviours and our personal values. It might be helpful to ask ourselves: were we too encouraging when our client spoke of reconsidering her decision to divorce her husband? Did we align too strongly with our adolescent client when they resisted parental demands and control? Were we too enthusiastic, curious or judgemental when our client shared their experiences with a dating application?

Becoming more aware of our own values, our clients' values and professional values will help us to note when these value systems are aligned and when parts of them are in conflict with each other. We can also note contextual and cultural similarities or differences and better understand how all the different value systems interact. This sets the stage for us to not just acknowledge the existence of values but actively work with them in a manner that can deepen the client's experience of therapy.

Intersections Between Client, Therapist and Cultural Values

Karen, a married female client in her early thirties is unhappy that her husband spends less time with her and shows little interest in being physically intimate. He is otherwise a good provider and a stable human being, who is supportive of her personal goals. Things at home are peaceful till she asks for more attention or intimacy. At this point, he gets upset and withdraws from her, expressing that he cannot give her any more than he already does. This leaves her feeling lonely and frustrated and wondering if she is asking for too much. She comes to therapy, feeling very distressed and uncertain about how she should respond. Should she push for more intimacy? Or accept him this way?

The client appears conflicted between valuing relational intimacy on the one hand and valuing stability and tolerance on the other. A therapist who values security could be inclined towards building her acceptance, while a therapist who values connection might really feel her distress and look at ways of building intimacy. If both Karen and her therapist had a shared position, valuing connection over security, their goals for therapy would also align more naturally. While this congruence can be beneficial, it could also constrain the space available to discuss contrary values, explore possibilities or suggest changes. We may never consider what could transpire if Karen explored another path—particularly if the therapist, however unintentionally, reinforces what feels most familiar or comfortable to them both. If Karen and her therapist held value positions that were not aligned, it would impact the therapy process differently, perhaps leading to more of a tussle around the goals of therapy. These alignments and divergences may not always be obvious to both therapist and client. As therapists, we know not to openly convey our personal values, but this does not mean that they stay out of the therapy process. Our values can manifest in subtle and non-verbal ways, sometimes as fleeing as greeting a client's idea with a nod and a smile, or choosing to remain expressionless while prompting them to continue.

It is always useful for the therapist to be aware of value differences vis-à-vis their clients, but all differences do not mandate the same response. Farnsworth and Callahan's (2013) description of the four ways in which value conflicts is a useful guide. They describe pre-emptive, adjacent, operational and unarticulated value conflicts; each of which requires a different action from the therapist. A pre-emptive conflict is an a priori value conflict which can make it seem difficult to engage in therapeutic work. For instance, when differing beliefs around religion or sexuality complicate the creation of goals that therapist and client can agree on. Adjacent value conflicts arise when client values clash with the personal values of a therapist but do not necessarily interfere with the goals of therapy. Operational value conflicts are those where the therapist and client share values but do not agree on the associated behaviours. Taking from the previous example, both Karen and her therapist can feel that security is an important value. However, Karen may wish to find security in the continuation of her stable relationship, while her therapist might want her to find security within her own strength. Finally, unarticulated value conflicts are those where one of our less conscious values are being violated. The therapist might experience a sense of unease or disquiet, unexplainable distance or otherness from the client, while unable to express or understand why. Even as we consciously strive to maintain neutrality, our emotions can inadvertently signal preferences, judgements or disapproval.

When we name and frame the client–therapist value conflict, recognizing the elephant in the room, this creates space for us to respond in a reflective and intentional manner. As therapists, we can experience internal value conflicts that pull us in opposite directions, while cultural injunctions about what is good, just or desirable exert additional influence. For instance, an adolescent seeking to individuate and leave home at the age of 18 would be considered healthy in some countries, but selfish and unmindful of family bonds and obligations in others. While individual autonomy is often emphasized in Western contexts, the concept of relational autonomy, which recognizes that identities and needs are inevitably shaped by relationships with others, holds greater significance in Asian and other collectivist cultures (Bhola & Chaturvedi, 2017). Therapists must create space for discussions that acknowledge the complexity of choices, particularly in situations where autonomy is influenced and sometimes constrained by relational and social contexts. This approach empowers clients to navigate their desire for autonomy in ways that can coexist with deep relational bonds, familial obligations and societal expectations.

Therapists can encounter both alignments and conflicts between their personal values, the principles upheld by the profession, and cultural expectations of behaviour. Often, cultural and professional values are adopted unquestioningly as implicit rules, reflecting the influence of a dominant discourse that shapes norms and expectations within the profession.

Pause and reflect...

One Part Woman, a novel by Indian writer Perumal Murugan is set in the 1940's and centres around the lives of a couple Kali and Ponna who are in a loving, committed marriage. It has been 12 years of prayers, potions and temple visits, but they do not have a child. The societal pressure, that holds the family's highest purpose as that of having children and places responsibility for conception on the woman, is tremendous. This pressure, both subtle and overt, intensifies. The couple reluctantly agree that Ponna engage in sex outside her marriage, as part of a temple ritual celebrating the *half-male, half-female* god *Maadhorubaagan* – *in order to conceive a child. This conflict between the patriarchal social values and personal values have a deep emotional impact on Kali and Ponna, with tragic consequences on their relationship.*

Reflect on your experiences as a therapist. Do you recall a time when socio-cultural values, your professional values and/or personal values suggested opposite courses of action? How did you engage with this value conflict?

While it is important to understand values contextually, we cannot assume that all clients and all therapists who belong to the same broad culture share the same world view. Like the blind men and the elephant, we may encounter unique value combinations that suggest different perspectives on how we can respond. The recognition that there are no absolute truths that can be applied across clients, therapists or contexts is what sets the stage for a reflective and curious engagement with value positions.

The Blind Men and the Elephant: Attending to Values in the Therapy Room

Working with Client Values in the Session

A gentle, sensitive stance can create openings for clients to share what is important and meaningful to them. Since value conflicts often lead to emotional distress, it is common for clients to openly and explicitly discuss these conflicts in therapy. As therapists draw clients into reflective conversations, this helps them articulate and understand their core values and choose when to make these legitimate targets of change in therapy. Merely naming and validating a value is insufficient; it is essential to create an environment that encourages exploration and critical examination. Helping clients create distance from societal or others' expectations and articulate their core values can foster greater internal clarity. Actively connecting this thinking to their feelings and choices, and feelings about their choices can make for a more complete conversation. If this step is overlooked, therapists might find themselves working at cross purposes with their clients. For example, after struggling to encourage a client to be more emotionally contained, a therapist may realize she values deep emotional experiencing more than emotional safety. Such moments can help clarify whether therapy goals align with client values, and whether clients are moving towards greater congruence or incongruence within themselves.

At times, therapists help clients recognize unstated value conflicts by reframing emotional struggles in terms of underlying values. This act of naming and reframing can shift the meaning of the choices being made, offering newer perspectives. However, the therapist's own convictions inevitably influence how value conflicts are framed. To minimize potential bias, it is helpful to adopt a tentative stance and reference a range of values rather than focusing on a single one. For instance, a therapist could say, "On the one side, we have autonomy, excitement, stimulation, exploration and on the other we have safety, security, prudence, being smart or playing along with societal rules. Is this how you would see your situation?" Once clients are aware of their value conflicts, these can be addressed directly by looking at underlying emotions and examining alternatives and consequences. Before initiating this, it's important to ask if the client will benefit from the discussion. Will it meet a therapeutic goal? Does the client want or need to know … or care?

Addressing values is most effective when the conflict is integrated into a comprehensive understanding of the client's needs in therapy, and when the client shares this understanding. As the process of value negotiation unfolds, clients can be encouraged to explore alternative values through behavioural change (Bonow & Follete, 2009). For instance, a therapist might encourage the client, "Why not try something else and see what happens?" In discussing behavioural options, the therapists acknowledge the possibility of operational value conflicts. While it is easier to find agreement on the more general values, disagreement tends to emerge around specific actions. Asking clients to clearly spell out their values, link them to particular behavioural choices and then examine the relationship between the two can help reduce misunderstandings between client and therapist.

A client's closely held values could enter the therapy room in ways that obstruct their own goals and even contradict the goals of therapy (Williams & Levitt, 2007). For example, if a client's value of family cohesion and harmony prevents them from revealing family secrets, the therapist might find it harder to develop an accurate understanding of the client's experience within the marriage. We can enter this conversation in a gentle manner, acknowledging and validating the client's value, and suggesting different ways they can honour that value. For instance, we might say, "I can see that protecting your family is of utmost importance to you and this is something we can definitely work together on. However, it feels like this need to protect them also makes you reluctant to talk about some of the struggles at home. Ultimately, I worry that if we do not address these problems that could end up being even more harmful for your family". In some situations, challenging client values more directly and encouraging a re-evaluation of those values and related behaviours may be necessary. When doing so, it remains important to support the individual as a whole. For example, while understanding a client's difficulties, a therapist would also explicitly challenge the use of violence against a partner during interpersonal conflicts. This approach is recommended when client actions or goals are self-destructive, antisocial or unethical, clearly obstruct therapeutic change, contradict therapy values or infringe on the rights and safety of others (Bonow & Follette, 2009).

Matching Client and Therapist Values

At the start of therapy, therapists typically know very little about their clients' values, which makes precise matching difficult, if not impossible. This challenge is compounded by the fact that values do not exist in isolation but form an interconnected constellation. Much like Heisenberg's uncertainty principle, it is impossible to know the full range of a client's values simultaneously and accurately. Given these complexities, it is perhaps unsurprising that research on the importance and impact of client–therapist value matching on therapy outcomes has been inconclusive. Kelly and Strupp (1992) demonstrated the Goldilocks principle, with moderate levels of value similarity between therapist and client predicting therapy gains. Interestingly, another study by Hogan et al. (2016) showed that while clients' perceptions of value similarity influenced the strength of the therapeutic alliance, actual value differences within the therapist-client dyad did not affect either the alliance or therapy outcomes.

While similarities in therapist and client values can build a shared understanding, certain differences can enrich the therapy process, allowing clients to broaden their range of life possibilities. For instance, a therapist who values independence may gently encourage a client struggling with codependency to explore healthier boundaries in relationships. If the therapist does this without being judgemental or critical, the client can feel supported in their journey. Clients' acceptance of differences within the therapy room can also help them extend this to people and contexts outside this interaction. A client with rigid beliefs about success might initially find themselves at odds with a therapist who values balance. As the client appreciates aspects of this new perspective, they may reevaluate their beliefs about success and its metrics and explore diverse life choices in relationships and work. Difference and sameness are both important in relationships, and their dynamic interplay which fosters understanding, growth and connection.

Prioritizing Client Values in the Therapy Room

A *value-sensitive approach* privileges clients' values about goals and positions the client as the expert (Williams & Levitt, 2007). As tourists in the client's world, therapists can choose to keep the client's values intact, even if this means an incomplete resolution of their problems. When clients come to therapy with questions around their values, it can be tempting for therapists to respond by sharing their own. In this process, the two sets of values may become more similar or converge over the course of therapy. This is perhaps better termed *value conversion*, as it is usually the client's values that shift to resemble those of the therapist (Tjeltveit, 1986). Therapists must exercise restraint to ensure that clients' values are not influenced, either overtly or covertly, against their wishes or without their consent (Jadaszewski, 2017).

If it becomes apparent that a client's values differ from those of the therapist, there may be a tendency to overlook the difference or avoid addressing it directly. However, this is not always possible or desirable, and at times, direct conflict may arise. In such situations, being aware of one's own values can help resolve difficult dilemmas, especially when values conflict or require prioritization. Greater reflection on personal values positions the therapist to better support clients in exploring their own values, empowering them to make more informed choices.

In the process of working with value differences, therapists have many tools or methods that can be applied to different situations. When the value differences are not too vast or do not interfere with the therapy process, therapists need to bracket their values. This is a self-reflective process of intentionally setting aside or even compartmentalizing personal beliefs to focus more empathically on understanding the client's world view (Jackson et al., 2013; Kocet & Herlilhy, 2014). For example, imagine a client, Sarah, who wants to forgive a friend who betrayed her trust, hoping to restore peace and connection. Her therapist believes in setting boundaries but avoids imposing this view, instead encouraging Sarah to explore her own values. As the conversation unfolds, the therapist helps Sarah clarify what forgiveness could mean for her, without directing her towards or away from reconciliation. Through open-ended questions, the therapist supports Sarah in considering both her desire to forgive and her right to self-protection, allowing her to find her own balance between the two.

In the face of emergent value conflicts, Buddhist-inspired acceptance and mindfulness approaches recommend beginning with the acceptance that no two people can have the same values (Choudhuri & Kraus, 2014). Having a beginner's mind or an open and curious stance about the client's value system (Suzuki, 1970), and the mindfulness stance of being neither accepting nor rejecting but observing things as they are, can create the space to try to transcend differences and look for similarities beyond. For instance, consider a therapist and client who have differing ideas about what it is to lead a good life—one emphasizing responsibility and duty, the other valuing richness and variety of experience. These differences can be transcended by both acknowledging that a meaningful life is one where we are able to express our values…whatever they may be. This approach can protect the therapeutic relationship, allowing the work of therapy to continue. Acknowledging the existence of opposing value systems, without attempting to privilege one over the other, creates space for both client and therapist to remain present in the same room.

A Therapist Speaks: A Room of Her Own

Rathna Isaac

As my client Lavanya spoke of her struggles to move into a home of her own, I felt increasingly disturbed and angry. I was aware of her difficult childhood—her mother had died when she was not yet ten. Her father had been both physically and emotionally abusive, neglecting her basic needs for regular food or medicine when she was ill and failing to protect her from sexual abuse. Lavanya felt unhappy and frustrated, as he remained both uncaring and irresponsible. She seemed conflicted between her duties as a daughter and the independence she longed for.

This father challenged every personal value I ever held about parenting. As a systemic therapist, I valued reciprocity in relationships and her staying with her father seemed like a violation of the values of human dignity, respect and care. Still, having been socialized with similar cultural values as Lavanya, I also admired her self-sacrifice and willingness to put her duty above her personal goals. I shared these observations as well as my concerns for her safety and well-being. She appreciated this perspective and contrasted it with her extended family who believed that her place was with her father, and that as a single woman it was selfish to consider other options.

Therapy became a space to explore her feelings and different views about choosing to leave home or continuing to stay. As we spoke more about duty and reciprocity, she recognized that what she felt was not a responsibility towards her father but towards her mother. Taking on her mother's roles would keep her legacy alive, and this included looking after her father. Understanding each of the values that were influencing her and locating their origin (culture, individual beliefs and unique emotional experience) helped us discover a pathway. Together, we identified how she could balance her self-care with care for her father, thereby negotiating a balance between being her mother and being herself. My reflections taught me to slow down to explore rather than rush to make a list of pros and cons and reach a decision. This helped uncover personalized layers and meanings, the blend of thoughts and emotions that drove Lavanya. While sharing my values opened a new conversation, it was placing my perspective as just one of multiple possibilities, which left her free to find her own answers.

Dr. Rathna Isaac *is a psychotherapist, supervisor and trainer in India with over 20 years of experience. She practices both individual and couple therapy from an integrated perspective.*

Therapist Disclosure of Their Values

Therapists who seek to conceal their values should be aware that some of these can be inferred from their appearance, use of language, practice setting, as well as subtle non-verbal communication and emotional reactions. While these are inadvertent disclosures, therapists can also choose to open a dialogue about values by disclosing their own. Some clients may seek a more authentic connection with their therapist and can find the active discussion of values a deepening and enriching experience. Clients may also be openly curious about the therapist's values, particularly when they are questioning their own value system or fear being judged. For instance, a client may ask, "Do you think it is wrong to be an atheist?" or "What choice would you make if you were in the same situation?" Both responding and not responding to such questions can affect the therapeutic alliance. If we respond too fast and with too much information, this can overwhelm or upset the client. However, if we choose to remain silent, we will leave the client wondering what we are not telling them.

It is better to be cautious about self-disclosure in the initial phase of therapy, when both the therapeutic alliance and the understanding about the client's needs and vulnerabilities are still evolving. At any stage, the sharing of therapist values must be preceded by reflection on the potential impact of these disclosures. A therapeutic response is one that is tempered by an understanding of the relevance to therapeutic goals, keeping beneficence and non-maleficence at the forefront of the decision-making process. Post-modern approaches such as feminist therapy encourage appropriate and well-timed therapist disclosure as a way to reduce the power differential in the room. When a therapist chooses to share, especially around values that could inform the therapy process, this is also aimed at empowering the client. Before taking this step, it is important to pause and anticipate the impact of such transparency, hoping that the client will also feel safe to disclose their own values, without needing approval or fearing censure.

Using Supervision to Recognize and Address Value Conflicts

During sessions, Carmen noticed that her client Juan constantly spoke about money - his growing investments and car purchases, and how to make more. He worked hard to make this money and was focused and driven. Carmen believed that life

must be about more than money and looked upon this behaviour as greed- especially in a country where so many have so little. Although she considered herself a non-judgmental therapist, these value differences made her uncomfortable. She could focus on the tasks of therapy such as addressing his phobia of travelling by air, but found it harder to like him. Carmen struggled with her strong emotions and wondered if anyone needed to change their values and beliefs in this situation. Was this even something to mention to her supervisor?

Like Carmen, therapists may avoid bringing some of their more subtle value-related dilemmas into supervision, perhaps fearing being judged. Supervisors can create a compassionate and conducive space by encouraging and legitimizing discussions about values, including value conflicts, assumptions and biases. This can help supervisees become more comfortable articulating their values as they arise in the therapy room, even in the absence of major conflicts. They can learn to distinguish between value differences that are best bracketed and significant value conflicts that need to be addressed. Supervision can also focus on the supervisee's emotional responses alongside practical strategies for what to do in the next session. This kind of support helps the supervisee maintain a therapeutic connection, preventing withdrawal or anger towards the client while they navigate how to respond. For instance, a supervisee might feel quietly uneasy when working with a client who expresses strong views on gender roles or parenting styles that contrast sharply with their own. Rather than dismissing or bypassing these feelings, a supervisor might respond with gentle curiosity, saying something like, "That sounds like it was difficult to sit with. Would it help to talk through what felt most challenging about it?" This conveys that the supervisee's emotional response is understandable and important to reflect on. If a supervisee notices a recurring pattern of value conflict with certain types of clients (for e.g., violent individuals or restrictive parents), this too can be explored in supervision. Supervision is also a valuable space to reflect on one's theoretical orientation and whether it aligns with one's values and assumptions about human nature.

When strong emotions cloud a therapist's perspective and there are seemingly irreconcilable differences in values, this might lead them to consider referring the client to another therapist. This is not a decision to be taken lightly, and carries several ethical ramifications. In some situations, referral has been seen as a way to protect the client's right to competent care and uphold the moral principles of beneficence and non-maleficence (Tjeltveit, 1986). However, such decisions can be difficult to reconcile with core professional values such as justice and non-discrimination, especially when they involve referring select clients based on value conflicts. Deep reflection on beliefs and biases within scaffolded spaces such as supervision and consultation is essential before taking action. Referral should be considered only in select situations, and certainly not as the first-line method of resolution. Therapists can begin by searching for shared goals, trying to build a connection with the client despite the differences, or considering options such as including a co-therapist to balance the emotions and values in the room (Kocet & Herlihy, 2014). Referral is advised only if a careful assessment of risks and benefits indicates that this is best for the client. The therapist still has the responsibility to engage in a sensitive and compassionate process, one in which referral options reflect the client's preferences, and the client's values, beliefs or actions are not presented as the reason for referral (Farnsworth & Callahan, 2013). The process of reflection on feelings and conflicts does not end with referral. As we know, a difficult experience with a client can continue to be an impetus for growth even years after it is over.

Pause and reflect...

Take a moment and think about value conflicts you might have experienced while working with clients.

What are some of the ways in which you responded?

Which strategies did you find easier or helpful in resolving value conflicts with your clients? Which ones were more difficult or unhelpful?

Imagine you needed to advise another therapist about ways to handle value conflicts. What would you tell them?

Engaging with Sociopolitical Values in the Therapy Room

Conversations around sociopolitical issues seem to be all around us and their presence is being increasingly felt in the therapy room, both implicitly and explicitly. We bring a focus to these sociopolitical values and ideologies that are a central influence on what we think and feel about a range of policies and also about people, communities and relationships. Sociopolitical positions are about much more than voting preferences and encompass value-driven perspectives on a range of issues such as migration, armed conflict, the death penalty, religious expression, climate change, human rights and affirmative action. Terms like right-wing or socialist reflect a constellation of values and life choices and create a sense of belonging to a group of 'people like us'. The world is fraught with political tensions and upheavals emerging from local and global sociopolitical events and schisms, often accompanied by reverberations from historical events. While political differences have always existed between individuals, these have become increasingly divisive and polarizing in recent times.

Anecdotal reports suggest an increase in disclosures and conversations about political events and views across the globe, although much of the research is largely in the context of the political landscape in the USA (e.g., Solomonov & Barber, 2019). Both therapist and client may initially feel around to sense the other's sociopolitical position and experience a sense of relief and camaraderie if they are similar. Our overarching sociopolitical values may be inferred through conversations about other issues and through assumptions we make about each other. Of course, with the looming presence of political events, election results, community protests and conflicts, clients can bring sociopolitical issues directly into the therapeutic discourse, asking, "Did you read the headlines about the Supreme Court verdict?" or "Are you going to vote next week?" Perceived value alignment could facilitate more open conversations about political material and potentially strengthen the sense of connection between the therapist and client (McCarthy et al., 2022; Solomonov & Barber, 2019). In this felt safe space, clients can speak more openly about their experience of sociopolitical distress and what this means to them. They might share their experiences of marginalization, perhaps questioning the lack of accessible spaces for persons with disability or describing painful experiences of exclusion due to their sexuality. These experiences may be in the form of systemic oppression or everyday discrimination in private and public spaces. For instance, several airline announcements start with 'ladies and gentlemen' and leave no space for the range of gender identities. Such small 'p' politics, often referred to as the "micro-politics of everyday life" (Janks, 2012, p.151), encompasses the subtle, informal power dynamics that play out in daily interactions and relationships within families, educational and workplaces, social circles, public spaces and online communities. Clients also tell us about their sense of self, well-being and inclusion in the world when they express their views on big 'P' politics centring on electoral politics and systems of government, relating them to current affairs, ongoing legal proceedings or trending social issues. As therapists, we can think about how to invite these conversations into the therapy room, neither forcing them upon a reluctant client nor indicating that we find them irrelevant to a person's psychology. Therapists can sometimes open the door for clients to discuss their experiences by sharing their own political stance, especially when clients' identities or realities feel marginalized. However, it is often wiser to wait for clients to raise these topics first, and to keep the focus on their experience rather than the therapist's views. Deciding whether to disclose requires careful reflection on the therapeutic relationship, client needs and the potential impact on trust and safety.

There is no denying that divergent or polarized sociopolitical perspectives do carry the potential for negative effects on client–therapist interactions and the therapeutic process. A bracketing of views in service of the client and the therapy process allows us to see the person that lies behind the political. When differences are recognized even if unarticulated, they can still vitiate the atmosphere in the therapy room. Ongoing attention to subtle tensions is necessary, as setting aside personal values does not guarantee that clients remain unaffected by underlying value divergences. If the client does not get the response they expected and senses a misalignment or implied disapproval from their therapist, this can disrupt the therapeutic connection. In such situations, it is ethical and therapeutically effective to openly acknowledge differences and discuss them with the client. We try to navigate these differences in such a way that we respect each person's individual positions while maintaining emotional connection and care. This approach fosters a more honest atmosphere in the therapy room and models a healthy way for clients to address sociopolitical differences in their other relationships.

Pause and reflect...

If a client expresses their political views during therapy, do you invite them to share further or do you feel uncomfortable with such discussions?

Have you encountered a client who expressed a socio-political position you find offensive? Think back to how you felt and responded.

If a client brings up what seems like misinformation or fake news that is influencing their judgement, the therapist can feel impelled to correct their information, even using an expert position to educate them. It may be more useful to understand the emotional significance of their position than to engage in a political debate with the client. As long as the therapist remains focused on the client's relationship with their sociopolitical values, seeking to become aware of their place in the client's overall psychological system, this discussion can be fruitful. This keeps the focus on the client's emotional experience and can also help us manage our own. Sometimes, a client may say something so offensive or hurtful, such as hate speech or a strong statement about religion or race, that it becomes difficult for the therapist to ignore. Such comments can be deeply triggering or feel invalidating, particularly when they touch on the therapist's own lived experiences. Strong emotional reactions are common when political or ideological views feel incompatible, and it is essential to ensure these responses do not manifest as countertransferential reactions. Reflecting on these value clashes in supervision or peer consultation can help therapists explore how to continue valuing themselves without devaluing their clients.

With several therapists explicitly stating their political ideology and political opinions on social media or through their engagement in advocacy, clients are also able to gauge a therapist's politics before they choose to reach out to them. This could serve as a form of gatekeeping where therapists attract clients with similar values, forming echo chambers where this is little chance of encountering alternative viewpoints. If the therapy room begins to reflect the polarizing forces in our world, we wonder if this contravenes the core values of our profession that emphasize justice and equity and the idea of a shared world?

Sociopolitical values can evoke powerful emotional responses, sometimes making it difficult for therapists to remain reflexive. Expressions of these values may be seen as infiltrators distracting from the real work of therapy, particularly since they also carry so much disruptive potential. Instead, if political positions (like other values) are considered as a part of the entire person of the client, there can be much to learn. We can gain a deeper understanding of how our client engages with the world, the ways in which they feel validated or excluded by what is happening in their social contexts.

Perspectives on Training and Development

Development of Value-Sensitive Training Modules

We recommend a greater focus on values in psychotherapy programmes, involving both individual and group spaces. While professional ethical codes are embedded in values, this knowledge is not enough for us to address the nuances and complexities of therapist and client values. In our experience as trainers, the values wheel (Schwartz, 2017) is a useful introductory exercise to get in touch with core personal values. It can be used as a springboard for trainees to reflect on how their values are playing out in their therapeutic experiences and dilemmas. We also recognize that engaging with values is an evolving process, one that is not easy. Aponte (1985) suggested that this delicate work of negotiating and working with emergent value conflicts could be done in a small-group format, where case vignettes and role-plays provide trainees with the language and confidence to address values as they emerge in therapy.

While generic training related to value clarification and the recognition and resolution of value conflicts is important, we recommend a deliberate focus on specific sensitive areas such as religion, sexuality and sociopolitical values. In our experience as supervisors, trainees tend to struggle when they encounter clients whose choices and behaviours collide with their own strongly held values about sexuality and sexual behaviours. For instance, research indicates that some therapists may see open relationship formats such as polyamory or consensual nonmonogamy as pathological, view their clients negatively and persuade them to change their choices (Grunt-Mejer & Łyś, 2022). There are added complexities in couple and family therapy contexts, with the individual values of each person to consider alongside family values. As therapists, we may align more easily with the spouse who shares our values of how marriage/family should be (e.g., concerning child rearing or gender roles), leaving the other spouse feeling alienated or unheard. The alignment could manifest in giving the favoured spouse more airtime or prioritizing their concerns over those of their partner. This bias can impact how the problem is formulated, how solutions are arrived at and the order in which they are addressed. Ultimately, it affects how therapists hold space for everyone present in the therapy room.

The political elements of our work are rarely discussed or even acknowledged in training programmes, leaving therapists feeling unsupported and unprepared to address sociopolitical values in the therapy room. The way these issues are introduced and discussed during training can set the stage for the ways in which we will approach them through the course of our careers as therapists. Active debates on the sociopolitical and value-based underpinnings of psychological theory and intervention goals and methods can help trainees learn to be critically reflective.

Training to Negotiate Value Differences in Supervisory Spaces

Supervision offers a space to speak about our dilemmas about values and values conflicts and supervisors are expected to respond to these complex situations often without enough guidance or training. We recommend that supervisors begin with an intentional reflection on their own values and the ways in which they enter the supervisory space (e.g., "While listening to my young female supervisee discuss her reaction to a client's angry email, I became aware of my heightened sensitivity to power dynamics, especially concerning gender"). Supervision training programmes that include experiential exercises such as role-plays and case vignettes can help supervisors imagine how to initiate and deepen value-based discussions with their supervisees and respond to emerging value conflicts between supervisee and client.

Value conflicts can also arise between supervisor and supervisee, and it can be challenging for the supervisor to balance the needs for supervisee development and client welfare in addition to their own emotional reactions. Veach et al., (2012, p. 225) drew attention to value conflicts between supervisees and supervisors as low frequency but certainly high impact events, many of which centred on cultural, religious and sexual issues. The supervisor begins by normalizing differing values and related emotions and then invites the supervisee to explore and reflect on their values and their impact (Dunn et al., 2017). Supervisors are advised to be mindful of the power differential and refrain from pushing for discussions around supervisee values. If a supervisee's actions seem to be impairing their functioning and could result in potential unethical practices or direct harm to the client, it is imperative for the supervisor to step in and guide the supervisee's learning.

Of course, it can also happen the other way around and the supervisee may be the one who notices and is disturbed by a value conflict with their supervisor. The power differential between the two can make it difficult for the supervisee to bring up their feelings of unrest at the conversation. Training institutions and supervisors need to make space for the possibility that the supervisee is feeling genuinely offended or confused by what they perceive as problems within the supervisor's value system. They also need to provide a pathway for redressal and open dialogue on perceived value differences. This will encourage supervisees to bring up their issues for discussion, rather than covertly judging their supervisors. When both can speak to each other with sensitivity, respect and a willingness to enter into the other's perspective, both have the opportunity to grow through this interaction.

Conclusion

As we traverse the path of self-exploration during our professional journey, our values encounter other values. If values are excluded from therapeutic discussions, the interaction can come across as inauthentic and superficial. Values need to be explored, examined, negotiated and occasionally even challenged during therapeutic interactions. Therapy is fundamentally about creating possibilities for change, even metamorphosis, and our values cannot remain isolated or static during this process. This idea is echoed in the words of the thirteenth-century Sufi mystic Rumi, "Out beyond ideas of wrongdoing and rightdoing, there is a field. I'll meet you there" (Rumi, 1997, p. 36). This metaphorical field symbolizes a realm of possibilities where individuals meet not only to share their differences but also to discover common ground. The true wisdom of therapy lies in embracing differences, fostering open dialogue and welcoming shared and shifting perspectives.

References

Aponte, H. H. (1985). The negotiation of values in therapy. *Family Process, 24*, 323–338.

Bhola, P., & Chaturvedi, S. (2017). Through a glass, darkly: Ethics of mental health practitioner-patient relationships in traditional societies. *International Journal of Culture and Mental Health, 10*, 285–297.

Bonow, J. T., & Follette, W. C. (2009). Beyond values clarification: Addressing client values in clinical behavior analysis. *The Behavior Analyst, 32*, 69–84.

Choudhuri, D. D., & Kraus, K. L. (2014). Buddhist perspectives for addressing values conflicts in counseling: Possibilities from practice. *Journal of Counseling & Development, 92*, 194–201.

Duggal, C., & Sriram, S. (2021). Confluence of therapist personal and professional values: How therapist values become signposts for therapeutic trails. *Psychological Studies, 66*, 167–180.

Dunn, R., Callahan, J. L., Farnsworth, J. K., & Watkins, E. C., Jr. (2017). A proposed framework for addressing supervisee-supervisor value conflict. *The Clinical Supervisor, 36*(2), 203–222.

Farnsworth, J. K., & Callahan, J. L. (2013). A model for addressing client–clinician value conflict. *Training and Education in Professional Psychology, 7*(3), 205–214.

Grunt-Mejer, K., & Łyś, A. (2022). They must be sick: Consensual nonmonogamy through the eyes of psychotherapists. *Sexual and Relationship Therapy, 37*(1), 58–81.

Hogan, L. R., Callahan, J. L., & Shelton, A. J. (2016). A matter of perception: Patient and therapist value differences impact working alliance and outcome. *Revista Argentina De Clínica Psicológica, 25*(1), 5–16.

Holmes, V. (1996). Values in psychotherapy. *American Journal of Psychotherapy, 50*(3), 259–273.

Jackson, A. P., Hansen, J., & Cook-Ly, J. M. (2013). Value conflicts in psychotherapy. *Issues in Religion and Psychotherapy, 35*, 6–15.

Jadaszewski, S. (2017). Ethically problematic value change as an outcome of psychotherapeutic interventions. *Ethics & Behavior, 27*(4), 297–312.

Janks, H. (2012). The importance of critical literacy. *English Teaching: Practice and Critique, 11*(1), 150–163.

Kelly, T. A., & Strupp, H. H. (1992). Patient and therapist values in psychotherapy: Perceived changes, assimilation, similarity, and outcome. *Journal of Consulting and Clinical Psychology, 60*, 34–40.

Kocet, M. M., & Herlihy, B. J. (2014). Addressing value-based conflicts within the counseling relationship: A decision-making model. *Journal of Counseling & Development, 92*, 180–186.

McCarthy, K. S., Capone, C., Davidtz, J., & Solomonov, N. (2022). The association between political climate and trainees' supervision experiences and needs. *The Clinical Supervisor, 41*(2), 107–126.

Podolskiy, D. (2012). Value learning. In N. M. Seel (Ed.), *Encyclopedia of the sciences of learning*. Springer.

Rumi. (1997). A great wagon. In *The essential Rumi* (C. Barks, J. Moyne, A. J. Arberry & R. Nicholson, Trans.). Castle Books.

Schwartz, S. H. (2017). The refined theory of basic values. In S. Roccas & L. Sagiv (Eds.), *Values and behavior: Taking a cross cultural perspective* (pp. 51–72). Springer.

Solomonov, N., & Barber, J. P. (2019). Conducting psychotherapy in the Trump era: Therapists' perspectives on political self-disclosure, the therapeutic alliance, and politics in the therapy room. *Journal of Clinical Psychology, 75*(9), 1508–1518.

Suzuki, S. (1970). *Zen mind, beginner's mind: Informal talks on Zen meditation and practice.* Weatherhill.

Tartakovsky, E. (2016). The motivational foundations of different therapeutic orientations as indicated by therapists' value preferences. *Psychotherapy Research, 26*(3), 352–364.

Tjeltveit, A. C. (1986). The ethics of value conversion in psychotherapy: Appropriate and inappropriate therapist influence on client values. *Clinical Psychology Review, 6*, 515–537.

Tjeltveit, A. C. (2021). A brief moral history of psychotherapy. In M. Trachsel, J. Gaab, N. Biller-Andorno, Ş. Tekin & J. Z. Sadler (Eds.), *The oxford handbook of psychotherapy ethics* (pp. 31–46). Oxford University Press.

Veach, P. M., Yoon, E., Miranda, C., MacFarlane, I. M., Ergun, D., & Tuicomepee, A. (2012). Clinical supervisor value conflicts: Low-frequency, but high-impact events. *The Clinical Supervisor, 31*(2), 203–227.

Williams, D. C., & Levitt, H. M. (2007). A qualitative investigation of eminent therapists' values within psychotherapy: Developing integrative principles for moment-to-moment psychotherapy practice. *Journal of Psychotherapy Integration, 17*(2), 159–184.

Chapter 7
Engaging with Diversity in the Therapy Room

One Palace, one million doors
Countless windows in between
From wherever I look
The Beloved is before me
~ Shah Abdul Latif Bhittai, 18th-century Sufi poet

This verse is the central motif of Shabnam Virmani and Vipul Rikhi's meandering journey through the white desert sands of Kutch in eastern India searching for mystic songs in remote villages (Virmani & Rikhi, 2019). The poet Shah Latif's words span both sides of the border between India and Pakistan and reflect diverse literary and spiritual influences; the Qur'an, Rumi and Nath Panthi yogis.[1] Virmani speaks of finding songs and stories from the Bhakti,[2] Sufi[2] and Baul[2] oral traditions that cross borders without visas, reflecting the intermingling of voices from different religions, languages, geographical locations and different time periods. Each tradition is unique, speaking the same truth about human experience—with different words but in a shared language. There are parallels with psychotherapy practice—where when we talk about engaging with diversity, we are actually talking about the possibility of connection. Although we may enter through different doors or look out of different windows, it is possible for shared perspectives to emerge.

Each of us is different and has different ways of being in the world. The culture we belong to makes us who we are, shapes the way we think, moulds our personal identities and gives us a sense of belongingness. This amalgamation of knowledge, beliefs, values, attitudes, meanings, experiences and practices acquired by a group of people over generations binds us together and helps us reach individual and collective

[1] A heterodox spiritual tradition from the medieval period in India, whose itinerant followers engage in practices such as yoga and meditation to connect with the divine.

[2] Various medieval Indian sects that promote spirituality, devotion and a direct relationship with God over traditional caste and religious divides. Their teaching were often spread by wandering mystics and singers, who challenged inequitable social and religious structures.

P. Bhola et al., *Reflective Practice in Psychotherapy and Counselling*,
https://doi.org/10.1007/978-981-96-9732-8_7

goals. There is an inherent multicultural fabric in the world we inhabit, and there exist *cultures within cultures*. Our cultural beliefs and practices impact beliefs about health and illness and determine the way in which we understand physical and mental health, and how we express distress and make decisions about help-seeking. The therapeutic space is often viewed as a sanctuary, somehow insulated from ideas of difference that exist in society. In reality, the outside is inside, and the therapist and client both carry their diverse personal, cultural and social values into the therapy room. Every encounter between a therapist and client is potentially a multicultural encounter, one which calls for awareness, understanding and acceptance as we navigate the differences in cultural beliefs, practices and identities. As reflective practitioners, we need to be cognizant of forces that challenge the recognition, understanding and acceptance of diversity and its impact on therapeutic processes. Psychotherapy offers an opportunity to create a voice and a space for diversity, and perhaps this is more critical in the face of trends towards othering in political and social spaces across the globe.

In this chapter, we introduce concepts of multicultural competence and intersectionality and discuss their relevance to psychotherapy practice. The chapter draws heavily on the authors' experience of practicing in the Indian context—one which is comprised of many Indias. This is used as an exemplar of contexts with complex intersections of identities based on religion, ethnicities, socio-economic strata, caste, language, literacy levels and rural–urban domiciles. Practitioner narratives and experiential exercises are used to illuminate the influences of class, caste, gender and religion on therapeutic work. Through a reflexive lens, we bring these ideas into conversations with ourselves, clients, supervisors and supervisees, with the aim of facilitating psychotherapy that is sensitive, affirmative and responsive to diversity.

Our Cultural Roots

Culture is always in the room, even when unspoken. It can be understood through visible and invisible markers; through our customs, what we eat, how we dress, how we relate to others, how we make meaning, and what we believe in, value and stand for. A person's full name—comprising their first, middle and last names—serves as a core marker of cultural identity, reflecting both their heritage and sense of belonging. The relationship individuals have with their names often becomes evident when they enter a new social environment; for example, immigrants frequently change or modify their names to better align with the culture of their new country. In numerous cultures, women are expected to change their last names upon marriage, signifying new roles and a continuity of the husband's family legacy. In some communities, a change of the first name is also expected and reinforces the commitment to traditional norms and gendered expectations surrounding marriage. As exemplified in the German fairytale of Rumpelstiltskin, names are not merely labels but are imbued with meaning, power and cultural significance.

Pause and reflect…

Take a moment to consider what might happen if you changed your name?

Would you feel like you are losing or gaining an identity you value?

Do you think others might perceive you differently?

We tend to understand the world, ourselves and others through lenses of sameness and difference and this is true for the idea of 'culture' as well. In today's world, nationalist narratives and slogans like 'unity in diversity' are promoted as unifying forces, intended to bridge cultural divides within a nation. An alternative perspective is 'diversity within diversity'—the recognition that even within a single cultural group, there exists a rich variety of subcultures, beliefs and values. For therapists, this highlights the need for multicultural competence—an understanding that goes beyond familiarity with 'other' cultural backgrounds to include a deep awareness of how culture shapes each client's unique world. In the therapy room, this calls for an adaptive, nuanced approach—one that respects the distinctions and the layered diversity within and between cultures. Ridley et al. (2021) highlighted key questions and challenges in operationalizing multicultural competence and integrating this into training and practice. Do therapists need to become cultural experts and accumulate extensive knowledge about varied cultures and acquire specialized skills to work with different cultural and ethnic groups? Or is multicultural competence more about learning how to respond to each client's unique context with curiosity and humility, and navigate differences with an open, not-knowing stance? Sedgwick (2023) reflects on whether true cultural competence requires direct and prolonged immersion and questions the feasibility of this for therapists who may only encounter a culture indirectly. Culturally competent therapists are mindful not to interpret beliefs, practices and values through the lens of the dominant culture, or view individuals from a particular cultural context as part of a homogenized collective.

The concept of culture as a dynamic, ever-evolving entity contrasts sharply with older views of cultural identity as static and homogeneous. In our globalized world, interactions between different cultures lead to hybrid or hyphenated identities—a phenomenon of in-betweenness that cultural theorist Homi Bhabha discusses in the context of colonialism (Bhabha, 1994). Our cultural identities are often formed in liminal spaces, reflecting contradictions and ambivalences. Appadurai's framework of interconnected cultural flows or scapes demonstrates how global influences continuously transform local cultures, resulting in environments where identities and values are perpetually negotiated and redefined (Appadurai, 1990). The movement of people—whether as migrants, tourists or refugees (ethnoscapes)—alongside the distribution of media and information (mediascapes), the rapid advancement of technology (technoscapes), economic forces (financescapes) and the exchange of ideas, values and ideologies across cultures (ideoscapes) collectively create new imagined worlds in the context of globalization. Migration, displacement and exile evoke a profound sense of nostalgia for what has been left behind, leading to the creation of imagined homes that exist in memory and longing (Said, 2000). This experience is often accompanied by a struggle for belonging and feelings of alienation in a new cultural landscape. This sense of otherness is poignantly illustrated by the term alien permit/visa, commonly used in immigration contexts to refer to the status granted to foreign nationals or the spouses of citizens and residents. This linguistic framing carries connotations of estrangement and non-belonging, but continues to be used across several countries, even those that are marked by cultural diversity. It is important to acknowledge the unique experiences of clients who navigate life between multiple worlds that are often situated within complex geopolitical contexts. Therapists seeking to grasp the psychological and cultural dimensions of displacement should look beyond traditional psychological literature. Insights from writings on diaspora and exile provide valuable perspectives on the emotional and identity challenges faced by individuals in these contexts.

Pause and reflect...

What are the images, feelings, smells and sounds that evoke the memory of home.

When you imagine home, what are the foods, rituals, objects, traditions and customs that come to your mind?

Reflect on a time you felt 'at home' in a new or unfamiliar place.

What can therapists do to create spaces where others feel at home, especially those from diverse backgrounds? Shared meaning and relatedness do not always emerge spontaneously, and we need to work towards developing cultural sensitivity. This work begins with deepening our awareness of our own and our clients' realities and consciously learning to value differences between cultural identities. Through reflections on which cultural groups we relate to and work with easily and which pose more of a challenge, we can sense where we feel a difference or otherness and where we feel belonging. It can also help us monitor the emergence of assumptions, biases and stereotypes that could pose an empathic roadblock within the therapeutic dyad, or when a sense of similarity blinds us to potential difference. By recognizing that identities are influenced by global dynamics and structural inequities, we can better appreciate the unique cultural contexts of our clients.

Understanding Intersectionality, Power and Privilege

When we encounter a new person, we often start by decoding aspects of their identity to understand their background, beliefs, values and potential responses to situations. An individual's social location is defined by the various groups they belong to, influenced by identities such as age, gender, religion, race, social class, caste, sexual orientation and nationality. Each social location carries its own privileges and disadvantages, which influence how one navigates the world, shaping both how others perceive us and how we view ourselves. The intersectionality prism, first introduced by black feminist scholar-activists, helps us understand how the meaning of each identity shifts in relation to other identities (Crenshaw, 1989). This perspective enables us to appreciate the complexities of multiple marginalized identities and recognize the distinct ways they can impact individuals. For example, Black women may face particular disadvantages or forms of discrimination that differ from those experienced by Black men or white women. Intersections between social locations also carry potential for unearned advantages or benefits, including easier access to resources, opportunities and societal acceptance. The invisibility of privileges often allows them to go unrecognized, leading to their perception as givens. This diminishes awareness of the constraints others face, the reasons behind their choices and the reality that such choices may not be universally available. In *Can the Subaltern Speak?*, Spivak (1988) argues that marginalized and oppressed groups—the subaltern—often lack a genuine voice within dominant power structures that have historically silenced them. More importantly, even when they articulate their experiences, their voices may not be heard, represented or considered valid. These insights resonate deeply within the field of psychotherapy, particularly in examining power dynamics, voice and representation in therapeutic contexts. Spivak also highlights how colonialism has imposed dominant Western ways of knowing, often erasing indigenous knowledge and ways of being. Psychotherapists can address Spivak's insights by reflecting on power dynamics in therapy, incorporating clients' cultural practices and systems of knowledge and creating space for their voices.

Through regular interaction with clients, therapists are uniquely positioned for intimate encounters with diverse cultures. When we are hurried and do not pause to reflect on our work, we might inadvertently impose our own cultural perspectives and expectations, failing to recognize our client's struggles with systems of power. For instance, therapeutic interventions may suggest a certain 'right' way to parent or work, without considering the meaning and value they have for clients or the resources available to them. We can begin by asking ourselves if the images displayed in the clinic include diverse representations beyond just heterosexual couples and families? Additionally, have we evaluated whether our documentation procedures could be burdensome for clients with varying literacy levels? Do we remain silent when a colleague makes a sexist remark, disparages a particular community or advocates conversion therapy? It is the responsibility of each mental health practitioner to push for equity—the ramp for wheelchair access or changes in the language on the intake form—wherever possible. The more powerful a position we hold, the greater our responsibility towards creating just and inclusive systems.

Unpacking Identity Dimensions

While several intersecting identity dimensions are critical determinants of experiences of privilege and marginalization, this discussion focuses specifically on class, caste, religion and gender, exploring how these factors influence the experience and expression of emotional distress and impact help-seeking behaviours, therapeutic processes and mental health outcomes. Therapists looking to incorporate an intersectional perspective in their work need to 'ask the other question'. Feminist scholar Maria Matsuda (1991, p. 1189) explains this approach, "When I see something that looks racist, I ask, Where is the patriarchy in this?" Ultimately, by recognizing and examining these intersecting identities, therapists can provide more nuanced and effective support to their clients.

Social Class and Inequities in Mental Healthcare

Remembering a bus ride years ago, Vahali (2015), a psychoanalyst, mused on her experience of distance between the self and the other. A girl and her brother, both with matted hair and in ragged dirty clothes, got on to a bus and began singing songs. While they sang, some passengers smiled and looked at them with affection or pity, while others were indifferent, distracted or even hostile. The singing ended and the children asked each passenger for payment. Vahali went on to describe how she gave the girl a coin and instinctively touched her thin arm to draw her close. Although there were no words, the young girl moved away forcefully from this contact, with her eyes conveying anger and repulsion. While the two children slipped out of the bus, this encounter endured in Vahali's thoughts and dreams. Reflecting on some moments in her life when she had felt insignificant and rejected, she tried to connect empathetically to the emotional state of the little girl, sensing how she must have experienced the world as an outsider. Drawing parallels with encounters in the therapy space, we realize the effort it can take to bridge the distance between us and them and engage authentically with those who exist in marginal spaces. Words may not always create a bridge to our client's experiential world; what remains unspoken can be profoundly felt by the therapist, manifesting as fears, anxieties, loneliness, anger and alienation. Even when we see ourselves as sensitive and empathetic to the realities of our clients who are economically deprived or homeless, the differences in our class locations may cast the helper in the position of the historical oppressor. We may want to be class-blind, believing in the ideal of an egalitarian relationship, but it seems inevitable that the realities of class differences will impinge on us and our therapeutic work.

Markers of social class differences are evident in the therapeutic encounter, even when not articulated or addressed in conversation. Assumptions are made about each other based on the way we dress, the brand of the cell phone we use, how we speak and where we live, study and work. We do need to remember that assumptions about each other's class location may not match self-perception, and that where we feel we belong matters, along with where we appear to belong. Class differences can be quite apparent, especially when the gap between the therapist and the client is quite large. But even when subtle, they can significantly influence the alliance, therapeutic processes, goals and outcomes.

Pause and reflect...

When you look back on your sessions, do you recollect an awareness of a class disparity between you and your client?

In what ways do you think this disparity could have influenced your interactions and the process of therapy?

Reflect on the possible reasons around your choice to leave these differences unspoken or bring them into the therapy discussions.

As therapists we can find ourselves feeling overly sympathetic or overly impatient with clients from disadvantaged backgrounds. We need to ask ourselves some difficult questions about our beliefs and attributions about poverty and economic disadvantages. Do we believe that poor people are held back from advancing because of their attitudes and abilities? How much weight do we tend to place on cycles that perpetuate poverty and disadvantage across generations? How much responsibility would we attribute to government policies and programmes aimed at job creation, minimum wages, pay equity and food security? Connecting with any biases or assumptions about individual or dispositional causes for poverty can help reduce an empathy gap that would otherwise keep us disconnected from the reality of our clients' lives. Our biases can also leave us less sensitive to the client's possible internalized beliefs and any unacknowledged resentment or helplessness that can come with the feeling that their lived experience does not resonate with accepted cultural narratives of success.

Conversations around the needs and experiences of those who are more disadvantaged are more readily found in the discourse, but feelings and assumptions about clients who are wealthier and more privileged tend to be relatively neglected. If therapists idealize these clients or experience feelings of inadequacy in their presence, they may feel overawed and hesitate to question or challenge them. This can limit therapeutic engagement and potentially constrain the outcomes of therapy. If therapists carry internalized beliefs that wealth insulates people from difficulties, this could lead to a trivialization of distress and interfere with empathic and compassionate responses in therapy (Hokemeyer, 2012). We need to be able to respect the inner lives, hopes and fears of *all* persons and recognize their capacities for resilience, empowerment and change, irrespective of their class locations. Even as we respond to this challenge and recognize that persons across all classes are unified in being human, we also need to keep in mind that denial of class differences can constrain authentic engagement and responsivity to clients' needs.

Reflections on our own early experiences with money can illuminate how these might have shaped current beliefs about the meaning and value of money in our lives and those of others. We might recall struggles with scarcity, arguments about wants versus needs, a sense of contentment and abundance or the lack of any conversations about money. These memories can evoke difficult emotions such as discomfort and guilt about our privilege or shame and resentment about experiences of financial want. We may face uncomfortable realizations about the ways in which we too maintain social inequalities and power differentials, at work and in our personal lives. These reflections can help us be more genuine and open to conversations around class and its impact.

Pause and reflect...

What do you feel is the relationship between money and well-being?

How much money is enough? Is it possible to have too much money?

Have you experienced difficulties negotiating session fees with certain clients?

As a therapist, what do you think is the scope of your responsibility towards those who have limited resources?

We recommend the use of a critical lens to interrogate the fit between traditional psychotherapy models and the needs of clients from economically disadvantaged backgrounds. Is psychotherapy as usual responsive to real-life contexts, where some of our clients have no money for bus fare or food or cannot get admitted to a hospital because they will lose their daily wages? Raguram (2016) narrated the case of a farmer experiencing depression, who encountered crop failure after a combination of delayed monsoons and pressure to use genetically modified seeds that needed more irrigation. With rising debts and pressure from the local moneylender, the farmer faced the impending loss of his land, his only source of income for the family. As a psychiatrist, he wondered if addressing negative cognitions of helplessness and hopelessness would be an adequate or appropriate intervention in this context of oppression and limited opportunities. The onus of change may be put squarely on the shoulders of the individual while the locus of the difficulties is embedded in the socio-political matrix. As we work with economically marginalized or disenfranchised communities, our therapeutic frames would need to shift from insular positions and be more sensitive to structural inequities associated with mental health vulnerabilities.

We need to engage with the real-life struggles of our clients and create space for them to share their concerns and constraints around money, education or employment. Plans for change are feasible only when they incorporate an awareness of the opportunities, resources and choices currently available to the client. Else, even when clients feel respected or cared for, they can end up finding therapy less relevant. For example, an international student working nights to support herself may not have the option to quit, even if it would benefit her mental health. The therapist would need to explore other options to reduce her stress or workload. Sensitivity to these realities can help us be more tentative in our language, do more check-ins about what the clients feels about our plans and interpretations and acknowledge the limits of our understanding. An open discussion of what the client feels we don't quite get about their circumstances can reveal new layers to their concerns. These can then become legitimate targets in the therapeutic process.

We ourselves may feel overwhelmed and powerless in the face of these seemingly immutable realities and prefer to skirt around the client's feelings of helplessness or rage about their situation. Perhaps we can reimagine the role of the psychotherapist in such a situation and expand our scope to not just to help a client look within themselves, but also to look around them with more clarity. We can introduce this perspective to clients and together explore who or what really needs to change for the client to find some relief from their distress. This approach can help clients to locate their problems in the system (if that is where they belong) and also understand how they interact with this system, the beliefs they have internalized and the behaviours they allow themselves. Finally, we should note that if we believe that clients from economically disadvantaged communities do not value talking treatments, lack the emotional or intellectual resources for therapeutic work and only need material and practical solutions, we can exclude them from the therapeutic process, thereby also denying them a possible vehicle for change and support.

There are also larger questions about the organization of mental healthcare systems and delivery of responsive and equitable services to persons and communities that are economically disadvantaged. A revisioning of therapeutic frameworks could involve a flexible approach to session fees and schedules, with sliding scales for fees, more infrequent sessions or sessions held after work hours to make therapy more accessible. The development of community-based initiatives co-located with primary health services or innovative digital services, are other ways to bring treatment closer to the client's reality. In resource-poor countries with large treatment gaps and a shortage of trained mental health practitioners, it may be particularly challenging to provide psychotherapy services using traditional one-on-one models. The Friendship Bench is an innovative programme developed in Zimbabwe that trains grandmothers in brief problem-solving-based counselling for depression (*kufungisia* or thinking too much) on wooden benches situated discreetly around mental health clinics (Chibanda, 2017). Later in peer-led support groups (*Circle Kubatana Tose* or holding hands together), members build close connections and are also involved in revenue-generating activities. Such culturally contextualized task-sharing approaches have the potential to be scaled up and provide more equitable access to mental healthcare. If we wish to address structural inequalities at their roots, we need to be willing to step out of the therapy room to play an expanded role in championing policies to reduce income inequities and mitigate risk factors contributing to psychological distress. We can think about how psychotherapy fits into other systems of care like economic policies, welfare schemes or health insurance and advocate for change where required. Creating a more equitable society, with fewer class differences and a smaller income gap is a large endeavour that will require interdisciplinary cooperation as well as long-term commitment. Psychotherapists have an important role to play in this conversation as our insights into the impact of inequality and discrimination on the human psyche can be translated into action points for societal change.

Caste and Mental Health Practice

A long history of social stratification and status differentiation, based on fixed traditional occupations, has created hereditary and hierarchical caste groups across several countries in South Asia such as India, Nepal, Bangladesh, Bhutan and in the diaspora. Individuals from dominant castes have historically enjoyed numerous privileges, while those from underprivileged caste groups have faced social and economic marginalization, oppression and disadvantage (Mosse, 2018). The practice of untouchability in India, which deems contact with members of the Dalit community as polluting, manifests in various forms, such as restrictions on entry into public worship places, limited access to community spaces and resources, segregation in living arrangements, seating and eating and low rates of inter-caste marriages, along with numerous other prohibitions. Although such forms of social exclusion and discrimination have been legally abolished, caste continues to wield significant social, economic and psychological influence in both rural and urban India, often overriding other identities. This pervasive reality means that the experience of untouchability impacts everyone in India, shaping lives as survivors, challengers, beneficiaries, perpetrators, bystanders or witnesses (Navsarjan Trust & Robert F. Kennedy Center, 2010, p. 3).

A Social Psychologist Speaks: **Breaking Structures of Indifference**

Yashpal Jogdand

Solitary imprisonment is generally regarded as the ultimate punishment for humans. It is emblematic of the threat that we, as a social species, find most damaging. It effectively denies social connectedness and social support – the elements critical for a healthy body and mind. The lives of Untouchables in India – the class of people considered impure on account of being born in an untouchable caste - constituted the caste society's version of solitary imprisonment where one barely existed while facing the cruellest mental tortures and forceful, unpaid, and unrecognized labor. Manu-Smriti, the law book of Hindus, composed between the second century BCE and third century CE, elevated Brahmins to divine status and prohibited education of Untouchables while prescribing the severest punishments for any attempt to gain knowledge and wealth. Dr B R Ambedkar, thinker, lawyer, and maker of modern India, instilled a radical hope among the Untouchables and taught them to differentiate between mere survival and survival with social dignity. Inspired by Ambedkar, the Untouchable men and women began to speak of their lived experiences and formulated their perspective on society and nation. They rejected contemptible and paternalistic names such as *Harijan*,[3] *Achhut*[4] and chose to call themselves Dalits. Daya Pawar, revolutionary Dalit writer and activist, invoked the metaphor of *Kondwada* – suffocating dungeon – for the Hindu social order and asked, "Shilekhali haat hota, tari nahi phodla hambarda, Kiti janmachi kaid, kuni nirmila ha kondvada" (translation: The hand was crushed under the boulder, yet no outcry was heard, How many generations of imprisonment? Who created this suffocating dungeon?). The question asked by Pawar continues to resonate deeply within the hearts and minds of the new generations of Dalits.

In 1950, the Indian constitution made a radical move of abolishing untouchability as a part of securing the fundamental rights of citizens and paved the way for eradicating caste inequity by ensuring social, economic and political safeguards for the oppressed castes. As we complete the first quarter of the twenty-first century, instead of diminishing its influence, caste-based inequalities are also increasingly shaping social attitudes and beliefs. The entrenched disparities in education, employment, health, and land ownership among caste groups and religious communities are fueling competition and negative social attitudes and beliefs towards each other. The social sciences have put a significant effort into comprehending the persistence of caste-based social attitudes and beliefs. While fields such as sociology, anthropology and lately economics are leading the battle front, new frontiers such as the Dalit studies and the critical caste studies are expanding the epistemological and ontological limits of theorizing and researching the impact of caste on society and individuals.

Despite the obvious importance of mental aspects in shaping caste attitudes and beliefs, the psychological disciplines, including psychology, psychiatry, and psychotherapy, have maintained an indifferent stance toward the issue of caste. Indifference is undoubtedly one of the most detrimental human attitudes. Hatred may be a terrible attitude, but it at least acknowledges the existence of the target and recognizes their agency. An indifferent attitude is rooted in contempt and completely disregards the social bond. Unsurprisingly, indifference, contempt, and disgust are correlates of dehumanization and violence. The Holocaust historian Ian Kershaw wrote about how, the road to Auschwitz was built by hate but paved with indifference. Not only has the indifferent attitude led to the invisibility of Dalits in the psychological disciplines, but the discipline itself has at times collaborated or remained complicit in legitimizing caste-based inequality. Consequently, the new generations of psychologists, psychiatrists, and practitioners have limited knowledge and resources to understand and address the impact of caste based inequality. There is little reflexive awareness about how their caste identities and that of their clients and the public affect professional engagement. The psy-disciplines must do the right thing and play their part in liberating the social mind imprisoned by the caste system.

Addressing caste in the psy-disciplines is a complex task because these fields are still predominantly influenced by theories and methods rooted in Euro-American

[3] The term Harijan was used by Mahatma Gandhi and translates to children of God in Sanskrit.

[4] The term Achhut is a Hindi and Sanskrit word meaning untouchable or impure.

culture. A special issue of the journal Caste: A Global Journal of Social Exclusion, edited by me, deserves attention as it marks the first systematic and collective effort to bridge the gap between caste and psychology (Jogdand, 2024). The special issue adopts a critical perspective and emphasizes the significance of posing the right questions about caste inequity. To paraphrase Marx, the issue is not just of explaining caste inequity but of removing it. I argue that the indigenous psychologies developed in the anti-caste tradition by ancient thinkers such as Buddha, Dignaga, and Dharmakirti, as well as by modern thinkers like Dr. Ambedkar and Mahatma Phule, have laid the foundation for establishing a new field of inquiry called critical psychology of caste. The contributions of Sukhadeo Thorat, Gopal Guru, Ramaswami Mahalingam, Sushrut Jadhav and some of my own work has provided new directions for theory and research. Scholars such as G.C. Pal, Divya Dwivedi, Rahul Sambaraju, Suryodaya Sharma, Meena Sawariya, Angel Sophan, Gayatri Suresh Babu, Iram Fatima, and many others from various social backgrounds are actively contributing to the expansion of the critical psychology of caste. Furthermore, addressing caste also requires challenging psychological frameworks that medicalize oppression and pathologize marginalized communities. Psychologists, psychiatrists, and practitioners need to recognize that even under the most powerless conditions, Dalits resist their oppression. Dalits reject society's imposed definition of their identity. Instead, they construct their own self-definitions through their struggle for meaning and dignity. Therefore, being Dalit does not imply being oppressed and crushed under the weight of casteism. Instead, it signifies being awake and aspiring for individual excellence, fighting for the radical transformation of Indian society, and working towards the liberation of humanity from suffering.

Yashpal Jogdand, *PhD is faculty at the Department of Humanities and Social Sciences, Indian Institute of Technology Delhi. His research examines the issues of prejudice, stereotyping, humiliation, leadership, caste/casteism, and coping/resistance.*

Dalit individuals face unique and compounded challenges due to their caste identities and persistent structural inequalities, which can deeply affect their mental health and well-being. They often endure a double stigma, facing marginalization both due to their caste status and as perceived beneficiaries of affirmative action (Deshpande, 2019). This dual prejudice frequently results in their academic or career achievements being stereotyped, undervalued, and dismissed (Dhanaraj, 2018). Internalizing this societal gaze can foster feelings of powerlessness, eroding personal dignity and self-esteem, while also giving rise to complex emotions such as anxiety, fear, anger, and psychological fragility (Jadhav et al., 2014). In the therapeutic space, it is essential to recognize caste as a critical social determinant of mental health and actively engage with its pervasive influence. Therapists must be informed and responsive to the enduring effects of caste dynamics, creating a space that validates these lived experiences while working to dismantle oppressive power structures that perpetuate inequality and marginalization.

Therapist reflexivity is a crucial starting point for addressing caste dynamics in mental health practice. This involves a deep and ongoing process of self-introspection, particularly for therapists from dominant castes, to explore and dismantle any internalized beliefs of superiority, power, or caste prejudice they may hold. Understanding caste as a social location in mental health practice requires deep reflexivity about how caste identity operates within ourselves, our families, and the broader social spaces we inhabit—our neighborhoods, social media platforms, educational institutions, and even newspaper matrimonial columns. This reflective practice challenges the notion of being caste-blind, which often perpetuates rather than disrupts caste hierarchies. As Yashica Dutt, author of *Coming Out as Dalit*, highlights in an interview with Hampapura (2020), "But most likely, if you can afford to say, 'I'm so progressive that I don't know my caste,' then you probably are upper-caste." By confronting these realities, therapists can move beyond privilege guilt or defensiveness to actively engage in creating equitable and inclusive therapeutic environments that acknowledge caste as a critical determinant of mental health.

Sawariya's powerful writing (2021) offers a compelling framework for understanding the complexities of therapeutic encounters shaped by caste dynamics. Their work highlights three possible dyads representing caste differences: the non-Dalit psychologist and the Dalit client, the Dalit psychologist and the non-Dalit client, and the Dalit psychologist and the Dalit client. Each dyad may experience challenges with regard to relational and power dynamics, but at the same time there may be unique opportunities for meaningful engagement. It is important for the therapist to be sensitive to historical social inequities and cultivate a therapeutic environment that does not replicate social power dynamics inside the therapy room, while supporting clients in their healing journey. This work requires courage and commitment, as the hesitation or discomfort surrounding caste discussions often risks silencing dialogue. In this context, therapy becomes a space to hold and honor the range of emotions and experiences that may emerge. The Diploma in Anti-Caste Mental Health Practices, offered by the Narrative Practices India Collective and The Blue Dawn, marks a pioneering step in addressing the erasure of caste in mainstream mental health practices and curriculums. This program bridges a critical gap by foregrounding the history of resistance and the lived experiences of marginalized communities, enabling a nuanced understanding of both trauma and resilience. By incorporating anti-caste counseling techniques, it challenges dominant frameworks and reimagines mental health training and practice as a space for transformation.

Individuals marginalized by their caste identities often face numerous challenges when accessing therapy. These challenges encompass limited access to mental healthcare services due to geographical or economic constraints, discriminatory practices that restrict access to government healthcare benefits, and the poor quality of healthcare services frequently provided to them. Addressing these systemic barriers requires innovative approaches, such as community-driven initiatives. An exemplar is The Blue Dawn, a support group and facilitator of affordable and accessible mental health services for Bahujan communities (Scheduled Castes, Scheduled Tribes, Other Backward Classes, Nomadic Tribes and Decriminalized Notified Tribes across religions). The goal is to bridge clients with mental health practitioners who not only comprehend structural oppression, particularly caste-based discrimination, but also embrace an anti-caste, queer-affirming, and disability-inclusive approach. The Blue

Dawn also provides online support for individuals seeking a safe space and sponsors therapy sessions for clients unable to afford services.

Psychotherapists must critically reflect on their role in improving access to mental health services for marginalized clients while advocating for more robust community-based and state-led interventions. Although recommendations for incorporating caste sensitivities into therapeutic practice exist, these efforts often risk falling into tokenism. To avoid this, a more deliberate and nuanced approach is necessary—one that ensures the meaningful integration into professional standards and practices, fostering just and accessible mental health care.

Religion in the Therapy Room

Religion and spirituality are related concepts that share an appreciation of that which is sacred, transcendent or set apart from the ordinary. Each of us have our own relationship with religion, spirituality and God—one which is either central or peripheral to our way of being in the world. When these relationships are more central, they strongly influence our choices and actions and can become the lens through which we view the world, evaluate ourselves and make meaning from our life experiences. Some of us may be spiritual rather than religious, while others may focus more on the social and scientific rather than the sacred. Whatever our personal orientation, we all have some perspective on God and religion and the role they play or should play in human life.

In as much as religion offers us a way to make sense of life, it can also provide a language and a lens through which to express and understand emotional distress. Suffering can be understood as God's test of our faith or as being a result of karma[5] and impacts what we see as the cause as well as the correct response to life's difficulties. Not all clinicians are comfortable with a religion-based explanatory model, that potentially conflicts with a biomedical model, and our training does not always equip us to navigate this territory with ease. Clients could feel diffident about bringing in their religious-spiritual beliefs and perspectives, even when they carry tremendous personal significance. Therapists who do not easily relate to such metaphors and meanings will need to put effort into connecting with the underlying emotional experience that is being described. If therapists demonstrate that care will continue even if worldviews happen to differ, this can leave clients feeling more confident and in control to express their real beliefs.

There are several spiritual practices that promote self-soothing, self-awareness, connection with community and of course spiritual growth, along with religious

[5] In Hinduism and Buddhism, the sum of a person's actions in this and previous states of existence or previous births are viewed as deciding their fate in future existences. The current experiences of distress and illness are often explained as an outcome of previous actions.

systems that offer direct succour and treatment for mental health concerns. Frameworks like dharma,[6] the Ten Commandments[7] or Sharia[8] all suggest ways of living that can be experienced as socially and personally fulfilling. The pathways to care do not lead straight to mental health clinics and people may seek treatment with healers or spiritual gurus in dargahs,[9] temples, churches and other spaces. Kakar (1997) argues for the coexistence of shamans, mystics and doctors, advocating for an integrative approach that recognizes the value of both traditional healing practices and modern medicine. In India, formal efforts to bridge medical models of treating mental illness with religious beliefs have led to collaborations of healing systems, such as the government supported Dawa–Dua programme (Dawa = treatment; Dua = prayer/invocation), between faith-based healers and allied mental health professionals (Shields et al., 2016). By exploring ways to connect and integrate religion and mental health services as healing forces, it becomes possible to support clients without making them feel they need to choose between them.

Engaging with the religious or spiritual lives of clients can be important, but this does not mean that we open these conversations or infuse spiritual components in the therapeutic process with all our clients. When a client makes a passing or subtle reference to their beliefs or uses a religious metaphor, only some of us may feel enthused by this information and respond by enquiring more deeply. However, when a client makes frequent references to religious or spiritual ideas or speaks of the centrality of these beliefs, these are cues that the therapist definitely needs to delve further. Therapists vary in their religious/spiritual beliefs and what they feel about religion entering the therapy room. While some therapists may find a natural integration of religious faith and therapeutic work, others might not experience this alignment and may feel uncertain, uncomfortable or disconnected when addressing these topics. This discomfort should not prevent the therapist from engaging with what matters to the client, whether in terms of religious behaviours and beliefs or the concomitant needs for safety and meaning-making. In pursuing these conversations, we recommend being guided by our client's seeking and not by our own beliefs.

Entering our clients' worldviews can be achieved by asking where they draw their strength or how they find comfort in times of suffering. When religious or spiritual beliefs are important to clients, it is beneficial to explore the role of faith in their lives and how it can be integrated into their therapy plan. Clients with religious or spiritual inclinations often find solace in their faith, especially during personal crises, challenging illnesses, or end-of-life issues. A therapist's willingness to bear witness to these experiences can be valuable in itself.

---

[6] In Hinduism, is regarded as a cosmic law underlying right behaviour and social order. Following dharma leads to happiness and adharma leads to misery.

[7] A set of religious precepts and guidelines for right living sacred to Judaism and Christianity.

[8] The Muslim concept of divine guidance that helps one to live a righteous life in accordance with God's wishes.

[9] A Persian word, meaning a shrine built over the grave of a revered religious figure, often a Sufi saint.

Wisdom from religious texts can be introduced to discuss ways of being in the world, make possible reinterpretations of difficult experiences and seek meaning and comfort. For instance, teachings from the Bhagavad Gita, a central Hindu text, have been advocated for the resolution of inner conflicts through discussions on the inevitability of the birth and death cycle, the immortality of the soul and the performance of dharma (Pandurangi et al., 2014). While this approach may resonate with some clients, it requires therapists to have more than a superficial understanding of religious and spiritual concepts. Therapists who commit to a deep and critical engagement with both the words and the meanings of religious/spiritual teachings can use their knowledge with select clients in their practice.

Pause and reflect...

Reflect on an experience where you experienced a divergence in religious/spiritual beliefs or practices between you and your client.

How did you respond at that time?

Would you like to do anything different in future encounters?

As therapists, we often do not consciously acknowledge the emotional significance of our religious or spiritual beliefs until they arise in the therapy room. When clients directly inquire about our beliefs in God, prayer or specific practices, we may feel thrown off balance, especially if we perceive a divergence from our clients' perspectives. Religious values are linked to other social and political values and can evoke strong emotions when activated during therapy. Differences in religious values can be most disturbing in controversial areas such as suicide, abortion and euthanasia or when clients' life choices seem to be constrained by their religious beliefs. It can be an effortful process to refrain from questioning clients' beliefs and assumptions, particularly if they seem harmful. As therapists, we walk a fine line between respecting a client's beliefs (religious and otherwise) and avoiding potentially important areas for fear of appearing disrespectful. If a client in a very abusive marriage insists on staying in the relationship because divorce is a sin, we do need to look for ways and windows into challenging this belief. We could look for alternate perspectives, that are more psychologically affirming, from within the same religious frame. The fractures in the sociopolitical climate are evident in the manifestations of overt and covert prejudice and discrimination against persons belonging to particular religions. There has been an undeniable increase in marginalization and discrimination against certain religious communities in several parts of the world. There are prejudicial statements made about them in our homes, offices and social media feeds—these beliefs are in the air and can settle under the skin of therapists and clients alike. Our clients can come in with stories of discrimination, telling us how they hesitate to use their last name in social situations or professional circles, sharing their struggles in getting a home on rent, their experiences of online trolling and hate speech or even outright violence. It is our responsibility to recognize and respond to the intense emotions—sorrow, outrage, anger or helplessness—that are evoked within us (and the client), both within and outside the session. There is also the possibility that we become inured to these stories and do not pause enough to create a safe space for further sharing and discussions. Intentional reflection may uncover times when therapists have made assumptions about their clients, imposed their own perspectives or engaged in microaggressions themselves. Even small gestures like raising an eyebrow at a belief we find outlandish, or glossing over things clients say that do not align with our own perspective, can add to their experience of marginalization.

A Therapist Speaks: You Believe, I Believe, We Believe

Mehak Sikand

I am a woman in my late 20s who was registered as a Hindu at birth and grew up being respectful of all faiths and beliefs. As an adult, I chose not to identify with or follow any religion. During my training as a psychotherapist at a tertiary mental healthcare facility, I began working with a Muslim man in his mid-20s. He believed that a *jinn*[10] was enticing him to engage in 'sinful' behaviour (masturbation) and struggled with overwhelming guilt and distressing psychosomatic symptoms. Early in therapy, he asked, "Are you a Muslim?" None of my clients had ever asked me about my religion, but I did realize that ignoring the difference between us would not work. It felt like my one answer would determine the level of comfort and safety in our relationship and impact the entire course of therapy. Pausing to take a breath, I answered, "No." In that moment, my client smiled and looked down. Taking the conversation further, I enquired about how he was feeling at that time. His response suggested disappointment and hopelessness about my ability to ever understand the gravity of the issue he was facing. It was true - I did not know much about his belief system. However, I knew how deeply distressed my client was and wanted to understand his concerns as *he* understood them.

Our differences were not erased, but a space was created for him to share religious beliefs without quick interruptions or alternative 'psychological' or 'biological' causal frameworks (which I was more inclined to believe in). My readings about Islam and jinns helped me connect more deeply with his experiences of guilt and fear of punishment from these diabolical creatures. This helped me find a language to speak about this in sessions. Gradually, the space expanded to incorporate *both* our models, and we were able to delineate and work on goals that could be managed by a mental health practitioner. None of my endeavours were made with the assumption that I could know all about Islam or all about my client's distress. It was merely an effort to put one block at a time while building a bridge between us.

---

[10] As per the divine scripture of Islam, jinn (also known as djinn) is one of Allah's creations. The Quran states that they were created from smokeless fire before the creation of mankind and were given choice and free will. While some of them are believers, the disbelievers or the devils are believed to misguide or punish mankind.

Dr. Mehak Sikand *is a clinical psychologist and mental health researcher and teaches at a university in India. She works within an eclectic framework and building a strong alliance is at the heart of her practice.*

The therapy room is meant to be a space that accommodates differences, but religious biases and prejudices can find their way in. An inward look at our own responses to markers of our client's religious affiliations and beliefs is critical. It can be hard to acknowledge our potential biases and harder still to challenge them, but essential work for a therapist. Engagement with religion as a social location calls for therapists to be sensitive to experiences of marginalization or oppression among clients from minority faiths. Without building this awareness and competence, we may come across as insensitive or ignorant of client realities. There can also be times when we feel hurt or triggered when clients overtly or covertly express their religious prejudices. We can allow ourselves to acknowledge these painful feelings and take them to safe supervision spaces. As we engage with religious and spiritual themes in a reflective manner, we can use the possibilities they offer more effectively in our therapeutic work.

Gender and Psychotherapy

We learn gender through social relational contexts (parents, peers, teachers, media) and through existing social structures and systems (schools, workplaces). This socialization process provides a blueprint for gender-related cognitions, attitudes and behaviours that determine the roles we adopt and impact our relationships and world views. Rules for how to 'do' gender seem to persist even in the face of sociocultural changes and continue to reinforce ideas about difference and inequality between genders. Gender-sensitive practice involves the acknowledgement of gender as a powerful determinant of client realities and a willingness to explore social determinants of mental health (Stone, 2020). Whether a client identifies as a man, woman, transperson or as non-binary, therapists can have gendered biases that blind them to a fuller understanding of their client's experience. Building an awareness of how gender impacts identity, opportunities and choices can help therapists understand themselves and clients in a more holistic and realistic manner. Therapists need to shift between looking *at* gender and looking *beyond* gender, as they seek to engage with the universal and unique experiences of the client.

Beliefs about gender can impact the understanding and interpretations of client's presentations of emotional distress. When both men and women exhibit similar emotional behaviour, this tends to be perceived as reflecting women's emotional disposition, whereas situational attributions are more likely for men (Barrett & Bliss-Moreau, 2009). This suggests that when a woman shows anger, this is attributed to her demanding personality, but when a man shows anger, we search more actively for reasons in the environment. Therapists may also be slower to recognize depression in a man, as symptoms may be masked or enacted differently from what is expected. Women are three times more likely to be diagnosed with borderline personality disorder than men, even though recent epidemiological research indicates conflicting findings about gender-specific prevalence rates (Bozzatello et al., 2024). These trends can result in significant health inequities and delays in access to mental healthcare.

Pause and reflect...

How do you feel when a man cries in a therapy session? Do you notice any discomfort or internal reactions?

When a woman client expresses anger or aggression, do you experience it as less acceptable or more unsettling than if a man did?

Does aggression from a man client feel more threatening or intimidating than from a woman client?

In what ways do you think your own gender identity shapes your emotional responses and therapeutic stance with different clients?

There can be subtle and insidious manifestations of therapists' internalized beliefs and biases in the therapy room. They can manifest in who has the opportunity to speak more, who is addressed first or whom we tend to listen to more. Do we expect that women clients will deprioritize their own needs and instead accommodate to relationship demands? Do we challenge men less, seeing them as more fragile or in need of ego protection? Are we slightly disappointed in men who do not take on traditional financial responsibilities or in women who express ambivalence about motherhood? Even seemingly benevolent beliefs about the virtue or innocence of women, or those that suggest that women need to follow more traditional roles to be well adjusted and gain male protection and affection, can be harmful (Glick & Fiske, 2001). Without critical reflection, the restrictiveness of such beliefs might be harder for us to identify in our own lives, our client's lives and in the therapy room.

The issue of interpersonal violence, a prominent risk factor for women's mental health, brings gendered beliefs into sharp focus. Women around the world experience gender-based disadvantages due to patriarchal social structures. They are encouraged to take on a subordinate role and identity, have limited access to resources like education, finance or healthcare and are discouraged from making independent decisions or even moving about on their own. As we engage with the lives and stories of our female clients, their narratives reveal a range of gendered expectations, privileges and restrictions. In the Indian context, gendered expectations of women as 'mothers, sisters and daughters', dowry[11]-related harassment and experiences of discrimination, abuse and violence, increase mental health risks and impact access to mental healthcare (Bhattacharya et al., 2019). In honour cultures (prevalent in some parts of the globe), the personal reputation and social image of an individual are to be

[11] A payment, such as property or money, paid by the bride's family to the groom or his family at the time of marriage.

protected at all costs. A man's ability to control the behaviour of the women in his family is valued, and his violence is often justified, minimized or even respected in this context. When therapists understand the social structures that perpetuate gender-based violence and limit women's choices, they will be more careful not to lay all the responsibility for change on the victim alone. Approaches that take into account the profound effects of systemic oppression are generally more effective and acceptable.

Therapists' action or inaction in challenging existing gender-power hierarchies could stem from their own unexamined or unarticulated beliefs. If therapists believe that they must be neutral, they may not critically examine their client's choices. Further, in situations like interpersonal violence, if neutrality is expressed as silence, clients can interpret this as an acceptance of the status quo. We do need to speak up and clearly acknowledge that violence is unacceptable, punishable by law and cannot be construed as an expression of love. Therapist neutrality is better expressed in encouraging the client to find their own solutions at their own pace. Anxieties about the difficult consequences of leaving the coercive situation could sway the therapist towards urging the client to 'adjust' or wait for a while. It is even more harmful when the therapist sees the woman as complicit in her victimization and works on ways for her to monitor and alter behaviours that are framed as provoking violence from the partner (Thapar-Björkert & Morgan, 2010). In some situations, the therapist might experience feelings of anger about the constrained choices of women and persuade their client to escape from or terminate their unequal and violent relationship. Intense emotions can blind therapists to the complexities of decision-making in such situations, lead them to suggest actions that the client may not be prepared for at that time, or even to act on their behalf. Working with interpersonal violence from a gender lens can really challenge us as therapists, as we balance between providing guidance and support to our clients and empowering them.

Understanding the needs, sensitivities and preferences of men clients in the therapeutic process is also important. Adherence to traditional masculine norms can deter both mental health help-seeking and the expression of emotions and vulnerabilities during therapy (Vogel & Heath, 2016). For instance, it is recommended that practitioners recognize that men clients might have fears around being seen as failures. A focus on their strengths and resources, for example, self-reliance, heroism or fatherhood can open more positive perspectives on masculinity (Seidler et al., 2018). When men find it difficult to express emotions, the therapist can first help them develop their affective vocabulary, titrating the use of emotional language based on the client's readiness. A collaborative relational and action-oriented style and the normalization and validation of discomfort or hesitation regarding therapy, can also facilitate engagement. Unpacking the dominant discourses around gender roles, masculinity, power and the ways in which they perpetuate notions of being strong, self-reliant or achieving at work can be useful in helping men identify their internalized imperatives (Stone, 2020). The online resource for men with depression, HeadsUpGuys, is an exemplar of a gender-sensitive approach that uses men-friendly messaging and male role models, builds a laddering approach to normalize help-seeking and strengthens pathways to self-management (Ogrodniczuk et al., 2018). As we reflect on how to change therapy to better fit men and boys, it is important to remember that men and women do not differ in all aspects, and of course, that all men are not the same (Liddon et al., 2019). Gendered expectations and behaviours are evolving globally, and the tough and rugged *Marlboro man* is no longer necessarily the masculine ideal. Men accessing therapy are often looking to lead more emotionally fulfilling and connected lives, suggesting that while some aspects of masculinity endure, others are being redefined.

The costs of non-conformity to binary notions of gender are high and cisgender therapists need to cultivate an awareness of the challenges and constraints encountered by people who identify as transgender and gender non-conforming (TGNC). These challenges include experiences of intolerance, discrimination and violence, all of which have cascading effects on mental health and well-being. Many of these struggles remain unseen, leaving individuals unsupported, as mental healthcare facilities are often unaffordable or perceived as exclusionary. Practitioners cannot burden their clients with the responsibility to educate them on transgender concerns and experiences. Gender-sensitive practices include staying updated with best practice guidelines for safe and affirmative approaches with transgender and gender diverse people in a range of healthcare settings (Coleman et al., 2022). There is much to learn from TGNC individuals' experiences of how gender was approached in the therapy context (Compton & Morgan, 2022). While some felt gender was like the elephant in the room, there were others who felt that the therapist overemphasized their gender identity and experiences of oppression. While there were some difficult moments when they felt devalued and put into boxes, some also recalled feeling heard by sensitive therapists who saw gender as fluid. TGNC clients really appreciated therapists who focused on developing an empathic, trusting alliance, opened respectful conversations around gender expression and identity and actively attended to issues of power.

Most therapists are women, and therapy is often regarded as a feminine pursuit. Currently, a minority in a field that is almost a poster child for the 'feminine' qualities of communication and emotional caring, men therapists can sometimes feel isolated. They may struggle to find space for their masculinity in the therapy room and their femininity outside of it. At times it may be difficult for men therapists to break through gender stereotypes to be emotionally attuned and care for their clients. Both men and women clients can be more comfortable with a woman therapist, seeing her as more understanding and less challenging. Whatever our gender, we can explore the client's comfort with expressing their intimacy and dependency needs and enquire into their preference for a therapist from the same or different gender and their reasons why. This can bring gendered beliefs to the fore and enable us to address them in therapy.

As therapists, it's essential to remain aware of how we process and communicate gender, staying fluid and responsive with women, men and non-binary individuals in our therapy rooms. How we 'speak' gender is less about being politically correct—though it can be a political act—and more about recognizing that our language shapes perception, either accentuating or narrowing the gender-power gap. Learning to use gender-inclusive language and appropriate pronouns shows respect for clients' realities. At times, however, gender-neutral language can obscure essential gender-related issues, making it necessary to bring gender more visibly into our discourse.

This process also involves unlearning, such as moving away from diagnostic labels like 'gender identity disorder' and questioning how dominant biomedical models may pathologize women's lives and suffering. Even one word can convey gendered expectations. For instance, whether we refer to a woman's relationship status as single or unmarried reflects how we view women—either as complete in their own right or as waiting for marriage to fulfil them. Similarly, the shift to using gender-based violence to include violence against men and gender non-conforming individuals recognizes that women are not the only victims of patriarchy, particularly in contexts where the violence is related to gender identity or presentation. Gender-sensitive approaches that recognize and address the specific needs, roles and experiences of different genders have evolved into gender-transformative approaches that use a critical reflective lens to address the structural roots of gender inequity. These initiatives mobilize collective action among boys, girls, women and men to redistribute power and effect deep changes in gender-related norms and dynamics within individuals, social structures, policies and systems.

A Therapist Speaks: Reshaping Conversations about Women's Lives

Prabha S. Chandra

Roxane Gay, a feminist author, wrote, "There is anxiety in being yourself, though. There is the haunting question of 'What if?', always lingering. What if who I am will never be enough?" These lines just about sum my professional life. As a woman psychiatrist in a male-dominated specialty in India, I do not think I had any doubt that women's voices needed to be heard in the mental health space. Yet after 30 years, I still think it is not enough. My role as a mother and woman has always defined me in my work, and I have remained authentic, sometimes at a cost. Talking to trainees about the inter- section of gender, caste and other inequalities and encouraging them (especially the men among them) to think contextually about what a mental illness actually means to a woman is an interesting journey. I have seen them gradually emerging out of their metaphorical strong cloaks to actually revealing stories about their mothers, sisters and girlfriends, and being vulnerable about their own helplessness when they felt they couldn't do much.

Motherhood has been the most challenging and rewarding experience for me as it probably is for so many of us. My strong connections to my body when I was pregnant with my daughter and then later to see her grow—part of me yet not entirely—has been a magical journey. It was early in my residency that I realized that the experience of motherhood was different for most women I saw in the hospital. I heard stories of early marriages, unwanted pregnancies and being torn away from everything that was familiar and supportive, and then having to care for your baby, when all you needed was someone to care for you.

With my team, I started the first perinatal mental health service and mother–baby psychiatric unit in Asia, where the mother–infant dyad is provided holistic and multidisciplinary care at a vulnerable time in their lives. Training psychiatrists, obstetricians, ANMs[12] and ASHAs[13] in gender-sensitive care and maternal mental health have been a critical part of the process. It was not enough to provide a hospital bed or antipsychotics, the healing process required so much more. One had to dig deep into the women's confused conversations and into oneself to have the patience to unravel their lives.

Long conversations on patriarchy and the power imbalance have, I think, yielded some sensitivity among trainees (men and women alike). I often worry that I get too agitated when sweeping statements are made about women's sexuality, their 'mad and emotional' behaviour or their responsibility to keep themselves safe in an unsafe world. I vacillate between the personal, political and medical, to try and get it all together into a coherent gestalt—sometimes failing, but often succeeding.

Dr. Prabha S. Chandra, *Senior Professor of Psychiatry at NIMHANS, Bengaluru, is an advocate for women's mental health, and a researcher on gender and mental health. As a teacher and clinician, she tries to ensure that recognition of social and gender determinants form part of all her work.*

Mapping Across the Intersections: Using the Wheel of Power and Powerlessness

Our privileged and marginalized identities are interlocked and continually shape our lives and therapeutic interactions, strategies and goals. The Wheel of Power/ Privilege presents a nuanced framework to understand privilege, marginalization and intersectionality (Duckworth, 2020). The wheel depicts different identity markers as separate slices of a pie. Within each slice some groups are closer to the power centre and others are at the margins. The combination of all identity markers together presents the unique social location of the person. Some social identities, such as relationship status, can change over time. Other identities like religion or ethnicity come into sharper focus based on the changing context, such as when an individual immigrates to another country. Reflecting on a visual representation of one's place in the world can be a powerful experience indeed.

The adapted Indian Wheel of Power and Powerlessness presents a way to map social positions of people living in an Indian context (The Listeners Collective, 2022). Social locations can carry varied meanings and salience across geographies and cultures, and contextualizing the power wheel in this manner keeps it relevant to where it is being used (Fig. 7.1).

---

[12] An Auxiliary Nurse Midwife (ANM) is a female health worker in India's National Rural Health Mission, who is based at a health sub-centre or primary health centre.

[13] ASHAs (Accredited Social Health Activists) are an all-female cadre of community health workers in India's National Rural Health Mission.

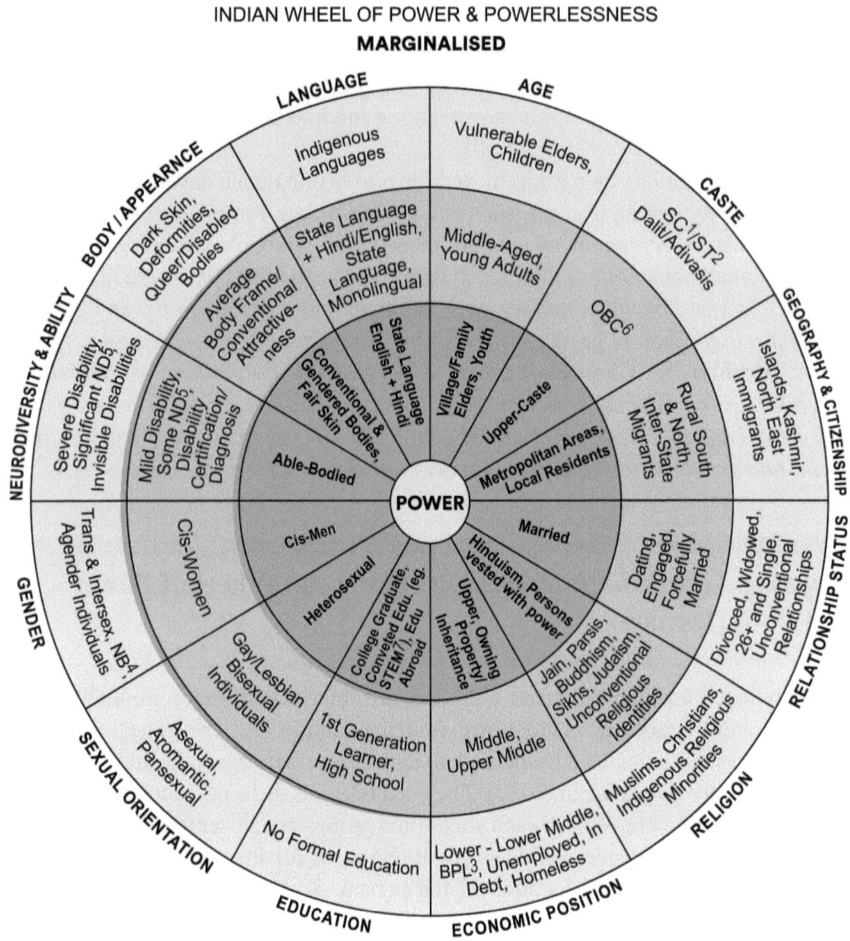

Fig. 7.1 The Indian wheel of power and powerlessness. The Listeners Collective (2022, July 30). Adapted from Sylvia Duckworth, Canadian Council for Refugees, and Olena Hankivsky, PhD. https://thelistenerscollective.org/

Expansion of terms: SC[1]- scheduled caste; ST[2]- scheduled tribe; BPL[3]- below poverty line; NB[4]- non-binary; ND[5]- neurodivergent; OBC[6]- other backward castes; STEM[7]- science, technology, engineering and mathematics.

The Listeners Collective provides guidance on how to read the power wheel.

- The centre of the wheel represents POWER and the closer you are to this centre, the more power you experience. As you move towards the margins of the circle, you move away from power/ privilege and towards marginalization.
- Your individual experience of powerlessness is intersectional; you can experience more power in one area and less power in another.

- Context and culture can impact the power structure of each factor.
- There is subjectivity in experience and this wheel cannot encapsulate the entirety of human experiences.

The Power Wheel can be used as a reflective tool for trainees and practitioners to unpack their own unique social location, bringing awareness of both privilege and experiences of being on the margins. While some may belong to many privileged groups, for instance, being educated and heterosexual and married, others may experience disadvantages across the various domains of their lives. Participants in workshops and reflective teaching sessions often share that they have never intentionally mapped or thought of their identities in this way before. Some identities such as age and gender tend to be discussed more easily within these groups, while conversations about others like skin colour or caste emerge more gradually. We recommend the use of a range of reflective prompts to stimulate and structure deeper explorations: Which identities do you think about most often? Which ones rarely cross your mind or seem difficult to speak about? Which of your identities would you like to learn more about? Which identities have the strongest effect on how you perceive yourself and which ones impact how others perceive you? Identifying our social location and the matrix of power and marginalization it represents, can help us see ourselves and our clients in a more nuanced manner.

The Wheel can also be brought into therapy sessions to facilitate an exploration of the intersections of our clients' identity markers and understand their world. Some client identity markers are more evident or might have been brought into therapeutic conversations, while others may not be known to us or thought about deeply. Clients may bring up experiences related to their social locations, perhaps hoping/wishing that their realities are heard and understood by their therapist. The therapy room needs to be a space where such articulations are not just possible but also invited by the therapist. These conversations can create an opening for clients to process the ways in which oppression (and resilience) impacts their lives and strengthen skills to recognize and respond to inequitable social structures. We need to be mindful not to use the language of intersectionality to make assumptions about clients' inner lives or outer realities based on their position at the nexus of intersections, or box them into a place of perpetual vulnerability.

Pause and reflect...

Think of the last client you met in a therapy session. Using a *Power Wheel* or similar framework, map your own and your client's relative social locations—consider factors such as race, caste, class, gender, age, ability, education, religion and more.

Reflect on the pattern of similarities and differences in your relative social locations.

Where do you hold more power or privilege?

Where might your client have access, experience or knowledge you do not?

In what ways might these similarities and differences influence the use of language, the therapeutic approach or the interactions in the therapy room?

An assessment of social locations is recommended for all clients, not just those from marginalized or minority groups. This sets the stage for becoming aware of any stereotypes, biases, or assumptions linked to each intersection, allowing therapists to be as sensitive to privilege as they are to marginalization. By understanding the role that social location plays in a client's narrative, therapists can better determine when to introduce and explore related discussions and how to develop integrated case conceptualizations and responsive interventions. Proctor (2022) notes that conflicts can arise between different social locations, such as the tension between queer identities and the heterosexism present in certain religious doctrines. Navigating and reconciling these complex intersecting conflicts may require an exploration of internalized beliefs about one's identity, as well as the societal expectations that shape these struggles. Therapists should also consider how clients may make assumptions based on the therapists' visible identity markers. It is important for them to reflect on these dynamics, and determine if, when and how to incorporate discussions about their own identities into the therapeutic conversation. Finally, using the power wheel can also sharpen the awareness of the implicit and explicit power dynamics—both within the therapy room and in how these dynamics are mirrored in the client's life. The Power Wheel holds significant potential for the therapeutic process as a tool for exploring inner and outer worlds and as a catalyst for change.

Perspectives on Training and Development

Interrogating Psychotherapy Models

Training institutes should periodically update their psychotherapy curricula to include sociocultural processes that influence the development and expression of psychopathology. Currently, factors such as political and social instability, war, conflict, displacement, economic disparities, urbanization and climate change are among the complex realities that significantly impact mental health. Trainers should also interrogate existing psychotherapy models to identify and examine those that have integrated intersectionality-informed frameworks. By foregrounding these therapies, trainers can play a crucial role in developing socially and culturally responsive formulations and interventions in psychotherapy training programs. Trainers can identify and forefront therapies that have integrated intersectionality informed frameworks. These can be used to build socially and culturally responsive formulations and interventions, so clients do not feel that both the problem and the solution are located within themselves. The recent integration of an intersectional lens into Time-Limited Dynamic Therapy (TLDP) represents an expansion from the traditional focus on individual psychological processes and dynamics within the therapeutic relationship (Farber & Motley, 2023). This shift aligns with a broader trend in psychotherapy that increasingly acknowledges the importance of social identities and systemic issues in shaping mental health.

Another critical question centres around whether and how therapies developed in Western contexts can be transplanted or translated to Eastern cultural settings. This inquiry goes beyond mere cultural adaptations, as it raises essential issues related to racism, colonialism and both historical and contemporary processes of marginalization. When we engage with these topics, we are compelled to examine how we, along with our professions, are implicated in perpetuating these dynamics. Decolonizing perspectives challenge Western and Euro-centric diagnostic and treatment frameworks that often neglect, invisibilize and pathologize the experiences of marginalized communities (Mills, 2014). This movement seeks to reclaim the knowledge, wisdom and healing practices of indigenous communities. This shift represents a broader movement towards collective healing, acknowledging the need for therapeutic approaches that honour cultural heritage and foster community resilience. Decolonizing perspectives can be integrated into the training curriculum in a meaningful way, moving beyond superficial adjustments like occasional lectures or an expansion of the reading list (Phiri et al, 2023). The toolkit developed by the University of London's Decolonising SOAS Working Groups (University of London, 2018) serves as a valuable resource for educators seeking to challenge traditional paradigms and create more inclusive learning environments. It describes ways to question and expand both content and pedagogies and invites reflections on which forms of knowledge are valued and who might be represented as an 'other'. Additionally, it emphasizes the inclusion of non-English resources, attention to the classroom environment and student engagement dynamics, more inclusive assessment methods and the development of a liberation-oriented educational framework. Although these initiatives are significant, it is crucial to also engage with the experiences and impacts of colonial histories from the perspective of the colonized (Phiri et al., 2023).

Methodologies for Diversity-Informed Training in Psychotherapy

Training programs can intentionally incorporate reflective and experiential methodologies to help trainees engage with questions around both therapist and client positionality. Through experiential exercises and personal reflective work, therapists-in-training can explore their own social identities and examine the assumptions and biases they may have internalized as members of specific social groups. Granular attention to the effective integration of diverse perspectives into decisions about the selection and timing of therapeutic techniques and goals, along with careful consideration of relational and power dynamics in therapy, is essential. During training, both trainees and teachers may inhibit open and honest discussions about their actual experiences and uncertainties, ultimately leaving less space for the grey. Establishing a safe environment where doubts can be voiced, and candid conversations can occur, is vital for authentic learning and critical reflection.

Shifting from a micro view of inside the room power dynamics, trainees can explore meta-perspectives of different power structures and systems and the ways in which they impinge on how therapy is understood and experienced. Ideas about how we should live, love, work, who is considered productive and who deserves to be heard are powerful and often oppressive, limiting the possibilities for both clients and therapists. In the process of mapping the different social, political and economic systems in which therapeutic practice and training is embedded, it becomes possible to identify the discourses, biases and assumptions associated with each.

Striving for cultural competence can at times devolve into a skill-driven endeavour, placing pressure on trainees and practitioners to demonstrate specific competencies as measurable outcomes. This idea of having the skill to be effective with those who may be different from us only furthers the notion of a singular way of knowing, perpetuating a top-down approach to determining what is necessary to understand the world and the lived experiences of others. In contrast, the concept of cultural humility, which emphasizes self-reflection and critical reflection and an openness to ongoing learning, offers a more ethical framework that is increasingly being advocated (Zhang et al., 2022).

Strengthening Equity in Access to Mental Healthcare Services

It is crucial to shift the focus from solely what occurs within therapy rooms to how individuals can access these services, particularly in low-resource contexts. This involves delivering care directly within communities and integrating mental health support into public health frameworks. Each training institute could benefit from a dedicated community development programme with mental health initiatives co-developed along with community health workers, traditional healers and local organization. Exposure to real-world challenges and a deep understanding of the pathways and barriers to care can enable trainees to navigate the complexities of designing equitable service delivery models at the grassroots level. Telehealth and digital mental health interventions, while promising, must be balanced with equitable access considerations, as many individuals may lack internet access or digital literacy. For instance, in regions with limited resources, task-sharing models where trained lay health workers deliver mental health interventions, have shown promise in broadening access and improving outcomes. This approach not only increases workforce diversity but also ensures that services are delivered in culturally and contextually relevant ways (Patel, 2022). Such initiatives are often developed though research funding and the real challenge is how to take them to scale while keeping equity, access and sustainability at the centre. To address this, we need robust research and clinical audits to evaluate the scope, quality and impact of low-intensity interventions provided by non-specialist workers. While expanding the workforce is essential to improving care access, it is equally important to establish systems that assess capacity and readiness for mental health tasks, foster competency, provide ongoing accessible training and ensure supportive supervision.

Building Competencies for Allyship and Advocacy

Therapists who choose to become allies commit to supporting clients facing oppression by actively leveraging their privileges to advocate for change. This role extends beyond traditional therapy and includes social actions such as raising public awareness, educating peers and creating access to supportive resources like safe spaces and job opportunities. Effective allyship requires self-reflection on one's own privileges and biases to ensure that these actions are meaningful and not merely performative or rooted in rescue fantasies.

Advocating within the therapeutic space involves identifying clients' strengths, understanding how issues of oppression impact their well-being and growth and equipping them with skills for self-advocacy. To do this effectively, therapists need a range of cognitive, interpersonal and professional competencies including contextual knowledge about laws and government policies. In training programs, internships with non-profits and immersive outreach experiences with community organizations can significantly help trainees explore ways to contribute to social justice. These opportunities not only aid in selecting relevant research topics but also enhance their understanding of real-world issues affecting diverse communities.

Conclusion

Diversity in the therapy room, community and the world is an undeniable aspect of life. As therapists, our willingness to immerse ourselves in and critically reflect on the structures underlying the society can open new doors in the minds of our clients as well. Conversely, our silence can in itself perpetuate and support existing disparities. When we engage openly and honestly with issues of diversity, it is no longer a threat but an opportunity for growth. It is through meeting the 'other' that we can truly meet ourselves.

References

Appadurai, A. (1990). Disjuncture and difference in the global cultural economy. *Public Culture, 2*(2), 1–24.

Barrett, L. F., & Bliss-Moreau, E. (2009). She's emotional. He's having a bad day: Attributional explanations for emotion stereotypes. *Emotion, 9*(5), 649–658.

Bhabha, H. (1994). *The location of culture*. Routledge.

Bhattacharya, A., Camacho, D., Kimberley, L., & Lukens, E. P. (2019). Women's experiences and perceptions of depression in India: A metaethnography. *Qualitative Health Research, 29*(1), 80–95.

Bozzatello, P., Blua, C., Brandellero, D., Baldassarri, L., Brasso, C., Rocca, P., & Bellino, S. (2024). Gender differences in borderline personality disorder: A narrative review. *Frontiers in Psychiatry, 15*, 1320546. https://doi.org/10.3389/fpsyt.2024.1320546

Chibanda, D. (2017). Reducing the treatment gap for mental, neurological and substance use disorders in Africa: Lessons from the Friendship Bench in Zimbabwe. *Epidemiology and Psychiatric Sciences, 26*(4), 342–347.

Coleman, E., Radix, A. E., Bouman, W. P., Brown, G. R., de Vries, A. L. C., Deutsch, M. B., Ettner, R., Fraser, L., Goodman, M., Green, J., Hancock, A. B., Johnson, T. W., Karasic, D. H., Knudson, G. A., Leibowitz, S. F., Meyer-Bahlburg, H. F. L., Monstrey, S. J., Motmans, J., Nahata, L., Nieder, T. O., … Arcelus, J. (2022). Standards of care for the health of transgender and gender diverse people, version 8. *International Journal of Transgender Health, 23*(Suppl 1), S1–S259. https://doi.org/10.1080/26895269.2022.2100644

Compton, E., & Morgan, G. (2022). The experiences of psychological therapy amongst people who identify as transgender or gender non-conforming: A systematic review of qualitative research. *Journal of Feminist Family Therapy, 34*(3–4), 225–248.

Crenshaw, K. (1989). Demarginalizing the intersection of race and sex: A black feminist critique of antidiscrimination doctrine, feminist theory and antiracist politics. *University of Chicago Legal Forum, 1*, 139–167.

Deshpande, A. (2019). Double jeopardy? Stigma of identity and affirmative action. *The Review of Black Political Economy, 46*(1), 38–64.

Dhanaraj, C. T. (2018). *I'm a Dalit woman, and my mental health matters*. Retrieved March 29, 2021, from https://medium.com/skin-stories/im-a-dalit-woman-and-my-mental-health-matters-4001055e4a2

Duckworth, S. (2020). *Wheel of power/privilege [Infographic]. Flickr.* https://flic.kr/p/2jWxeGG.*CC BY-NC-ND 2.0.*

Farber, E. W., & Motley, V. J. (2023). Integrating intersectionality into time-limited dynamic psychotherapy. *Journal of Contemporary Psychotherapy, 53*, 325–331.

Glick, P., & Fiske, S. T. (2001). An ambivalent alliance Hostile and benevolent sexism as complementary justifications for gender inequality. *American Psychologist, 56*(2), 109–118.

Hampapura, V. (2020). *Does upper caste society acknowledge the private reservations it has had for years?* Scroll.in Retrieved from https://scroll.in/article/951818/does-upper-caste-society-acknowledge-the-private-reservations-it-has-had-for-years-yashica-dutt

Hokemeyer, P. L. (2012). Treating wealthy patients and their families: A guide for competent psychotherapeutic care. *The Journal of Wealth Management, 15*(1), 9–11.

Jadhav, S., Davar, B., & Jain, S., & Shinde, S. (2014). *Caste, stigma and mental well-being: From transition to conversion.* Conference on the politics of diversity: pluralism, multiculturalism and mental health. McGill University, Canada. Retrieved from https://www.researchgate.net/publication/262932092_Caste_Stigma_and_Mental_Well-being_from_transition_to_conversion

Jogdand, Y. (2024). Laying the ground for a critical psychology of caste. *Caste: A Global Journal on Social Exclusion, 5*(2), 49–72.

Kakar, S. (1997). *Shamans, mystics, and doctors: A psychological inquiry into India and its healing traditions.* Oxford University Press.

Liddon, L., Kingerlee, R., Seager, M., & Barry, J. A. (2019). What are the factors that make a male-friendly therapy? In J. Barry, R. Kingerlee, M. Seager, & L. Sullivan (Eds.), *The Palgrave handbook of male psychology and mental health.* Palgrave Macmillan.

Matsuda, M. (1991). Beside my sister, facing the enemy: Legal theory out of coalition. *Stanford Law Review, 43*(6), 1183–1192.

Mills, C. (2014). *Decolonizing global mental health: The psychiatrisation of the majority world.* Routledge.

Mosse, D. (2018). Caste and development: Contemporary perspectives on a structure of discrimination and advantage. *World Development, 110*, 422–436.

Navsarjan Trust & Robert F. Kennedy Center (2010). *Understanding untouchability: A comprehensive study of practices and conditions in 1,589 villages.* http://navsarjan.org/Documents/Untouchability_Report_FINAL_Complete.pdf

Ogrodniczuk, J., Oliffe, J., & Beharry, J. (2018). HeadsUpGuys: Canadian online resource for men with depression. *Canadian Family Physician, 64*(2), 93–94.

Pandurangi, A. K., Shenoy, S., & Keshavan, M. S. (2014). Psychotherapy in the Bhagavad Gita, the Hindu scriptural text. *American Journal of Psychiatry, 171*(8), 827–828.

Patel, V. (2022). Scale up task-sharing of psychological therapies. *The Lancet, 399*(10322), 343–345.

Phiri, P., Sajid, S., & Delanerolle, G. (2023). Decolonising the psychology curriculum: A perspective. *Frontiers in Psychology, 14*, 1193241. https://doi.org/10.3389/fpsyg.2023.1193241

Proctor, G. (2022). Diversity in counselling & psychotherapy. *European Journal of Psychotherapy & Counselling, 25*(1–2), 198–209.

Raguram, R. (2016). Ethics in therapeutic practice: Culturally universal and valid? In P. Bhola & A. Raguram (Eds.), *Ethical issues in counselling and psychotherapy practice: Walking the line* (pp. 187–197). Springer.

Ridley, C. R., Mollen, D., Console, K., & Yin, C. (2021). Multicultural counseling competence: A construct in search of operationalization. *The Counseling Psychologist, 49*(4), 504–533. https://doi.org/10.1177/0011000020988110

Said, E. W. (2000). *Reflections on Exile and other essays.* Harvard University Press.

Sawariya, M. (2021). Caste and counselling psychology in India: Dalit perspectives in theory and practice: bluestone rising scholar honorable mention 2021. *CASTE A Global Journal on Social Exclusion, 2*(1), 189–201.

Sedgwick, J. M. (2023). Therapy and diversity—An (un) therapeutic relationship? *European Journal of Psychotherapy & Counselling, 25*, 29–52.

Seidler, Z. E., Rice, S. M., Ogrodniczuk, J. S., Oliffe, J. L., & Dhillon, H. M. (2018). Engaging men in psychological treatment: A scoping review. *American Journal of Men's Health, 12*(6), 1882–1900.

Shields, L., Chauhan, A., Bakre, R., Hamlai, M., Lynch, D., & Bunders, J. (2016). How can mental health and faith-based practitioners work together? A case study of collaborative mental health in Gujarat, India. *Transcultural Psychiatry, 53*(3), 368–391.

Spivak, G. C. (1988). Can the subaltern speak? In C. Nelson & L. Grossberg (Eds.), *Marxism and the interpretation of culture.* MacMillan.

Stone, G. (2020). Working with men: A gender-sensitive practice model. *Masculinities and Social Change, 9*(1), 28–52. https://doi.org/10.17583/MCS.2020.4277

Thapar-Björkert, S., & Morgan, K. J. (2010). "But sometimes I think … they put themselves in the situation": Exploring blame and responsibility in interpersonal violence. *Violence against Women, 16*(1), 32–59.

The Listeners Collective. (2022). The Indian Wheel of Power and Powerlessness. Adapted from Sylvia Duckworth, Canadian Council for Refugees, and Olena Hankivsky, PhD. https://thelistenerscollective.org/

University of London. (2018). Learning and teaching toolkit for programme and module convenors. https://blogs.soas.ac.uk/decolonisingsoas/learning-teaching/toolkit-for-programme-and-module-convenors/

Vahali, H. O. (2015). Could I become human by engaging with your un(der)stated life? Struggles from a psychoanalytical perspective on listening to the mentally ill poor person and the homeless poor. *Psychology and Developing Societies, 27*(2), 231–253.

Virmani, S., & Rikhi, V. (2019). *I saw myself: Journeys with Shah Abdul Latif Bhitai.* Penguin India.

Vogel, D. L., & Heath, P. J. (2016). Men, masculinities, and help-seeking patterns. In Y. J. Wong & S. R. Wester (Eds.), *APA handbooks in psychology®. APA handbook of men and masculinities* (pp. 685–707). American Psychological Association.

Zhang, H., Watkins, C. E., Jr., Hook, J. N., Hodge, A. S., Davis, C. W., Norton, J., Wilcox, M. M., Davis, D. E., DeBlaere, C., & Owen, J. (2022). Cultural humility in psychotherapy and clinical supervision: A research review. *Counselling and Psychotherapy Research, 22*(3), 548–557.

Chapter 8
Navigating Therapy Practice in the Digital World

In the film *The Sea that Thinks*, Dutch director Gert de Graaff explores our relationship with reality through the medium of optical illusions. The film uses imaginative visual techniques to illustrate how our sense of reality is shaped by our perceptions rather than objective external truths. It is in the melding of our internal and external worlds that we make meaning of life. Extending this notion, we posit that our interactions with the digital world both mirror and reshape reality, creating experiences that feel real even as we remain aware that they are mediated by screens and algorithms.

Increasingly, the virtual world is being experienced as inseparable from the real world. It *is* the world in which we live, relate and experience ourselves and others. From relationships and identity to shopping, entertainment and even healthcare, digital spaces influence so many aspects of our lives. Many clients, and therapists, have grown up as digital natives, immersed in online interactions that influence their sense of self, emotional well-being and social connections. While some engage with these spaces in deeply meaningful ways, others find themselves caught in patterns of compulsive use, constantly responding to the beeps, buzzes and notifications that permeate not just their daily lives but even therapy rooms. As therapists, we cannot treat the digital world as a separate force operating outside our work. To truly understand our clients, we must engage with their experiences in digital spaces.

As much as we recognize the value of online connection, we also need to be cognizant of potential pitfalls. In particular, the impact of social media on mental health has become an urgent concern—one that has now entered the realm of legal and policy debates. Growing lawsuits and public outcry have put social media platforms under scrutiny for their impact on young users' psychological well-being. In response, a few countries have begun implementing legally enforceable age restrictions on certain social media platforms and calling for age verification systems and more regulations to protect vulnerable populations (e.g., Australian Government eSafety Commissioner, 2025). As therapists, we may increasingly be called upon to navigate these complexities—not only in supporting clients struggling with social media-related distress but also in reflecting on our own positions. How do we, as

P. Bhola et al., *Reflective Practice in Psychotherapy and Counselling*,
https://doi.org/10.1007/978-981-96-9732-8_8

mental health professionals, engage with digital spaces ourselves? In what ways do we integrate an awareness of these debates about technology into our clinical work?

For therapists, this is a new playing field—one we are still learning to navigate. Our responses to the digital world vary widely, from wholehearted embrace to caution and mistrust. This ambivalence reflects a broader tension between viewing technology as a powerful tool and as a force that feels dehumanizing or beyond our control. As therapists, we must remain attuned to the tensions and synergies between humans and machines, continually reflecting on their implications for psychotherapy practice and mental healthcare.

In this chapter, we explore key dimensions of the evolving landscape of digital mental health. We begin by examining how the therapeutic alliance is negotiated in digital spaces, where technology can act as both a bridge and a barrier to connection. We also discuss how therapists can attune to the subtle nuances of online engagement and deepen their understanding of relational dynamics in virtual settings. The chapter also reflects on how digital visibility and online encounters invite a rethinking of therapeutic boundaries and ways of knowing each other, opening new dimensions in the client–therapist relationship. With the growing influence of social media figures, we examine how mental health discourse is shaped within the broader media ecology and how this, in turn, informs the expectations clients bring into therapy. Further, we explore the integration of artificial intelligence into mental health services—from chatbots to AI-driven platforms—and consider the implications of introducing such technologies into such a deeply human experience. Finally, we address emerging guidelines for telepsychotherapy, highlight the importance of clear social media policies and offer insights into ethical and responsible engagement in the digital realm.

Meeting on the Bridge: The Therapeutic Alliance in Telepsychotherapy

The traditional notion of therapists and clients sitting together in a therapy room was disrupted by the COVID-19 pandemic, which forced a massive global shift to online practice. Technology, once external to the therapy process, became a silent third presence in a shrinking therapeutic space, where fragmented representations of the therapist and client exist within small on-screen boxes. This transition raised concerns about whether therapists and clients would perceive each other as real, and whether a deep sense of connection could be fostered without physical presence. Therapists, in particular, questioned whether co-regulation—so central to therapeutic attunement—would still occur without sensory cues and the embodied presence of the attachment figure. While research suggests that a strong working alliance can indeed be formed online, therapists also reported feeling less present, more vulnerable to distractions and potentially less attuned to their clients' needs (Aafjes-Van Doorn et al., 2023). As both therapists and clients adapted, they learned to create a shared space in virtual therapy rooms, albeit with undeniable changes in the relational frame and process.

During online therapy, a therapist's responsiveness to a client's internal state is shaped not only by clinical expertise but also by the reliability of the Wi-Fi signal. Ruptures in audio and video links, pixelated emotions and frequent "Are you there?" check-ins can disrupt the flow of communication, leaving therapists and clients frustrated and exhausted. To compensate, therapists may over-rely on words to convey emotions and meaning (Kashyap et al., 2020). This pressure to fill the space with words can make it harder to allow a moment of silence to flower into a thought or a deeply shared emotional experience. The drive to stay technologically and interpersonally connected can also interfere with the free-floating reverie that helps us situate the moment within the broader arc of the client's narrative. Meanwhile, clients might also struggle to feel connected—sometimes hyper-focusing on the therapist's face or holding the screen uncomfortably close, to create an intense but overwhelming intimacy. Looking away may be perceived as distancing, with both therapist and client wondering whether the other is distracted by something or someone off screen. Even seemingly minor changes, such as silencing notifications, adjusting lighting and screen positions or optimizing audio settings, can transform a session from feeling fragmented to feeling deeply connected (Geller, 2021).

The ways in which technical disruptions are managed can significantly influence the client's experience. Whether a therapist takes responsibility for poor connectivity, maintains composure or demonstrates flexibility, each of these responses can influence the therapeutic relationship. For example, subtle differences in phrasing—such as "Your screen froze just now", "My screen froze just now" or "The screen froze just now"—each carries distinct connotations that clients may be sensitive to. While therapists can use these moments to model patience and flexibility, it is validation of the client's emotional response that is crucial. These technical breakdowns can be loaded with emotional significance for some of our clients, evoking feelings of rejection, abandonment or shifts in power dynamics. Indeed, such moments of disruption can be a gateway to exploring deeper themes related to attachment, trust and vulnerability, allowing for valuable insights into the client's emotional world.

The creation of the virtual therapy room, physically, emotionally and relationally, introduces a new layer of complexity to the therapeutic process. Some clients may struggle to find a private, uninterrupted environment for sessions, particularly in smaller homes or shared living situations. The absence of physical boundaries can lead to feelings of self-consciousness or even evoke resistance from others in the space who feel excluded from the process. These challenges are often intensified for clients with histories of violence or trauma, who may have an increased need for both physical and psychological safety in order to access or regulate their emotions during sessions. Any indication that the therapist is in a shared space or that conversations might be overheard can lead clients to question the privacy of the session and the exclusivity of the therapeutic relationship. Therapists can help reinforce the sanctity of the therapeutic space, by taking active measures such as locking doors, using visual cues, or by explicitly reassuring clients that the space is protected and confidential.

The complexity of creating a coherent therapy space increases in relational therapies, where family members or partners must decide whether to join sessions from the same device or from separate spaces. Managing dynamics, such as drawing out a reticent partner or supporting a more vulnerable one, can feel harder to navigate across a screen. During in-person sessions, therapists often use subtle shifts in gaze or body position to facilitate communication or de-escalate tension, but these tools are less accessible online, where directionality is ambiguous. Similarly, the physical arrangement of a therapy room often helps maintain neutrality and balance by ensuring everyone is equally positioned and visible. In online settings, differences in framing, lighting or device setup can cause some participants to appear more dominant or audible than others, inadvertently introducing hierarchies within the therapeutic space.

Since clients may no longer have access to the physical therapy room as a refuge, it becomes essential to co-create a sense of safety within the virtual space. Establishing a secure and consistent therapeutic environment online requires both therapist and client to engage in intentional practices. Clients may find it helpful to designate a specific therapy space at home, and small actions, such as placing a comforting object nearby, keeping water or tissues within reach or choosing a seat near a window, can contribute to a supportive setting. Assisting clients in negotiating privacy with family members or housemates also presents an opportunity to foster boundary-setting skills and affirm the value of self-care. The therapist, in turn, plays a crucial role in creating a sense of safety, consistency and privacy, mirroring the secure frame of in-person sessions. Maintaining a stable, real background can subtly convey that both therapist and client are grounded in their spaces, present and showing up as their authentic selves. While virtual backgrounds may offer visual appeal, they can feel impersonal and even distracting, particularly when parts of the person's body or surroundings distort or disappear. In contrast, a real background that conveys warmth through subtle, distinctive details can enhance the therapist's presence. One might also choose a plain, uncluttered wall as a neutral and unobtrusive alternative.

Pause and reflect...

If you practice online, how do you plan your background for sessions?

What do you think your background conveys to your clients, and how do you imagine they experience it?

Have you ever changed the location of your online sessions? How did your client respond to the change—did they mention it, seem affected or remain neutral?

Therapists are becoming more attuned to the significance of beginnings and endings in online therapy, recognizing the vital role of rituals in framing the therapeutic process. In traditional in-person settings, the act of arriving at and leaving the therapy room naturally facilitates transitions, giving clients time to mentally prepare for and process their sessions. In contrast, online therapy lacks these built-in cues, making it essential to create intentional openings and closings. As therapists, we must intentionally cultivate micro-boundaries to sustain a consistent therapeutic frame. This includes guiding how sessions open and conclude, pacing interactions in text-based therapy and signalling entry and exit from digital spaces. Even minute details, such as who initiates or ends the call, who waits for whom and who logs out first, can reflect our attunement to clients' preferences and enhance their experience of the therapeutic process. Discussing with clients how they prepare for and debrief from a session can also support the development of new personal rituals.

Online psychotherapy also offers unexpected gifts and unique ways of connecting that are not possible in traditional in-person settings. While being seen is central to therapy, there are moments when a sense of invisibility can provide solace. Some clients find it easier to open up when they do not have to meet their therapist's gaze, feeling protected from perceived scrutiny or judgement (Taylor et al., 2023). For instance, a client struggling with body image concerns may find it liberating to speak without the self-consciousness triggered by their own reflection. The option to switch off the camera can reduce inhibition, creating a space where vulnerability feels safer and disclosure more natural. We can support this by inviting open conversations about comfort with visibility, offering the flexibility to turn the camera on or off as needed and normalizing these choices as part of the therapeutic frame. At times, an online therapeutic space can even feel more intimate—free from physical distractions, where words and emotions take centre stage. The client may feel grounded in reality, yet the experience might be just unreal enough to facilitate the exploration of inner wishes and fantasies.

Pause and reflect....

Can you recall a moment in an online session when you felt a deep sense of connection or a moment of disconnect with a client?

What have your experiences in telepsychotherapy taught you about fostering a strong therapeutic alliance?

A Therapist Speaks: Finding Presence in Distance

Simran Chatha

It is remarkable how easily we overlook the familiar. Throughout my psychotherapy training and the initial three years of my professional journey, I navigated the bustling corridors of numerous hospitals, each with its own hectic outpatient department. In these settings, it was the norm to seamlessly manage three to four tasks concurrently, all while conducting sessions throughout the day. Amidst the mental juggling act, interruptions were constant: individuals seeking directions, doctors from other specialties on the lookout for something, trainees in need of assistance, or the need to relocate due to space constraints. These interruptions became a part of the daily routine, so much so that their significance went unnoticed.

However, the onset of the pandemic and the ensuing shift to remote work brought about a revelation. It was only then that I became acutely aware of the multitude of interruptions I had become accustomed to, the inherent chaos of my previous work environment, and how these factors had prevented me from being fully engaged as a therapist. I remember not having to rush for meals at home, which made me realise that I might have neglected my basic needs during those years. Unsurprisingly, the transition to working from home was a welcome change, bringing immense relief.

I found myself becoming deeply engrossed in my sessions, experiencing a new sense of fluidity. I could feel myself letting go of my own mental checklist, fully entering my clients' worlds, embracing whatever they brought, all the while attuned to how my body responds to them, and it felt exhilarating to have these moments of synchrony. Through this newfound presence, it seemed as though the distance between my clients and me lessened. I felt a profound sense of closeness with my clients, even though we were working online. I gave it a few months, and perhaps stemming from my initial cynicism toward online therapy, I decided to inquire about my clients' perspectives. Interestingly, they echoed a similar sentiment: provided they had uninterrupted privacy during our sessions, they felt more secure delving into deep emotional work from the comfort of their homes without having to worry about their surroundings or when they step out of a clinic. Many shared that they felt very seen, even through a screen. What then struck me deeply was this realization that safety within the therapeutic relationship transcends physical distance or proximity. True safety seems more anchored in the profound ability to be fully present and to meet the other person wherever they may be.

Time flew by, stretching into many months. At home, I found a haven where I could carefully orchestrate my surroundings, minimizing distractions during working hours. And on days it was unavoidable, I became acutely attuned to moments of interruption, such as awaiting a delivery or anticipating a phone call from a family member. In the serene confines of my home environment, I observed a fascinating shift: as external disturbances subsided, my internal dialogue became more pronounced, filling the silence with my own voice.

While I have felt intimately acquainted with my own helplessness, fears, and pain in the therapy room, there was little or no escape at home. The decision to start recording my sessions, while initially unclear in its motivation, whether born from a deepening awareness of my own pain or a desire to advance my training, marked a significant shift in my approach. This new practice heightened my awareness of moments when I felt overwhelmed or helpless. While reviewing these recordings, I was able to relive some of these experiences. This also provided valuable insights into understanding what I found myself doing in the therapy relationship, in moments when my vulnerabilities were triggered. Over time, I became more aware of the connections of my own history with the discomfort I felt and that helped me grow more comfortable with experiencing my own discomfort alongside my clients. Being in the familiar environment of my home played a significant role in fostering this sense of safety and willingness to embrace discomfort.

I like to think that transitioning my work online gifted me a deeper understanding of therapeutic presence and opened the door to a more profound inward journey. It feels as though I've developed a kind of muscle memory of presence and my own blocks to empathy that I can access during sessions, whether they are online or in person. Could I have reached this depth in an in-person setting? Maybe. Yet, I am certain that the online platform, with its ability to reduce distractions and simplify recording, accelerated and supported my process. This discovery felt deeply validating and enriching for me as a therapist, and I hope it benefited my clients as well. It made me feel truly seen, more authentic and better understood in my role.

Simran Chatha *is a clinical psychologist, researcher and supervisor with a deep interest in facilitating emotional change and congruence within individuals and in couple relationships. She uses Emotion Focused and Accelerated Experiential Dynamic Psychotherapy approaches in her private practice in India.*

The therapeutic relationship has always been an interplay between knowing and being known. In online therapy, this dialectic takes on new dimensions, as the digital medium enables forms of knowing that may not be accessible in traditional in-person settings. Meeting online offers therapists an intimate, immediate window into their client's world, while also introducing a subtle shift in which the therapist is also known in new ways. Clients may choose to build the relationship by inviting their therapist into their space by giving a virtual tour of their home, introducing a beloved pet, or sharing the view from their window. At times, we may see more than we typically would or even want to. Clients who are at ease in their own environments might attend sessions in nightclothes, eat a meal, or step away momentarily to answer the doorbell. This redefinition of traditional boundaries can also create powerful opportunities for intimacy and trust. One client, speaking from home, emotionally walked their therapist through the spaces where their grief had unfolded. As they moved from room to room, they narrated memories and marked the presence of a family member lost to suicide. In those moments, the home was not just a physical space, but a container for grief, memory, and connection, making the act of sharing even more powerful.

At the same time, online therapy allows clients to carefully curate what is shared. They can obscure their background, reposition their screen, or choose to conceal parts of their environment. The act of hiding carries meaning, prompting reflections about what is kept out of view and why. Is it an effort to downplay differences in class or lifestyle? A hesitation about sharing too much too soon? Or a fear of being judged for their space and, by extension, their lives? Therapists might also be left to wonder if clients are doing something else while the session is on or if there is someone else in the room overhearing the conversation.

Establishing shared agreements on session etiquette such as expectations around privacy, minimizing distractions, and maintaining presence, can provide structure while allowing for reasonable adaptations based on client needs. If a therapist experiences discomfort regarding a client's behavior in an online session, addressing it through open dialogue rather than imposing rigid rules can foster mutual understanding. Do these actions necessarily represent boundary crossings or a lack of respect? Or might they reflect a sense of comfort and trust, where clients feel safe enough to present themselves authentically? Our initial reactions, whether discomfort, curiosity, or a sense of connection, act as mirrors for our internalized beliefs about therapeutic boundaries. Rather than viewing this shift as a threat to the integrity of therapy, we might see it as an invitation to reflect more deeply. Honest engagement with questions of containment, connection, and separation in online spaces can expand the scope of therapeutic work. Perhaps the virtual space creates a shared, liminal zone. Here neither therapist nor client is entirely at home, but both inhabit a third space that lies between their private lives. In grappling with the loss of the world as it once was, we are also beginning to learn the rules and rhythms of this new game we find ourselves playing.

Knowing Me, Knowing You…

Clients and therapists alike construct digital narratives in online spaces, which may differ from, or even contrast sharply with, their offline expressions of the self. Accidental encounters can happen online—through algorithm-driven friend suggestions, tagged photos or even something as mundane as a restaurant review. Both clients and therapists, often driven by curiosity, can also find themselves tempted to explore each other's online presence. With just a few keystrokes, an entire digital footprint can unfold—professional achievements, personal interests, even wedding photos or details of past relationships. What happens when a client stumbles upon a personal blog post from their therapist discussing burnout? Or when a therapist, mid-session, struggles to ignore something they have viewed online about their client's weekend activities? The availability of this information alters the dynamic, raising critical questions: When does curiosity become an intrusion? And how does knowing or being known outside the therapy room change the work itself? Traditional notions of carefully considered self-disclosure are challenged in an era where visibility is often beyond one's control.

Beyond the practical desire to confirm a therapist's credentials or values, clients' searches can be driven by deeper, often unarticulated needs. Clients might wonder, "Do I matter to my therapist? Are they thinking about me outside of sessions?" The act of searching may reflect a desire to bring the therapist into the client's world, offering comfort that the therapist exists somewhere, even during periods of absence (Kaluzeviciute, 2020). Fantasy plays a significant role in the therapeutic relationship. Clients inevitably imagine aspects of their therapist's life that remain unseen, filling in gaps with hopes, fears and projections. Searching online can be an attempt to make these fantasies more tangible, to validate or challenge imagined narratives. The need to know their therapist better is not always about deepening or extending the therapeutic relationship. For sensitive clients, especially those with histories of abuse or marginalization, seeking to understand their therapist's values and way of relating can arise from a desire for safety. Online communication, through comments on posts, text messaging or emails, could also serve as an indirect way for clients to express emotions they struggle to voice in therapy. A client who feels shut out in session may find it easier to send a late-night email, expressing the frustration or sadness they could not articulate face-to-face. Another may subtly test the therapist's availability by liking or responding warmly to posts, hoping for some level of personal engagement in return.

Yearning for connection, frustration, envy or the wish to be seen as special are all rich, powerful emotions that rightfully belong in the therapeutic process. When such feelings are communicated outside the therapy room through emails, comments or other forms of engagement, it is important not to overlook them simply because the channel is not traditional. Instead, therapists can gently bring this material into the session, encouraging clients to express these emotions more directly, explore their meaning and work through them together. For example, "You shared something with me over email that hasn't come up in our sessions. I'd really like to understand that. What made it feel easier to express in writing?" By making space for these expressions, therapists ensure that meaningful therapeutic material is not left unexamined simply because it arrived through a less conventional route.

Pause and reflect…

Basuki sat in his office, looking at the empty chair across from him. Zahra had missed her session. No email. No message. Just silence. Even when she did come for sessions, conversations seemed incomplete with important topics sidestepped and details left unsaid.

A thought suddenly surfaced—Is she safe?

His fingers hovered over the keyboard. A quick online search might fill in some of the gaps.

Have you ever searched for a client online? If so, what were you hoping to find?

And if you have resisted the urge, what stopped you?

Many therapists acknowledge having searched for current, former or even prospective clients on the internet, motivated by concern, curiosity or a desire to feel prepared for sessions. These searches are rarely disclosed to clients or colleagues, hinting at an implicit awareness of their potential to disrupt the therapeutic alliance. Interestingly, while therapists may feel uneasy or even violated when they themselves become the targets of online searches by clients, they often minimize, justify or rationalize their own similar behaviours (Gupta et al., 2016; Trub & Magaldi, 2021).

When the impulse to search for a client online arises, it can signal an important opportunity for therapist reflection. Instead of acting on this impulse immediately, therapists might choose to pause and explore what is unfolding within themselves. The urge may stem from discomfort with not knowing, doubts about the client's capacity to reveal what matters or even a subtle desire to take ownership of the client's story by filling in the gaps. In such moments, supervision can offer a crucial holding space where these internal responses can be thoughtfully examined and understood. Feelings of protectiveness, mistrust, exclusion or vulnerability may also emerge, and attending to their origins can deepen the insight into what is being enacted within the therapeutic relationship. Reflective questions such as, "What would it mean to sit with not knowing?" or "Could this concern be explored in the session rather than managed outside it?" can help re-anchor us in our role.

What therapists encounter online can evoke a wide range of emotional and professional responses. A client who speak about financial hardship during sessions might be seen vacationing at a luxury resort on social media, prompting feelings of irritation, suspicion or confusion within the therapist. In some cases, what is discovered may raise serious clinical concerns: a cryptic post hinting at suicidality, or images suggesting undisclosed substance use. At other times, therapists may come across dimensions of a client's identity, belief systems or lived experience that have never been spoken about in the therapy room, such as impassioned political views or expressions of sexuality and gender. Even seemingly benign discoveries can disrupt the therapist's understanding of who the client is, and how much of themselves they are willing or able to bring into the space.

Even when an online search yields relevant or clarifying information, it introduces a complex ethical dilemma. The therapist is left holding knowledge that was not offered within the therapeutic frame, raising important questions about how, or whether, it should influence the work. Sharing this information may disrupt the client's sense of privacy and safety while withholding it may create a sense of dissonance within the therapist. Ethical guidelines provided by professional bodies such as the American Psychological Association (APA, 2017), the British Association for Counselling and Psychotherapy (BACP, 2018) and the UK Council for Psychotherapy (UKCP, 2019) advise against searching for client information online without explicit consent, except in situations where there is a clear concern about risk or harm. Resisting the impulse to check in on a client via social media helps preserve the foundational principle of therapy about the clients control over what and when to share. It is through the exploration of what is revealed in the therapeutic space that therapists can support clients in becoming more aware of their patterns of relating and responding. Searching for client information online offers a kind of knowing about which is an externally derived and often decontextualized picture. The real work of therapy is grounded in knowing with, a relational, unfolding understanding co-constructed in the room.

The Many Selves of the Therapist in Online Spaces

The motivations behind online sharing are layered and complex, often creating tension between overlapping, and sometimes conflicting, identities and goals. A therapist's digital presence might reflect a desire to connect, be seen, validate their expertise, share knowledge, advocate for change or build a professional brand. When using multiple platforms, therapists face additional decisions, such as whether to share the same content across all spaces or tailor it to the unique audience and norms of each. These decisions are not only strategic but also reflect personal boundaries, values and the degree of self-disclosure each therapist is comfortable with. Some therapists, of course, choose to maintain a minimal or anonymous online presence, keeping their personal and professional worlds separate. Navigating these digital spaces requires careful reflection on how to balance authenticity with professionalism, and visibility with containment (White & Hanley, 2025).

Pause and reflect...

Which aspects of your therapeutic self feel constrained, or unexpectedly liberated, when you engage online?

Have you discovered something about yourself—your needs, values, or ways of relating—through the process of creating content online?

For clients, social media offers a window into a therapist's personality, therapeutic orientation and stance on various mental health issues. This kind of transparency enables more informed decisions that are not just based on credentials, but on whether a therapist feels warm, serious, relatable or aligned with a client's worldview. In this way, the online persona becomes an extension of the therapeutic process, offering glimpses into who the therapist is beyond the clinical setting.

A User-survivor and Media Creator Speaks: Restoring Sanity to Therapy Content on Social Media

Tanmoy Goswami

I am a survivor of life-threatening mental health conditions and started speaking publicly about my experiences about a decade ago. At the time, such self-disclosure was nowhere nearly as normalised as it is today. During a particularly nasty bout of illness, I began writing an unfiltered Twitter diary of my daily struggles. This went somewhat 'viral', brought me unexpected solidarity from strangers online, and changed my life. The community also enabled me to find purpose, encouraged me to exit my mainstream journalism job where I no longer felt fulfilled, and pivot to writing full time about mental health. I chose the mental health sector's potent intersection with social media as one of my core focus areas.

The topic acquired unprecedented momentum during the pandemic, when therapists emerged as critical health care workers. I observed how the discipline, which had traditionally lacked a public profile, started boldly putting itself out there. Therapists, together with lived experience experts, took the lead in creating critical psychological education using innovative info-tainment formats on social media. In the process, they transformed the image of therapy from a little-understood, insular discipline to one right at the centre of the public discourse. However, the pandemic also commoditised mental health content. My research showed that mental health stories in the global English-language media more than doubled in this period. With this glut has come serious concerns about the quality and ethics of mental health content, including therapist-created content on social media.

To begin with, as therapy goes inexorably online and fuses with internet culture, there has been rising anxiety and competition over engagement and reach, fueled by the narrative that therapists must also turn influencers. As technology threatens jobs, there is growing restlessness among early-career therapists, with many viewing social media followings as a shortcut to quickly gain clients. The psych academia has failed to educate students on balancing therapeutic stillness with the post or perish mechanics of social media. In the absence of regulation, anyone can broadcast content and build a following with little accountability—so long as they keep up with shifting trends. Therapist communities on social media are increasingly fractured by 'my qualification or modality is better than yours' rhetoric—often gamed for outrage. Thoughtful voices, wary of these dynamics, frequently see their reach limited by platforms that appear to reward only the provocative or pseudoscientific.

Even meaningful content has its side effects. Amplifying social justice themes has been a powerful contribution of #TherapistSocialMedia. Therapists, the majority of them women, routinely risk abuse and harassment on social media by standing up for their beliefs (or simply existing). In parallel, I have heard muted conversations among practitioners, academics, and (prospective) service users questioning whether ideologically charged content, framed in the language of activism, risks losing nuance and compassion —elevating a person's politics over their patienthood. Those who do not align with therapists' strongly articulated public views could feel judged, dehumanised, and undeserving of therapy. This can cut them off from transformative care and further deepen polarisation.

In my discussions with the community, the following thorny issues repeatedly come up:

- What can go wrong when you expect your therapist to be your friend or comrade because of the illusion of accessibility and shared struggles that social media creates?
- What happens when your patient becomes your 'follower', drawn by the aura of social media celebrityhood? How does the power asymmetry between a 'famous' therapist and an 'ordinary' patient affect therapy dynamics?
- How do we foster more nuanced conversations on the intersection between therapy and activism, and balance systemic and structural critique with ideas such as recovery and healing that every individual deserves?

To be sure, we do not need simplistic answers to these questions. Technology and social media are irreversible forces, and they are capable of great good, when used with constant reflection and governed by a community-approved code of conduct. To this end, in April 2025 I hosted PostCode, a first-of-its-kind online learning forum where experts from multiple disciplines came together to co-develop a manifesto for therapists navigating social media ethics.

Here is the consensus we evolved:

- Therapists need a clear sense of *why* they are on social media. Are they primarily interested in being therapists, or is their main goal turning content creators and influencers? Creating a personal charter that answers this will help them find the right tone, cadence, and values for their content.
- Algorithms are the raw material of the modern world. Therapists must understand how they manipulate attention and recognise how content—whether consciously or unconsciously optimised to appease them—can impact both their personal standing and the perceptions of those seeking care.
- Professional training needs to address livelihood anxieties among early career therapists and re-establish the importance of growth fueled by real-world professional networks.
- We need to build sandboxes where ethically minded creators and influencers (not limited to those from psychology) can share their learnings with therapists.
- Finally, therapists need to use social media to practice their profession's most fundamental skill: listening. Therapists would do well to tap into stories about the kind of support patients and caregivers need and continuously develop skills that help them meet these needs in the clinic (or Zoom room).

At its purest, therapy is a life-saving form of communication between people desperate to be heard and experts trained in the healing use of words — and silence. Protecting the sanctity of this work from the assault of the algorithms ought to be the business of every stakeholder in the mental health movement.

Tanmoy Goswami *is the creator of Sanity, an independent mental health storytelling platform based in India. He is a fellow of the Reuters Institute at the University of Oxford and an advisor to the Centre for Global Mental Health at King's College London and the London School of Hygiene and Tropical Medicine.*

Tensions often surface in online spaces around topics such as diagnostic language, therapist self-disclosure, sociopolitical events, or professional turf wars. In the absence of tone, context, and the containment offered by the therapeutic frame, such conversations can escalate quickly. Importantly, these interactions unfold in highly visible spaces and may be witnessed by peers, members of the professional community, current and former clients, prospective clients, and the general public. Our language, tone, and manner of engagement carry added responsibility. We are not only individuals expressing personal views, but also representatives of the profession and its ethical commitments. A key discipline in navigating online conflict is the capacity to pause before engaging. This helps us discern whether a response is likely to contribute to meaningful dialogue or merely amplify noise. Grounding oneself in core therapeutic values can help transform digital tensions into opportunities for modeling respectful engagement and emotional regulation. Drawing from the Crucial Conversations framework (Patterson et al., 2022), therapists may benefit from recognizing when a conversation becomes emotionally charged and potentially conflictual. Signs such as rising emotional intensity, polarizing language, or a sense of personal defensiveness often indicate a need to pause, self-regulate, and respond with intention. A simple reflective question, "What am I hoping to achieve here?", can offer clarity and curb impulsive engagement. Language that invites dialogue rather than debate, such as "I would be curious to hear more about your view, "I see it differently based on my experiences," or "Here is how I have approached this in my work". helps sustain openness and mutual respect. Appreciating others' contributions, even when disagreeing, can also model respect. If a comment triggers strong reactions, it is important to pause and reground before responding. Not all disagreements require sustained interactions and knowing when to disengage is part of maintaining professional and relational boundaries. How we choose to respond (or not), can reflect and reinforce the values we hold as therapists.

Decentralizing Expertise: Mental Health in the Age of Influencers

While scrolling through a social media platform, a young viewer paused on a video about trauma. This was not from a therapist, but from a favourite influencer. Personal and engaging, the video offered mental health advice that felt both relatable and grounded in real insight. This seemingly ordinary moment highlights a broader shift in how mental health information is consumed online. Recognizing this trend, researchers at the Harvard T.H. Chan School of Public Health (2023, August 9) launched an innovative collaboration with some of the internet's most influential creators, some with audiences of over twenty million, to address the growing spread of mental health misinformation. Influencers and experts came together through virtual panels and a live summit, covering topics from trauma and the mind–body connection to evidence-based approaches to well-being. The goal was to amplify reliable psychological knowledge through voices people already follow and trust. In doing so, the project highlighted the power of likes, shares and personal stories as tools for credible mental health advocacy.

As therapists, we are witnessing a paradigmatic shift in which mental health discourse is increasingly decentralized, democratized and digitally mediated. Therapists are no longer the sole, or even primary, interpreters of psychological life. Influencers, content creators and individuals sharing from lived experience have become central voices in shaping how the public understands suffering and healing. Peer-led initiatives like *The BPD Bunch*, a video podcast and social media collective created by individuals with symptoms of Borderline Personality Disorder, exemplify a form of digital solidarity. They offer a model of community grounded in lived experience, mutual support and the active dismantling of stigma through storytelling and collective influence. Such opportunities to find your tribe—those who speak a familiar emotional language and offer resonance without judgement, can be profoundly validating.

This transformation raises pressing clinical and relational questions. How do we respond when clients reference influencers or bring in social media narratives? What do we do when viral content about trauma, diagnosis or healing resonates deeply with their lived experience? These shifts reflect a redistribution of epistemic authority.

Trust is now placed not only in professionals, but also in those who speak with immediacy, emotional resonance and authenticity. Rather than positioning ourselves in opposition to such content, it can be approached as a meaningful entry point. When a client cites a viral post about cutting off toxic people as self-care, we might respond with curiosity asking what the message evoked and explore how the idea might fit with their experiences in their current relationships. In doing so, we honour the emotional resonance of the material, acknowledge the significance of the client's engagement with it and invite further reflection. However, this participation raises a sobering question about the ways in which distress tends to be interpreted through a diagnostic or pathological lens. What then happens to the ordinary aches and contradictions of human life? In this new landscape, digital narratives not only shape the discourse on mental health but can also influence how therapists engage with the complexities of human experience.

Algorithm or Authenticity? Balancing Technology and Humanity in Mental Health

Mia struggles with anxiety and has been on a therapist's waitlist for weeks. To bridge the gap, her therapist recommends an AI-powered app that tracks her mood through daily journal entries and offers real-time natural language processing-driven support. Once she begins therapy, Mia brings insights from the app and her smartphone to every session—patterns of her stress levels, sleep disruptions and emotional triggers. Between sessions, when distress strikes late at night, she turns to the app's chatbot, which mirrors her therapist's voice and offers coping strategies and grounding exercises. During online sessions with her therapist, Mia asks if she can record their conversations for later reflection, just as she revisits her interactions with the chatbot.

Digital technology and AI-powered psychotherapy tools are transforming mental health practice by enhancing accessibility, improving early detection of symptoms and personalizing treatment approaches. As technology continues to influence mental healthcare, therapists are increasingly integrating it into their practice and responding to clients who bring it to sessions in various ways. One key emerging trend is the use of machine learning algorithms to predict psychotherapy outcomes and identify key predictors of success (Taubitz et al., 2022). These predictive models can help match clients with the most suitable therapeutic interventions, optimize treatment plans and identify individuals at risk of dropout or poor response, allowing for timely modifications to care. Another advancement is digital phenotyping, which captures real-time behavioural and physiological data including sleep patterns, physical mobility, social interactions, mood fluctuations and social media usage, through personal electronic devices. By analysing a person's digital footprint, researchers and clinicians can track changes in psychiatric symptoms and intervene proactively to prevent relapses (Oudin et al., 2023). With the growing use of wearables for health tracking, some clients are already sharing weekly trends with their therapists. As this technology becomes more prevalent, it raises important questions about whether therapists should receive this data directly to monitor client health and how it intersects with clinical intuition. The sheer volume of granular information can be overwhelming, and therapists might miss the forest for the trees. Additionally, the increasing reliance on big data for digital phenotyping brings significant ethical and privacy concerns, particularly regarding consent, data security and the risk of algorithmic bias.

The integration of digital phenotyping with machine learning models has the potential to refine mental health predictions and enhance AI-driven support systems, such as chatbots. A growing number of chatbots leverage Conversational AI to deliver just-in-time support for experiences of depression, anxiety and stress. By offering a private space for free-text conversations and support via messaging platforms, these systems help reduce perceived stigma and lower barriers to seeking help. The Healthy Moms initiative in Kenya is an exemplar of an AI-powered intervention used to expand access to treatment for perinatal depression in the community (Green et al., 2020). Zuri is positioned as a health coach for pregnant women and new mothers, with the tagline—'Zuri is not a person, so she can respond to you day or night. She doesn't need sleep!' While conversational agents show promise, sustaining user engagement remains a challenge, especially in maintaining long-term interest. Mental health apps are becoming more sophisticated, using interactive features and personalized responses to foster deeper user engagement. Some now leverage artificial intelligence to analyse language patterns and activity levels, detecting subtle shifts that might indicate distress. When a user withdraws or their tone changes, the app may send a gentle check-in, suggest a grounding exercise or encourage connection with a support network. This early intervention helps identify those who may need more intensive care, improving retention and therapeutic outcomes. Many platforms also include built-in escalation systems, ensuring that users in crisis are swiftly connected to a therapist, crisis hotline or emergency services when needed.

For AI-driven mental health interventions to truly make an impact, they must be built with the people they aim to support. Meaningful collaboration among mental health professionals, service users and policymakers is essential, and a co-design approach ensures that these tools are not only effective but also culturally relevant, ethical and widely accepted. A compelling example comes from Cullingham et al. (2024), who developed an AI-supported intervention for anxiety in autistic children. Rather than imposing a top-down solution, they engaged autistic young people, adults, parents, clinicians and researchers in every stage of development. This neurodiversity-affirmative approach ensured that the intervention was inclusive and attuned to the real needs of the community. The process also sparked critical discussions about power dynamics, ensuring that service users had an equal voice in decision-making. Lessons from various proof-of-concept studies underscore the value of iterative testing and user feedback in refining chatbot interventions before they scale. However, as AI-driven mental health tools gain traction, they face a pressing challenge: balancing ethical, user-centred design with the commercial interests of tech startups. True co-design, sustained engagement and responsible implementation require investment in the participatory processes that make these tools genuinely effective.

Just like Goldilocks searching for what feels just right in a strange and unfamiliar world, we are tasked with finding the optimal level of engagement and interaction in this rapidly evolving space of AI-powered psychotherapy applications. Each choice involves finding the delicate balance between harnessing technological advancements and maintaining the human connection that is essential to effective therapy. One of the central questions is around how closely AI needs to mimic human empathy, appearance and communication to create a sense of connection.

Pause and reflect...

The *Turing test* or Imitation Game is a test of a machine's ability to exhibit intelligent behaviour that is equivalent to, or cannot be distinguished from that of a human (Turing, 1950).

Do you think that Conversational AI needs to pass the Turing test? Are human-like responses and understanding essential in order to contribute meaningfully to mental healthcare?

Making virtual representations more human-like is not necessarily better. The *uncanny valley effect* first mentioned by Japanese roboticist Masahiro Mori (1970) describes the uncomfortable feeling when robots or other audio-visual representations quite closely resemble humans but are not convincingly real. To avoid this, developers must strike a delicate balance by creating systems that are human-like and personalized enough to foster rapport and make users feel understood, yet not so life-like that they create misleading expectations of emotional depth, care or reciprocity. Transference may emerge during interactions with AI-enabled therapeutic services. Users could express feelings of idealization and attribute human-like qualities to the system or conversely express disappointment or frustration which might mirror patterns from past relationships. Holohan and Fiske (2021) raise an intriguing question about the potential benefits of intentionally fostering transference in the design of AI-enabled therapy apps, encouraging users to project their emotions, experiences and relational patterns onto the AI. While AI systems respond to patterns in user interactions, such scripted and programmed responses do not allow for the delicate interplay of transference and countertransference, which allows human therapists to gain deeper insights into their clients. It is difficult to envision how AI-powered dynamic algorithms could fully replicate the nuanced processes of navigating closeness and distance in therapy sessions, the interpretation of silences and the unspoken language of embodied emotions. We wonder how AI-enabled therapeutic spaces can be designed to respond to experiences that reside in the unthought known, those that are felt, inferred or sensed rather than articulated.

Concurrently, the increased accessibility of AI-mediated support introduces complex relational dynamics. While such technologies may enhance a sense of availability and responsiveness, features like unsolicited information and frequent notifications or check-ins may come across as intrusive. With emerging technologies like digital phenotyping, designers must carefully consider when close monitoring enhances care and when it risks feeling like digital surveillance.

Pause and reflect…
Have you reviewed the privacy policies of the digital tools that you use or might recommend to clients?

What steps do you take to ensure clients understand how their data is stored, used and protected when using digital tools?

Therapeutic spaces are designed to encourage open disclosure, including discussions of controversial ideas and politically sensitive topics. However, if users are concerned about data security, could they begin to self-censor—restricting not only what they share but even what they permit themselves to think? Striking the right balance requires AI systems that are both informed and responsive while ensuring that individuals retain control over their level of engagement and the personal information they share. One valuable resource for practitioners looking to evaluate AI tools is the comprehensive guide provided by the American Psychological Association (2024) which focuses on key areas such as functionality, clinical and data security.

As AI-driven tools become an integral part of therapeutic spaces, we are faced with crucial questions about their design and inclusivity. At the heart of this debate is a key question: how do we design avatars and chatbots that truly reflect the diversity of human identity.

Pause and reflect…
Should a mental health app's avatar or chatbot be designed to mirror a user's personal identity?

If so, which aspects—race, gender, cultural background or emotional expression—should shape this personalization?

Who gets to decide what is appropriate, and on what basis?

We must also consider how well AI-driven therapy tools address the complexities of linguistic diversity, neurodivergence and varied communication styles. This goes far beyond surface-level adjustments, such as changing skin tones or facial features. The real question is: how well do these tools account for the intricate ways people express distress, communicate their needs or process emotions? Are they truly capable of capturing the full spectrum of human experience, or do they risk reducing it to predetermined algorithms? To move beyond superficial representation, we must engage in a deeper exploration of how AI systems interpret, respond to and, crucially, adapt to diverse lived experiences, cultural contexts and the ways people in which navigate their emotional landscapes.

When developers design interfaces that steer users toward specific choices, we must consider the implications of nudging them toward particular representations. For instance, an app that defaults to a light-skinned avatar or enforces binary gender categories may unintentionally exclude users who do not see themselves reflected. A chatbot designed to offer culturally sensitive mental health support can be valuable but relying on rigid scripts risks oversimplifying individual experiences. For example, the chatbot might assume that seeking spiritual guidance is a preferred coping strategy in certain communities, or that family involvement is always beneficial in collectivist cultures. In these cases, well-intentioned design choices could inadvertently alienate the very users they aim to support. Understanding user expectations, engagement patterns and experiences in virtual environments is critical to creating ethical, inclusive spaces that genuinely reflect and support the diverse tapestry of human identity.

Partnerships between mental health practitioners and technology developers and evangelists are crucial as future developments in the digital space expand the portfolio of therapeutic services. As AI tools proliferate, there are concerns that more long term, complex interventions might get left behind, along with individuals who cannot access devices or the internet. AI-enabled digital platforms typically provide low-intensity interventions, although it can be argued that this experience could be a steppingstone to more intensive interventions. Psychotherapists need not imagine this as yet another competitive race between online and offline services, where one will win and must have a prize. Our reflections today will influence the direction of technology tomorrow, allowing us to leverage digital innovations in our practices and mental healthcare systems.

A Digital Mental Health Clinician Speaks: Holding Space in the Cloud

Smriti Joshi

When I first began exploring AI-driven mental health solutions, my scepticism ran deep. With 21 years as a clinical psychologist, I valued the intimacy of face-to-face therapy—body language, subtle emotional cues, and genuine, lived empathy. The idea that an algorithm could provide meaningful emotional support seemed not just improbable, but almost absurd.

In 2016, when we started developing Wysa, our intention was - and still is - to offer permissionless, non-judgemental mental health support to scale. Yet, as a clinician accustomed to personalized interactions, I struggled deeply with the challenging task of crafting scripts for an AI chatbot. Imagine asking "How are you doing?" to a million users, each potentially giving a unique response. The challenge was to craft a single universally empathetic reply. It felt like writing a deeply personal letter addressed "To Whom It May Concern."

A turning point came when our team at Wysa received an email from a 13-year-old girl who said simply, "It was Wysa that helped me hold on to my life." Her brief but powerful message reshaped my perspective entirely. Suddenly, we were not merely building technology—we were creating lifelines. Early user interactions provided critical insights into AI's potential and limitations. AI design, especially in mental health, requires a delicate balance. It should not feign human traits like empathy or compassion, as this may mislead users into believing they are receiving genuine human understanding. Instead, AI must be trained to respond empathetically and consistently within clear boundaries—remaining transparent about its algorithmic nature and avoiding any inaccurate mimicry of human emotions.

This distinction between human-like and humane AI is increasingly important. Humane AI is not about AI saying, "I understand exactly how you feel." Instead, it is about honestly reflecting its limitations, like, "I think I understand," or "That sounds really hard." Humane AI creates an authentic, safe space by asking reflective, open-ended questions, gently encouraging introspection and personal discovery without overstepping emotional boundaries. Carefully trained AI prompts like, "What's making you feel this way?" or "What small step could help you feel better right now?" encourage valuable introspection without falsely promising human-level empathy. These gentle, reflective prompts can empower users to recognize their insights, possibly motivating them to reach out for professional support later. Like Freud's famous couch, the invisibility and anonymity of text interactions create a uniquely safe space. Even though someone is present, the lack of direct visual observation helps users feel less vulnerable, allowing them to engage more comfortably in free association and openly explore their thoughts and emotions. I vividly remember a user from Korea who carefully used a dictionary to craft her messages, investing immense effort to clearly articulate her innermost feelings and struggles. With over 500 million text-based conversations across 90 + countries, it reminds us about how meaningful this space can be for someone in distress.

Yet, despite these encouraging numbers, I remain deeply aware of potential pitfalls. The creation of human-like personas in digital mental health spaces with a focus on engagement or user acquisition is not just ethically questionable but potentially harmful. Mental health support hinges on trust, and when the boundaries between AI and human professionals are blurred, even unintentionally, that trust is at risk. Users may mistakenly believe they are interacting with trained therapists, leaving them emotionally vulnerable to confusion, disappointment, or even harm. From experience, prioritizing safety, accountability, and transparency is not just an ethical imperative—it is also valued by users and healthcare payers alike. Having faced resistance while advocating for these ethical boundaries, I understand the importance of continuously educating users and maintaining stringent ethical standards.

We have expanded our offerings to include skilled mental health professionals to complement our AI chatbot, particularly for situations requiring more intensive support. Our human-delivered therapy and mental health coaching services are available in English, Spanish, Hindi, Marathi, and other Indian regional languages, through text, audio, and video. Importantly, our therapists enjoy substantial freedom and autonomy, allowing them to deliver mental health support in alignment with their individual therapeutic styles and schools of thought. We consciously refrain from interfering with their unique approaches, enabling them to bring their authentic selves into their work with clients. At the same time, strong safeguards—including standard operating procedures, structured frameworks, clinical guidelines, and supervision—are in place to maintain consistency, ensure clinical safety, and uphold the quality of all interactions.

Reflecting deeply, I believe our future lies in honest collaboration between transparently defined AI tools and trained human clinicians. My initial scepticism has evolved into a cautious yet passionate belief, continually reaffirmed by witnessing authentic connections unfold - one thoughtful message at a time.

Smriti Joshi *is a clinical psychologist, thought leader, and digital mental health advisor contributing to ethical practices in online mental health service delivery. She currently serves as Chief of Clinical Services and Operations at Wysa and is also on the company's Board of Directors.*

As AI-driven tools become increasingly integrated into mental health care, it is important to reflect on the aspects of AI-powered therapeutic support that seem most promising. At the same time, we should consider any concerns or reservations we might have. Our reflections can evolve over time as we engage with both the possibilities and limitations of AI's emerging real-world applications.

Beyond Guidelines: A Dynamic and Dialogic Ethical Process

Guidelines for Telepsychotherapy Practice

Telepsychotherapy guidelines help therapists navigate complex professional landscapes, providing structure for ethical and effective remote practice. Frameworks such as McCord et al. (2020), synthesized five telepsychology guidelines into a model with nine core practice domains; including administrative skills, assessment, psychotherapy, ethics and law, multicultural competence, research and evaluation, risk assessment, supervision and technical skills. While these offer valuable direction, their application must be context-dependent, shaped by factors such as the delivery modality (e.g., video, phone, email) and the therapeutic setting (e.g., individual therapy, group therapy, crisis intervention). These guidelines are not rigid roadmaps but evolving frameworks that must be continuously examined and adapted to accommodate emerging technologies, shifting clinical needs and the diverse realities of remote therapy.

Ethical perspectives are shaped by practitioners' theoretical orientations, social locations, and systemic factors. What one therapist deems ethical may differ from another's convictions and realities. In regions with limited access to care, rigid exclusions risk withholding vital support from those who need it most. For example, a rural therapist with scarce mental health resources may view online therapy as a necessary means of accessibility, even for clients with moderate risk. Meanwhile, an urban-based practitioner with abundant resources may adhere more strictly to guidelines discouraging remote treatment for high-risk individuals. Context also shapes the delicate balance of risks and benefits in teletherapy. For a therapist working with survivors of domestic violence, online sessions can be a crucial form of support that offers privacy and safety. Yet, this also comes with risks, especially if the abuser is monitoring communication. With experience, therapists gain a keen sense of who benefits most from online therapy and when greater caution is needed. Insights from research and the collective voices of therapists further refine this understanding. Hagyari-Donaldson and Scott (2024) highlight how virtual spaces can be a refuge for young people with anxiety or those on the autism spectrum. Meanwhile, younger children (under ten) or individuals with attention deficits often benefit more from in-person therapy, where non-verbal cues and sensory engagement are more readily accessible.

Despite the rise of teletherapy, its guidelines rarely address the relational nuances of non-verbal cues, attunement and presence that define the therapy process. While therapists are developing their own strategies, we hope that guidelines will evolve beyond their narrow focus on risk management to offer concrete guidance on fostering engagement. Some therapists have incorporated creative digital tools, such as shared drawing boards or gamified interventions, to sustain engagement while working with adolescents. Others have worked to support older adults with minimal digital literacy by providing pre-session technology coaching to help them feel more comfortable and empowered in the process.

A particularly pressing concern is therapist jurisdiction. Can therapists ethically and legally provide care to clients in another country? Are they accountable to the laws and regulations of the country where they live and work, or those of the client's location? In crisis situations, how does a therapist ensure safety when the client is geographically distant? As more therapists and clients connect across borders due to cultural compatibility, continuity of care or even the affordability of sessions, these questions become even more urgent. There is an urgent need for clearer directives that balance access, affordability and legal responsibility.

Most tele-mental health guidelines are rooted in Western contexts, assuming stable internet, private spaces and personal devices and often overlook the realities of low-resource settings. Limited attention has been given to diverse practice environments such as schools, elder care homes and hospices, where privacy may be compromised, access to technology can be inconsistent, and the involvement of caregivers or staff is often necessary (McCord et al., 2020). Guidelines must move beyond idealized assumptions and account for real-world challenges. By systematically gathering and integrating these practitioner insights, we can build a shared repository of knowledge that informs future guidelines and strengthens teletherapy practice.

Guidelines rightly prioritize client rights, but this focus creates an asymmetry that leaves therapist vulnerability relatively unaddressed. For instance, if clients record sessions without discussion and consent, this can expose therapists to the risks of misrepresentation, unauthorized sharing or even legal complications. A therapist's carefully worded intervention, meant to be understood within the broader arc of treatment, could be selectively shared in ways that distort its meaning. In extreme cases, recordings could be used to discredit or pressure therapists, adding another layer of risk to an already emotionally demanding profession. Moreover, such anxieties about digital surveillance may subtly shift how therapists engage in sessions. Telepsychotherapy guidelines need more than a surface-level approach. They must dive deep into the complexities of real world dilemmas, examining ethics from both the therapist's and client's perspectives.

Guidelines for Social Media

Various psychological organizations, including the American Psychological Association (2021), the British Psychological Society (2019) and the Canadian Counselling and Psychotherapy Association (2019), have crafted guidelines to help clinicians navigate the ethical challenges of social media. While these frameworks share common concerns about privacy, confidentiality and professionalism, each emphasizes cert distinct aspects of digital ethics.

Across various guidelines, clinicians are advised to review privacy settings and maintain a degree of separation between personal and professional profiles, although this can be challenging to implement in practice. The evolving nature of digital platforms and algorithms means that even with tight privacy settings, content can still be exposed through tags, shares or search engine results. The British Psychological Society (BPS) encourages psychologists to regularly audit their digital footprint, acknowledging that online presence can shape public perception, influence client trust and invite regulatory scrutiny. Similarly, the Australian Psychological Society (2019) highlights the permanence of social media posts, urging caution in advocacy, debate and personal disclosure, as past content may resurface, even years later, in disciplinary proceedings.

Clients may interpret a therapist's social media presence as an invitation to engage, underscoring the need for a clear policy to avoid ethical dilemmas and misunderstandings (Pirelli et al., 2016). Many therapists now include a social media clause in intake forms, explicitly stating they do not accept friend requests, follow clients or engage in online therapeutic conversations via certain platforms. It is also important to inform clients that email and text are not secure channels and should not be used to share sensitive information. Outlining typical response times for communications during working days, weekends and holidays can help set realistic expectations. Equally important is reminding clients that digital platforms are not appropriate for urgent or crisis-related matters and clearly specifying the steps to take in such situations. However, we must also be prepared for the reality that clients may still reach out in distress through these channels, despite clear policies.

Clients should be informed about digital communication and social media policies during the informed consent process, ensuring mutual understanding from the very beginning. While transparency matters, so does tone. A policy that sounds cold or overly legalistic can inadvertently create distance and affect the therapeutic alliance. Instead, using language that is clear and compassionate and highlights the importance of protecting confidentiality and the integrity of the therapeutic process, helps communicate boundaries without alienating the client. Generational differences and evolving digital norms further shape how clients interpret a therapist's online presence. Younger clients, accustomed to fluid and responsive digital interactions, may view limited availability or strict boundaries as signs of disinterest or inaccessibility. This gap in expectations calls for therapists to be more intentional when discussing digital boundaries. Clarifying these limits while staying attuned to the client's perspective can help build trust and understanding.

Pause and reflect...

What guidelines have you established for interactions with clients on social media?

How do you navigate requests from clients to connect on social platforms?

Engaging with the ethical challenges of sharing client stories in online spaces is crucial, as digital platforms amplify the reach and permanence of therapeutic content. While guidelines generally advise against sharing real client stories without explicit, informed consent and urge substantial alterations to protect confidentiality, there remains ambiguity around how to create composite or hypothetical examples that are both ethical and meaningful. The ethics of storytelling in psychotherapy go beyond consent and disguise and touch on deeper questions of ownership, representation and relational responsibility. Bringing clinical material into public spaces, whether for teaching, supervision, webinars or conferences, raises deeper questions: to whom does the story truly belong? And what responsibilities come with telling it? In retelling, we inevitably view the client's experience through our own lens, sometimes unintentionally altering its meaning or emphasis. A client's consent may not carry the same meaning when a story can be clipped, reposted or resurface years later in entirely different contexts. The notion of informed consent needs updating to include a temporal and digital dimension that includes not just what is shared but where, how and for how long. Consent must also be seen as an ongoing conversation—one that explores the emotional weight of sharing, potential power dynamics and possible long-term implications. As therapists, we must consider if we genuinely have permission or if it is coming from our client's sense of gratitude, deference or a wish to please. Even a refusal can open a reflective space to explore the relational dynamics in therapy and the ways in which the client navigates trust, power, vulnerability and autonomy. Just as importantly, we must interrogate our own motivations for wanting to share the therapeutic process. Are we seeking to teach, to inspire, to be seen or to affirm our own competence? Navigating these questions with care and awareness is essential as we engage with the complexities of online spaces.

Guidelines for Online Psychotherapy Research

Imagine you are about to participate in an online study. A lengthy consent form appears, filled with dense legal jargon. Pressed for time, you quickly read through and hastily click 'I agree', not fully grasping the study's scope or potential risks. This scenario highlights a critical gap in the online consent process. Research by Geier et al. (2021) found that participants frequently skim online consent forms without a complete awareness of potential risks, their rights or the study's true objectives. Addressing this issue, Holtz et al. (2024) demonstrated that integrating interactive elements, such as quizzes or multimedia formats, can significantly improve comprehension. These methods encourage active engagement, ensuring that consent is truly informed rather than a mere formality.

Digital exclusion can skew research findings and reinforce existing disparities by systematically excluding entire groups of people. Consider an older adult struggling to navigate a digital consent form filled with tiny text and complex jargon, or a visually impaired participant trying to engage with a research survey that is not screen-reader compatible. These challenges do not just make participation difficult but sometimes even impossible for some individuals, effectively silencing their voices in research. Strategies such as hybrid consent models (e.g., phone-based or paper-based options), accessibility tools like screen readers and speech-to-text software and real-time technical support via helplines or live chat can help participants navigate digital obstacles. Emerging guidance on online recruitment emphasizes the importance of these strategies in fostering accessible and inclusive research practices (Iflaifel et al., 2024).

Unlike in-person studies, where a researcher can immediately notice signs of distress and intervene, online settings introduce a layer of distance that may leave struggling participants unseen and unsupported. What happens if someone becomes overwhelmed while answering sensitive questions? To address this, gathering emergency contact information, scheduling preemptive check-ins for high-risk participants and integrating crisis resources directly into research platforms are essential safety nets. Even small interventions that integrate pop-ups displaying helpline numbers, automated check-ins or follow-up messages, can provide timely support and help prevent participants from feeling isolated during moments of distress.

To conclude, ethical frameworks provide a critical foundation for guiding mental health professionals, but they must be regularly revisited to remain relevant. This involves keeping pace with technological advancements, shifting social norms and the increasingly blurred boundaries between personal and professional identities. As telepsychotherapy practice, social media engagement and online research continue to expand, practitioners require ethical guidelines that are both adaptive and grounded, and capable of supporting decision-making in complex, evolving contexts. Despite the growing integration of artificial intelligence into mental health services, current ethical guidance remains fragmented and largely provisional. While some professional mental health associations bodies have issued advisories, these emphasize caution and stop short of offering comprehensive or legally binding directives. For instance, one specific recommendation comes from the American Psychological Association (2023), which advises clinicians not to input client data into generative AI systems such as ChatGPT, due to significant concerns about privacy, confidentiality and data security. These emerging technologies call for a careful balancing act, leveraging innovation while upholding ethical responsibility. Yet what this balance looks like in practice remains an open and pressing question, one that must be addressed through interdisciplinary dialogue, reflection on clinical experience and continuous empirical inquiry.

Perspectives on Training and Development

Expanding Training Frameworks for Digital Practice

Current psychotherapy training, which still focuses primarily on traditional competencies, must expand to prepare trainees for the realities of modern practice. Rather than treating digital therapy as an afterthought, training programs should integrate digital practice from the start, asking how each intervention would work online. This approach ensures that trainees develop the necessary telehealth skills organically, rather than facing abrupt transitions or requiring additional upskilling later. Core telepsychology competencies, particularly technological proficiency, knowledge of legal and ethical guidelines, and the ability to adapt therapeutic techniques for digital platforms, must be explicitly embedded in curricula and evaluated for both pedagogy and outcome. Students can be encouraged to explore digital therapy communities, online peer support platforms, virtual reality spaces and a range of AI-driven mental health apps and critically examine their potential. However, we must also acknowledge that today's trainees are already adept at navigating digital spaces. Perhaps the real challenge is ensuring educators remain open to learning from their students, embracing innovative technologies rather than resisting them.

Mental health training programs need to acknowledge how issues like technology addiction, online gambling, cyberbullying and the complexities of digital relationships are becoming increasingly central to both diagnosis and treatment in the digital age. Therapists must develop a nuanced understanding of digital-age stressors and interactions. For example, recognizing the emotional impacts of doomscrolling and ghosting in relationships, the impact of social media algorithms on self-esteem and body image and the mental health risks associated with deepfake technology. Beyond individual treatment, training should prepare therapists to work systemically to collaborate with schools to design anti-cyberbullying programs, guide families on digital boundaries and link with policymakers for digital well-being and online safety.

The scope of work for a mental health professional has expanded, with companies developing AI and robotics looking for individuals with a more nuanced understanding of the brain, emotions and human interactions. Training programs must prepare therapists for AI-enabled services and startup environments by integrating technology into clinical work. This includes experience in writing therapeutic scripts for AI tools, critically evaluating and co-creating digital mental health platforms and collaborating with developers to refine emotion recognition systems used in wearable tech and virtual reality therapy. This shift demands a radical transformation in education, moving beyond traditional models to embrace interdisciplinary learning. For example, courses could include media studies (to explore how therapy translates into digital narratives), human–computer interaction (to refine AI-driven therapeutic conversations), ethics in AI (to address privacy and bias) or learning neuroscience-backed UX design.

Artificial Intelligence and Professional Training and Practice

The integration of AI into psychotherapy training raises critical concerns related to academic integrity, reflective engagement and the development of core therapeutic competencies. While AI-powered tools can assist with case conceptualization, practice simulations and theoretical understanding, they also pose risks of plagiarism, reduced critical thinking and over-reliance on algorithmic feedback (Campbell et al., 2025). One of the primary concerns is the potential for trainees to use AI-generated responses in assignments, case reflections or process notes without deep engagement. Educators must design training processes that encourage authentic engagement, such as oral case presentations and structured role-play exercises that require demonstrated therapeutic skills rather than just theoretical knowledge. There is emerging clarity on the ethical use of AI and appropriate attribution in academic work, with guidelines recommending disclosure about contributions of AI tools (OpenAI, 2023). Since AI-generated content is difficult to detect, a balanced approach combining ethical guidelines with trust-based learning is essential.

AI is emerging as a significant tool in psychotherapy training, offering innovative ways to develop and assess counselling skills. One application involves using AI models like ChatGPT to simulate client interactions, providing a flexible, low-risk training environment that is both controlled and repeatable (Maurya, 2024). AI can analyse large datasets, detect patterns in therapist-client interactions and offer feedback on therapist competencies. For example, a multimodal AI-based measure was developed to evaluate therapists' abilities to facilitate collaborative relationships (Aafjes-van Doorn et al., 2025). This proof-of-concept research underscores the potential for AI-driven assessments to complement traditional training and supervision by reinforcing structured interventions and ensuring fidelity to specific techniques. However, their effectiveness in cultivating more advanced competencies remains limited. Can these simulations capture a client's defensive withdrawal or the slightest flicker of uncertainty in their voice and prompt appropriate responses from therapists? There is still work to be done to determine how effectively AI simulations reflect and respond to the messiness of real-life therapy. A key consideration is whether reliance on AI-driven evaluations might place too much emphasis on measurable competencies while neglecting more nuanced, context-dependent aspects of psychotherapy—such as attunement, and the therapist's capacity for mentalizing or self-reflection. Training programs must find ways to integrate traditional training and supervision with these innovative methods.

The increasing integration of AI into psychotherapy raises pressing ethical and practical questions. Platforms now exist that can analyse therapy transcripts to assess the quality of skills and the therapeutic relationship, offering organizations a potential tool for quality control and monitoring. But how much should individual therapists rely on AI to evaluate what happens in the therapy room? Innovative AI-powered models are being developed to generate prompts or guidance for counsellors during their online sessions. CARE is an exemplar of an AI-powered tool designed to support online peer counsellors by providing real-time, context-specific response suggestions based on the Motivational Interviewing framework (Hsu et al., 2023). Such tools are typically positioned as being useful during simulated training for novice counsellors, but the impact on long-term skill development remains uncertain. While such real-time suggestions can enhance training by offering immediate feedback and reinforcing evidence-based techniques, it is crucial that these tools leave ample space for clinical intuition and flexibility.

Professional development opportunities are essential for trainees, academicians and clinical supervisors to deepen their understanding of generative and assistive AI, and to ensure its responsible use through ongoing evaluation, ethical oversight and a sustained commitment to high standards of quality.

Psychological Assessment in Digital Contexts

Digital adaptations of psychological assessment methods must demonstrate equivalent psychometric properties, with adequate standardization, reliability and ecological literacy before widespread adoption. There are some promising adaptations of self-report measures and task-based assessments such as the Wisconsin Card Sorting Test (WCST) and the Cambridge Neuropsychological Test Automated Battery (CANTAB). Projective assessments, such as the Rorschach Inkblot Test and the Thematic Apperception Test (TAT), involve nuanced human interpretation, nonverbal cues and qualitative analysis, making it more challenging to translate into a digital format. While efforts have been made to develop computerized scoring systems and automated linguistic analysis tools for storytelling tasks, these adaptations require further validation to ensure they preserve the depth and diagnostic richness of traditional methods.

Emerging technologies such as wearables for passive data collection of biorhythms as indicators of anxiety, stress or mood fluctuations and virtual reality (VR)-based assessments for assessment of social cognition in autism and schizophrenia, offer new possibilities for task-based evaluations. Furthermore, natural language processing (NLP) tools are being developed to analyse speech patterns in mood and psychotic disorders, providing objective markers for clinical assessment. Collaborative efforts between psychologists, neuroscientists and technology developers will be crucial to ensuring that digital adaptations maintain the clinical utility and depth of traditional assessment methods.

Future trends in digital psychological assessment include the transformation of traditional task-based evaluations into interactive digital games, which enhance both engagement and ecological validity. Artificial intelligence also holds promise for revolutionizing psychological testing through adaptive assessments, where test items adjust dynamically based on a respondent's answers. To advance the field responsibly, it is essential to conduct rigorous validation studies, involve clinicians in tool development and address critical factors such as digital literacy, accessibility and cultural bias.

Tele-Supervision as a Growth Area

The expansion of remote practice has positioned telesupervision as a crucial element in psychotherapy training, offering increased accessibility to expert mentors across geographical locations. However, effective telesupervision requires careful attention to technical aspects such as appropriate positioning, distance, lighting and eye contact to ensure supervisees are adequately visible and connected with each other (Nadan et al., 2020). To sustain engagement and learning, supervisors should incorporate structured breaks and strategies to mitigate screen fatigue. Research underscores the need for formal telesupervision training, as many supervisors adapted to online formats without proper preparation (Ratcliffe & Kaluzeviciute-Moreton, 2023). Emerging AI-driven telesupervision tools, such as automated session analysis and feedback systems, can enhance training efficiency by tracking speech patterns, generating frequency charts of therapist and client talk time and organizing client language into thematic categories, such as anxiety or relationships. Additionally, real-time transcription with time-stamped comments can support supervisors in delivering timely, accurate feedback, improving both the efficiency and quality of clinical training. These tools have the potential to further streamline session analysis and provide more precise, focused feedback (Maurya & DeDiego, 2025).

The ability to reach a supervisor from anywhere around the world has opened to doors to this support for private practitioners who might otherwise have struggled to access quality supervision. Therapists can now seek supervision that aligns with their specific theoretical orientations or areas of expertise, tailoring the experience to their unique needs. At the same time, supervisors benefit from a broader pool of supervisees, allowing them to form special interest groups that foster deeper engagement and professional growth.

Conclusion

As mental health professionals navigate an increasingly digital world, evolving modalities and pathways require reflection, adaptation and innovation. Yet, at its core, the essence of the work remains unchanged. Clients continue to seek understanding and guidance in their journeys toward change. Therapists still need to create strong alliances, attune to the subjective experience of others and respond to their needs with empathy and expertise. We now have a new and expanding toolbox—one that opens doors to new possibilities in therapeutic practice. It is exciting to imagine what we might build and how far we will go.

References

Aafjes-Van Doorn, K., Békés, V., Luo, X., & Hopwood, C. J. (2023). Therapists' perception of the working alliance, real relationship and therapeutic presence in in-person therapy versus tele-therapy. *Psychotherapy Research, 34*(5), 574–588.

Aafjes-van Doorn, K., Cicconet, M., Bate, J., Cohn, J. F., & Aafjes, M. (2025). Development of an artificial intelligence-based measure of therapists' skills: A multimodal proof of concept. *Psychotherapy*. https://doi.org/10.1037/pst0000561

American Psychological Association. (2017). *Ethical principles of psychologists and code of conduct* (2002, Amended June 1, 2010, and January 1, 2017). https://www.apa.org/ethics/code

American Psychological Association. (2021). *APA guidelines for the optimal use of social media in professional psychological practice*. American Psychological Association. https://www.apa.org/practice/guidelines/social-media-use

American Psychological Association. (2023). *APA urges caution about incorporating AI into clinical practice*. Psychiatric News. Retrieved from https://doi.org/10.1176/appi.pn.2023.08.8.57

American Psychological Association. (2024). *APA's AI tool guide for practitioners*. Retrieved from https://www.apaservices.org/practice/business/technology/tech-101/evaluating-artificial-intelligence-tool

Australian Government eSafety Commissioner. (2025). *Social media age restrictions*. https://www.esafety.gov.au/about-us/industry-regulation/social-media-age-restrictions

Australian Psychological Society. (2019). *Ethical guidelines on social media*. https://psychology.org.au

British Association for Counselling and Psychotherapy. (2018). *Ethical framework for the counselling professions*. https://www.bacp.co.uk/events-and-resources/ethics-and-standards/ethical-framework-for-the-counselling-professions/

British Psychological Society. (2019). *Guidance on the use of social media*. https://www.bps.org.uk/guideline/guidance-use-social-media

Campbell, L. O., Frawley, C., Lambie, G. W., Cabrera, K. S., & Vizcarra, B. D. (2025). Examining artificial intelligence policies in counsellor education. *Counselling and Psychotherapy Research, 25*, e12880. https://doi.org/10.1002/capr.12880

Canadian Counselling and Psychotherapy Association. (2019). *Guidelines for uses of technology in counselling and psychotherapy*. https://www.ccpa-accp.ca/wp-content/uploads/2019/04/TISCGuidelines_Mar2019_EN.pdf

Cullingham, T., Rennard, U., Creswell, C., Milton, D., Buckle, K. L., Godber, L., Gordon, K., Larkin, M., & Green, J. (2024). The process of co-design for a new anxiety intervention for autistic children. *JCPP Advances*. https://doi.org/10.1002/jcv2.12255

Geier, C., Adams, R. B., Mitchell, K. M., & Holtz, B. E. (2021). Informed consent for online research—Is anybody reading? Assessing comprehension and individual differences in readings of digital consent forms. *Journal of Empirical Research on Human Research Ethics, 16*(3), 154–164.

Geller, S. (2021). Cultivating online therapeutic presence: Strengthening therapeutic relationships in teletherapy sessions. *Counselling Psychology Quarterly, 34*(3–4), 687–703.

Green, E. P., Lai, Y., Pearson, N., Rajasekharan, S., Rauws, M., Joerin, A., Kwobah, E., Musyimi, C., Jones, R. M., Bhat, C., Mulinge, A., & Puffer, E. S. (2020). Expanding access to perinatal depression treatment in Kenya through automated psychological support: Development and usability study. *JMIR Formative Research, 4*(10), e17895. https://doi.org/10.2196/17895

Gupta, K., Sinha, A., & Bhola, P. (2016). Intersections between ethics and technology: Online client-therapist interactions. In P. Bhola & A. Raguram (Eds.), *Ethical issues in counselling and psychotherapy practice: Walking the line* (pp. 169–186). Springer.

Hagyari-Donaldson, P., & Scott, N. (2024). Online therapy for children: Yay or nay? Clinicians' insights from the COVID-19 era. *Child & Youth Care Forum*. https://doi.org/10.1007/s10566-024-09835-3

Harvard T. H. Chan School of Public Health. (2023, August 9). *Social media influencers, faculty connect to improve mental health content*. https://hsph.harvard.edu/news/social-media-influencers-faculty-connect-to-improve-mental-health-content/

Holohan, M., & Fiske, A. (2021). Like I'm talking to a real person": Exploring the meaning of transference for the use and design of AI-based applications in psychotherapy. *Frontiers in Psychology, 12*, 720476. https://doi.org/10.3389/fpsyg.2021.720476

Holtz, B., Mitchell, K., Adams, R., Grier, C., & Wright, J. (2024). Enhancing comprehension of online informed consent: The impact of interactive elements and presentation formats. *Ethics & Behavior*. https://doi.org/10.1080/1050842

Hsu, S.-L., Shah, R. S., Senthil, P., Ashktorab, Z., Dugan, C., Geyer, W., & Yang, D. (2023). Helping the helper: Supporting peer counselors via AI-empowered practice and feedback. https://doi.org/10.48550/arXiv.2305.08982

Iflaifel, M., Hall, C. L., Green, H. R., et al. (2024). Using online methods to recruit participants into mental health clinical trials: Considerations and recommendations from the RE-MIND study. *Trials, 25*, 596. https://doi.org/10.1186/s13063-024-08435-9

Kaluzeviciute, G. (2020). Social media and its impact on therapeutic relationships. *British Journal of Psychotherapy, 36*(2), 303–320.

Kashyap, H., Chandur, J., & Reddy, R. P. (2020). The loss of the shared space: Process issues in telepsychotherapy. *Indian Journal of Psychological Medicine, 42*(5), 469–472.

Maurya, R. K. (2024). A qualitative content analysis of ChatGPT's client simulation role-play for practising counselling skills. *Counselling and Psychotherapy Research, 24*, 614–630.

Maurya, R. K., & DeDiego, A. C. (2025). Artificial intelligence integration in counsellor education and supervision: A roadmap for future directions and research inquiries. *Counselling and Psychotherapy Research, 25*, e12727. https://doi.org/10.1002/capr.12727

McCord, C., Bernhard, P., Walsh, M., Rosner, C., & Console, K. (2020). A consolidated model for telepsychology practice. *Journal of Clinical Psychology, 76*(6), 1060–1082.

Mori, M. (1970). The uncanny valley. *Energy, 7*(4), 33–35.

Nadan, Y., Shachar, R., Cramer, D., Leshem, T., Levenbach, D., Rozen, R., et al. (2020). Behind the (virtual) mirror: Online live supervision in couple and family therapy. *Family Process, 59*(3), 997–1006.

OpenAI. (2023). *ChatGPT (March 14 version) [Large language model]*. OpenAI. https://openai.com/chatgpt

Oudin, A., Maatoug, R., Bourla, A., Ferreri, F., Bonnot, O., Millet, B., Schoeller, F., Mouchabac, S., & Adrien, V. (2023). Digital phenotyping: Data-driven psychiatry to redefine mental health. *Journal of Medical Internet Research, 25*, e44502. https://doi.org/10.2196/44502

Patterson, K., Grenny, J., McMillan, R., Switzler, A., & Maxfield, D. (2022). *Crucial conversations: Tools for talking when stakes are high* (3rd ed.). McGraw Hill.

Pirelli, G., Otto, R. K., & Estoup, A. (2016). Using social media in psychological practice: Ethical implications and a model for ethical decision making. *Professional Psychology: Research and Practice, 47*(5), 314–321.

Ratcliffe, K., & Kaluzeviciute-Moreton, G. (2023). Telesupervision in counselling and psychotherapy: A systematic review of the literature. *British Journal of Guidance & Counselling, 52*(5), 801–814.

Taubitz, F. S., Büdenbender, B., & Alpers, G. W. (2022). What the future holds: Machine learning to predict success in psychotherapy. *Behaviour Research and Therapy, 156*, 104116.

Taylor, L., Kegerreis, S., & Rohleder, P. (2023). Loss and survival: Experiences of psychoanalytic psychotherapists working remotely during the COVID-19 pandemic. *British Journal of Psychotherapy, 39*(1), 182–197.

Trub, L., & Magaldi, D. (2021). Secret powers: Acts of googling in the therapeutic relationship. *Journal of Clinical Psychology, 77*(4), 968–985. https://doi.org/10.1002/jclp.23107/

Turing, A. M. (1950). Computing machinery and intelligence. *Mind, 236*, 433–460.

UK Council for Psychotherapy. (2019). *Code of ethics and professional practice.* https://www.psychotherapy.org.uk/media/bkjdm33f/ukcp-code-of-ethics-and-professional-practice-2019.pdf

White, E., & Hanley, T. (2025). "What I share is not the same as therapy": Psychologist experiences of Instagram use as a mental health influencer. *Psychology and Psychotherapy: Theory, Research and Practice.* https://doi.org/10.1111/papt.12585

Chapter 9
Learning from Clients

In the fantasy novel *The Lord of the Rings* (Tolkein, 1994), we leave the safe and familiar Shire and journey on a long and dangerous quest with Frodo, the Hobbit. When Frodo is uncertain and reluctant, Gandalf the powerful and wise wizard helps him get started and is a constant guide and mentor. He persists on a quest to destroy the One Ring and save Middle Earth from the Dark Lord Sauron, saying—"I will take the Ring, though I do not know the way" (Tolkein, 1994, p. 264). Along the way, Frodo has many challenging encounters, experiencing inner struggles and powerful enemies, facing difficult choices and enduring a series of tests. Gandalf encourages him to have experiences outside his comfort zone and appears when needed, to lead him to safety. Gandalf seems like the central figure in Frodo's transformative journey. But really, *Frodo* is the hero. Even Gandalf is impressed with Frodo's will and choices, perhaps more than the mighty deeds performed by kings, knights and even himself. In a similar vein, Duncan and Miller (2000, p. 173) remind us, "It is time to recast the drama of psychotherapy, to retire the star therapist and place the heroic client in the leading role."

As trainees, we usually enter the world of psychotherapy through teachers, academic courses and books. This process opens our eyes to new ideas and is often an exciting experience of emotional and intellectual growth. It is no wonder, then, that when we first encounter clients, we may believe that we know far more than they do and want to share our insights, knowledge and understanding with them. In this rush, we might not heed what our clients are trying to tell us about themselves and their lives. Over time, most of us realize that like Frodo, our clients are on their own journeys, motivated by their own purposes. They have chosen to recruit therapists to help them with part of the way, but it is their desire to heal and grow that provides the real energy of therapy. Rather than seeing therapy as a process where treatment/therapist operate on the client to create change, Bohart (2000) suggests that we need to see the client as operating on treatments and theories to produce effects. What this means for us as therapists, is that we need to hold theory and technique as background, while foregrounding the client's frame, values and goals.

P. Bhola et al., *Reflective Practice in Psychotherapy and Counselling*,
https://doi.org/10.1007/978-981-96-9732-8_9

Therapeutic work often brings reality checks with moments when theory and technique fall short, and our clients lead and take us along in their journey. As these experiences are understood and integrated, humility grows alongside the growing awareness of our limitations. Conversely, a sense of confidence and competence can deepen, as we come to see our role more clearly. No two therapeutic encounters are the same, no two paths of self-discovery are similarly mapped, and no two sessions are alike. With each client we discover new ways of listening, relating and being, and somewhere along the way we change as therapists.

In this chapter, we reflect on the various ways we can enter the clients' world through enhancing our sensitivity to the language that they use, drawing out their theory of change and responding to their preferences. We examine the value of methods of eliciting, monitoring and processing client feedback to measure progress in therapy, through a process of shared reflection. Attention is also given to client voices beyond the therapy room, including narratives about their therapeutic experiences and insights from the user-survivor movement. The chapter concludes by considering how therapists themselves grow and change through their work with clients.

Stories that Teach: Learning from Client Narratives

As therapists, we often reflect and theorize about what might be going on with clients during sessions. However, what the client finds meaningful in each therapy session may not be what the therapist notices as significant. This is beautifully described in Irvin Yalom's book *Every Day Gets a Little Closer: A Twice-told Therapy,* where both the therapist and the client describe their experience of each therapy session. Reflecting on the experience, Yalom notes, "Often she values one part of the hour, I another" (Yalom & Elkin, 1974, p. 351). There is ample evidence for what he calls the subterranean life of the client—that clients do not share all their experiences, thoughts and feelings with the therapist. Ginny (the client) agrees with this saying, "At times I acted in his office, deliberately subduing my spirit to coincide with the therapy hour" (Yalom & Elkin, 1974, p. 378). As this story suggests, perfect attunement is not possible. However, we can come closer to our client's realities through listening, asking and reflecting together.

When we step back and see therapy (and therapists) through our clients' eyes, rather than through the lens of expert-led research or theory, there is much to learn about the gaps (and bridges) in the ways we provide therapy and what is valued by clients in the therapeutic experience. If our clients' voices are not heard and psychotherapy occurs within a closed system, we may remain oblivious to the fact that therapy can sometimes be harmful or ineffective.

Listen…

Preeti, a 58 year old woman client sought help for feelings of helplessness and anxiety. She discussed her family's financial struggles in recent years but struggled to explain her ongoing discomfort now that things had seemingly improved. Preeti described feeling like 'Gandhari'[1] *as she turned a blind eye to how her husband and son managed the family business and finances. She used this culturally powerful metaphor - of being blindfolded by choice so the deeds of others are not in our view - to communicate her situation to her therapist. As Preeti explored this metaphor with her therapist, it opened new possibilities for both to connect with her emotional experience in ways not previously possible. The therapist asked reflective questions about how Preeti's gender, family values and life experiences might have contributed to her being in this position. Together, they explored alternative responses and what it would mean for her to choose to open her eyes.*

There are several ways in which therapists can learn from clients. One of the most important aspects is allowing oneself to truly listen to what each client is communicating about their experiences and needs. This emphasizes the need for sensitivity to the full range of client communications, including their verbal and non-verbal language, the metaphors and idioms they use to express their distress, as well as the images, drawings, dreams or the arrangement of objects on a sand tray that resonate with them. Does the client call their partner by name, or do they refer to the relationship, as "my husband" or "my girlfriend"? What might this mean for the client, how they view their relationship and how they want you to view it? This sensitivity can help the therapist enter the inner world of the client and tune in to experiences that clients may not be able to fully articulate.

Pause and reflect…

Do you recall a powerful metaphor shared by a client that illuminated their deeper experience for you?

In what ways did it enhance your understanding of the client's experience?

How did you respond to the metaphor?

Therapists can support change by asking clients to imagine how their metaphors could be transformed, or even by introducing metaphors during the session (Wagener, 2017). Such a process allows for change that emerges from within the client's own frame or narrative. For instance, if a client describes their experience of depression as dragging a black hole behind them, we can ask what it might feel like for them

[1] Gandhari is a character from the Indian epic *The Mahabharata*, who chose to blindfold herself through her life when she found out that her to-be husband was born with a visual impairment.

to put that burden down or step away from the hole. Angus and Scott Mio (2011) tell the story of a couple who used the metaphor of armour to describe how the wife protected herself. The therapist shifting the metaphor for protection to soft pillows enabled the husband to see how he could gently move the pillows away one by one, rather than having to poke his way through the armour—thus paving the road for better intimacy.

Of course, the most straight forward and direct way to learn more about our clients is to ask them. By inquiring about their needs, expectations and preferences regarding therapy, we can better understand their unique perspectives and tailor our approach accordingly.

Ask…

When clients enter an often-unfamiliar therapeutic space, they may wonder what to talk about, worry if their problems are legitimate or feel emotionally inhibited and vulnerable. When the therapist gently enquires about and responds to what the client wishes for in therapy, and what they want to talk about, this can leave clients feeling safer and more trusting of the therapeutic space (Cooper et al., 2023). This process sets the stage for the development of a healthy therapeutic alliance, a sense of partnership that supports the work of therapy. While attention to client experiences and preferences may be particularly useful in the early trust-building phase of therapy, there will be several opportunities to have these conversations during the process of therapy.

A Client Speaks: Musings on a Partnership

Suman Bolar

I vividly remember my first visit to a therapist.

After I'd explained why I was there, I was instructed to lie down and clench and unclench my muscles from head to toe. I was irritated. I'd expected and wanted to be asked questions, hoping that a professional would help me understand my pervasive, inexplicable sadness. Instead, I was doing isometrics! When I left, I knew that I wouldn't return.

I now know that the therapist was trying to relax me prior to therapy. But to me, it was the equivalent of a first date with someone who orders on your behalf without being asked to. It might have felt different if there had been an effort to explain, but there wasn't. I struggled through several different therapists before I found one who was right for me. What made her different? She seemed to recognize that we were in a partnership.

In any partnership, clearly articulated expectations and boundaries are essential: What is each one's role? Like dancers, each partner must learn when to step up and when to step back. Above all, each partner must earn and keep the other's trust. My therapist trusts that I will be punctual, stay committed and pay promptly. I place faith in her professional ethics, trusting that she will pay attention, try to 'get' what I'm feeling and push me (but not too hard!) when necessary.

But this is not an equal partnership; only one partner (me) is making themselves completely vulnerable—and the imbalance is at first deeply unsettling. Over time, we have grown into this partnership, coming to trust, like and perhaps even admire one other. We've come to understand and appreciate each other's words, silences, patterns and rhythms. Whenever we're in sync, sessions are fruitful and productive, with actionable outcomes. Things are trickier when our priorities differ. I've learnt to pay close attention when my therapist veers off to something seemingly irrelevant. Sensing something that I haven't, she has seized the wheel, gently confronting me with uncomfortable truths or pushing me into expressing something I've been suppressing or avoiding. Even though I rarely understand where she is going or why, I'm able to acquiesce to her agenda because she always acknowledges that she's taking charge. Such sessions are exhausting, for both of us. There's no immediate payoff and I'm sometimes restless or agitated for days. But eventually, some tiny nugget shifts or widens my perspective, helping me respond to life experiences with composure and equanimity. We've both learnt to be patient with the therapeutic process, trusting that a planted seed takes time to sprout and longer to flourish.

A partnership cannot be one-sided. As a client, I offer my therapist access to a wider set of human experiences, more emotional high notes, low notes and octaves to draw from, and the chance to hone her craft. But more than anything else, I think that I contribute to giving her the one thing we all need as human beings: the sense that she matters.

Suman Bolar *is a school administrator from India who was diagnosed with treatment-resistant major depressive disorder at the age of 27. She shares her life with her husband, two sons, and beloved pets that live on in her heart.*

As therapists, we need to work consciously to ensure that clients feel comfortable sharing their preferences, whether these are about therapy methods or techniques, foci of conversations, preferred therapist style or goals of therapy. This is also a time for therapists to share what they need and expect from clients, and to respond to their questions about the therapy process, explaining what is possible to accomplish through therapy and clarifying the respective roles in this new relationship. During this interaction, clients might speak about their efforts to engender change or draw from their previous experiences in therapy – what worked, what did not work, and what they are looking for. This experience of choice can be an empowering experience, one that helps clients shift their frame of reference from "I need help" to "I am learning how to help myself."

When therapists reflect with clients on their preferences, it opens possibilities and, most importantly, creates hope that things can be different (McLeod, 2013). The client no longer tries to find the right answer and can be freed to find the answer that works best for them. It is easier to respond immediately to micro choices such as, "I would like you to ask me more specific questions about my relationship with…." While therapists are not required to acquiesce to every request, for example, a request for increased session frequency, they do remain respectful and seek to explore the reasons and meanings around the expressed need.

Pause and reflect...

Do you recall a time when you noticed and asked your client about a need or preference from therapy. What do you feel you learnt and how did it inform the therapy process?

Can you recall an experience when you regretted asking your client about their preference? How do you understand what happened?

We invite you to reflect not only on what to ask, but also on how and when to ask. What is the language that is most likely to encourage clients to express themselves. "What do you want from therapy?" may be too broad or vague a question for some clients to answer. We also need to remember that not all clients may know the answer to such a question straightaway. "Shall we begin by looking at your current situation or would you prefer to start with sharing your early life experiences?" may be easier for clients to respond to, even as it limits their choices to two. Each of us would have developed our own style of enquiry and it is useful to pause and think about how well our clients are responding to it.

While eliciting client preferences is useful, this does not mean that the therapist takes a back seat or becomes too passive. Clients who are feeling stuck or avoiding issues may wish for the therapist to guide them and perhaps even challenge them. In general, clients seem to prefer active therapists who lead the way, but do so in a warm and caring manner, giving them the space to explore themselves (Cooper et al., 2023). Based on their cultural background, clients may be more or less comfortable with taking the lead or even stating their preferences. In traditional hierarchical societies like India, therapists might need to work harder at inviting such discussions (Bhola & Chaturvedi, 2017). Clients with previous therapy experiences often have a clearer sense of what works for them and what does not, and could appreciate the opportunity to express their needs to a new therapist. Therapists also need to consider when clients will welcome the opportunity to take the lead and when they may prefer not to. A client who is already feeling emotionally overwhelmed, depressed, and apathetic may not be ready to discuss their preferences. Instead, they need to feel that they are with a therapist who knows what they are doing and can guide them out of their stuck place.

Client preferences and therapist understanding and appropriate response to the same, can keep evolving through the course of therapy. Both client and therapist can (and should) revisit this conversation whenever they feel the need to. For instance, a therapist could say, "I understand when you say you would prefer to keep a focus on your current relationship, and I am happy to keep our focus here. However, it may happen that I sometimes feel that your early life experiences are really impinging on the way you are feeling right now. In this case I might ask you if we can explore your those experiences as well. Would this be okay for you?" We also need to keep in mind that clients might need time to experience both therapy and the therapist, and their needs and preferences can change over the course of therapy. A client might initially seek focused behavioural work to address a particular issue, but as therapy progresses, they may become more aware of their emotional patterns and wish to explore those in more detail.

These conversations are often stimulated by a therapy interaction, but therapists can also use measures to help frame and kickstart conversations around client preferences in the therapy process. A structured tool, such as the popular Cooper–Norcross Inventory of Preferences (Cooper & Norcross, 2016), can be filled by the client before the start of therapy. It allows for several aspects of preferences to be gathered in a short period of time, and can ensure that several significant areas are covered. This inventory examines four key preferences: therapist directiveness versus client directiveness, emotional intensity versus emotional reserve, focus on past experiences versus focus on the present, and warm support versus focused challenge. The framework enables exploration of additional preferences, such as session length, therapy modality and orientation, as well as therapist characteristics. When strong preferences emerge, the therapist can mirror them back to the client, inviting a deeper exploration of their significance.

Each therapist will have their personal style of introducing the measure being used. We need to take time to introduce the idea and garner client acceptance before proceeding. Clients (especially those new to therapy) can worry that they do not actually know what they prefer—they may wish for the therapist to guide them, or they may need the freedom to change their minds. It is up to the therapist to support their clients in this process, and the way the interaction unfolds can set the tone for the nature of the therapist-client relationship…who leads, who follows, and how much support or space is extended.

When eliciting preferences (especially in such a structured form), therapists can also reflect on their own ability to meet client preferences. We cannot develop a sense of humour because our client wants that from us. It may not even be easy to shift our natural stance to one that is more directive or less intense. So, before we ask clients what they want from us, we need to conceptualise how we can actually deliver on these needs. Whether we accommodate the preference or not, the openness and flexibility we show in trying to meet client needs and tailor the therapy process towards their unique situation remains valuable. Therapy that aligns with client preferences leads to lower dropout rates and fosters a stronger alliance and better outcomes (McLeod, 2015). However, not accommodating preferences can also be beneficial, particularly when it encourages clients to explore new approaches to achieve their goals (Cooper et al., 2023).

As therapists, we distinguish between preferences and needs, going beyond the client's stated preference to understanding their story. We do not just ask the clients what they want but also explore why they want it. Through this uncovering of the meaning of a preference we can arrive at a deeper understanding of the client's psychological needs in any interaction. As we ask our clients about their lives and likes and listen for what they are trying to convey, a more complete picture of the human being sitting in front of us can emerge.

Interact…

Every client has a story about themselves – who they are, how they got here and where they wish to go. Embedded within this story, is their *theory of change*, or their ideas around what change means to them, what needs to happen for change to occur, what help they feel they need, and the pathway they sense will lead from where they are to where they wish to be (Duncan & Miller, 2000).

As therapists, we can elicit the client's theory of change by immersing ourselves within the client's world view and really attempting to get their experience at a visceral level. Some clients have thought through aspects of their concerns and share it actively, while others might use the therapy space to discover and crystallise their understanding. The process of developing this understanding can be described as piecing together a jigsaw puzzle. The client brings in the pieces, either together or one at a time, and with the therapist's help, finds a way to create a fuller picture.

Engaging more directly with clients about how they envision improving their situation or how they would like to proceed can open up valuable conversations. Enquiring about their previous efforts to overcome difficulties can reveal therapeutic possibilities that stem from their existing attempts to understand and help themselves. This approach elicits perspectives and processes that resonate with them (Duncan & Miller, 2000). Ideas that harness client strengths while directly addressing their concerns are particularly effective in activating their self-healing capacity (Bohart, 2000). Ideally, therapists support the client's frame, encouraging them to take the lead in developing and expanding their own theory. Sharing knowledge of different treatment models can help them find one that aligns with their personal narrative.

Leading from half a step behind, therapists adopt a position of respectful curiosity while applying their expertise to support the client's journey. When the client's social and cultural context is incorporated into the narrative, it broadens the shared reflective process. By using various lenses of personal experience, family practices, religion, and spirituality, the therapeutic dialogue can facilitate the expression of the client's unique insights. When we prioritize their local knowledge on these matters, more pieces of the puzzle fall into place.

A client may insist on focusing on their difficult childhood experiences, believing that their problems stem from the unconscious. The therapist, however, might feel that the client's difficulties are more rooted in their current environment or may lack training in psychodynamic approaches. How can such a situation be navigated? Wherever possible, it is helpful to privilege the client's perspective and remain flexible and open to their ideas. When therapists choose to work with the client's theory of change, they are making an effort to understand what the client believes they need from therapy. This approach not only helps in clarifying therapeutic goals and processes but also informs the therapist's role in the client's story. By treating the client as an equal partner, therapy becomes more of a collaborative and growth-oriented experience rather than a correctional one. When the therapist's formulation and interventions align with the client's own understanding of their distress, treatment is likely to be more effective.

As we listen to and engage with each client's theory of change, we can grow to be better therapists. We can bring our learning from each experience to gradually develop our theory of change. We painstakingly gather the building blocks of the skills and insights that seem to work in therapy, learning and unlearning with each new client we meet. Through our reflections, we might arrive at a better understanding of the real significance of our role in each of our clients' lives. We also learn about ourselves as therapists. How flexible can we be? Which perspectives do we find it easier to work with? How do we handle challenges or deal with a client who does not accept our clinical wisdom? The answers to these questions can shape the skills we choose to hone, the nature of the therapeutic relationships we form and ultimately, our identity as therapists.

Learning from Client Feedback

Privileging and responding to client perspectives is a process that continues through the course of therapy. Their viewpoint often emerges through subtle verbal and non-verbal cues during the nuanced moments of therapy, revealing layers of meaning that might otherwise go unnoticed. A client who slips from the chair to the floor when discussing how to organize her task list is conveying something very powerful—both about how she views her tasks as well as what she wants to talk about in therapy. The therapist can respond to these emotional signals, notice and validate what the client is experiencing in the moment and open a discussion on what she can and cannot bear as well as how she would like to address this in therapy. Therapists and clients often differ in how they share and receive feedback, with some placing greater importance on non-verbal or spontaneous cues, and others on verbal or intentionally elicited responses.

Incorporating a regular practice of asking reflective questions can support clients in engaging more actively with the therapy process. These might include prompts such as: What are your feelings about the session? What did you learn? What did you not like? What did you wish had happened? Such questions help draw the client's attention to what is unfolding in the session and signal that the therapist values their experience and is open to learning from it (Haber et al., 2014). Therapists can seek feedback at a micro level about specific interventions, as well as ask broader questions about therapeutic progress and the experience of the therapeutic alliance. It is also important for therapists to reflect on their own patterns when it comes to receiving feedback. We may become aware that we are more open to receiving feedback from some clients than others. Perhaps we are more receptive when the feedback comes from clients perceived as articulate, emotionally regulated or those from similar backgrounds or worldviews. In contrast, we might unconsciously dismiss or minimize feedback from clients who express themselves in ways we find more challenging. These tendencies can reveal valuable insights into our interpersonal dynamics, implicit biases and areas of comfort or discomfort. Importantly, such tendencies may also reflect broader power structures within society where some clients already have less of a voice, both inside and outside the therapy room. Therapists who acknowledge this are better positioned to make intentional efforts to ask, listen and remain open to the diverse realities, needs and perspectives of all their clients.

Therapists have access to a range of formal feedback instruments designed to systematically track clients' progress and therapeutic experiences. Some measures are robustly quantitative and came along with computer programs to help score and interpret them, while others are qualitative and flexible, relying more on context and conversation. Pragmatic considerations such as time, cost, human resources and relevance for our practice may influence which measures we use and how frequently we do so. Regular tracking of client's symptoms and concerns, using structured measures at multiple points, can lead to a shared understanding of the problems throughout the course of therapy. Routine Outcome Monitoring (ROM) is a method that allows therapists to graph and track each client's trajectory of change, identify those who are not on track and use this feedback to modify therapy goals and processes. While there are variations in the scope, length and targets of assessment, measures are typically brief to allow for repeated use. Two exemplars are the Outcome Questionnaire (OQ-45; Lambert et al., 2013) and the Partners for Change Outcome Management System (PCOMS; Miller & Duncan, 2004). These measures can be used to evaluate the progress of a particular client, and also to look at the standards of overall service provision within an organization. The OQ-45 tracks symptoms related to distress, emotional states, interpersonal relationships and social roles. This can be used in combination with a clinical support tool, the Assessment for Signal Clients, which measures in-session experiences such as alliance and motivation, as well as outside therapy experiences of social support and life events (ASC; Lambert, 2015). The PCOMS includes the Outcome Rating Scale and Session Rating Scale and is used to monitor treatment outcome, therapeutic alliance and client views on progress, with specific guidelines for how to intervene with clients who are improving, not improving or deteriorating (Reese et al., 2009). Personalized measures which require clients to describe and rate their problems, functioning and well-being can place more demands than tick the box forms. But this can be worth the effort, as learning about the client's world in their own words can open the door to an exploration of sensitive, hidden and important issues.

Some clients may be reluctant to repeatedly engage with paper-and-pencil surveys, perceiving them as too effortful or time-consuming. Beginning with a solid rationale can be helpful; for example, explaining how the feedback measure is part of an interactive process of building a partnership. Providing opportunities to ask questions and learn how responses will be used can enhance acceptance of this method. However, if there is clear reluctance to engage with a formal measure, it is essential to respect this preference while exploring the reasons behind the hesitation.

Once elicited, feedback needs to be integrated into the therapy process. Each session could begin with examining feedback from the previous session, noting areas where the scores are particularly low and discussing this with the client (Reese et al., 2013). Therapists often find it easier to respond to specific feedback (e.g., "I would like to talk more about my childhood experiences") where the required change is more accessible. They may feel less sure about how to respond to general dissatisfaction (e.g., "This therapy is not working for me"), sometimes taking the feedback seriously only if the client drops out (Brattland et al., 2018). Unsolicited or strongly expressed feedback can throw even experienced therapists. Like any frustrating experience, it can leave them feeling self-critical or guilty, annoyed with the client. Some may off their emotions just to get through the session. As we take the time to reflect on client feedback, we can become more aware of patterns within ourselves. Perhaps we are quick to blame ourselves rather than pausing to consider why the client said what they did or what it might reveal about the client's own needs and experiences. Feelings of anger or hurt may emerge when it seems that our care is not being received in the way it was intended. We could note a particular sensitivity to feedback from certain clients and not so much from others. Taking time to reflect on feedback or explore it in supervision can open up new perspectives on what to do next and create space for growth at our own pace. Such learning can inform our work with the current client, or it may be something we apply to new clients, eventually becoming a part of how we operate. Reflecting on the feedback received enables us to develop a meta-understanding of therapeutic process and practice, offering a scaffold to help us move beyond our theory or comfort zone.

Client feedback (whether specific or generic) is most useful when we treat it as a launchpad for further discussions. Acknowledging our impact on the client, or the fact that we sometimes don't get it, can be freeing for the therapist and validating for the client. The best response to client feedback is to explore why they want what they want, understand how this fits into their broader intra- and interpersonal systems and discuss ways to work toward a better experience and outcome. The act of asking for feedback itself seems to have a positive impact on clients, and the use of structured measures has several benefits. Using a feedback tool can open the door for clients to describe the needs they might be otherwise reluctant to do face to face. Overall, tracking progress can be empowering as clients learn the language and skills to express their needs (Oanes et al., 2015). The use of instruments like PCOMS and OQ has been proven to improve outcome in about two-thirds of clients, reducing deterioration and increasing the number of clients with clinically significant change (Lambert et al., 2018). However, feedback tools are not without their drawbacks. Feedback measures may need to be recalibrated and contextualized to what is meaningful and important in clients' lives and recovery journeys. For instance, tracking depressive symptoms tells us how our client is feeling, but how they are doing in interactions with their spouse or children might be more relevant for them. We need to assess whether feedback systems allow clients to express what they found helpful or hindering, if they felt understood and safe with the therapist, and if they felt free to disagree. Therapists can also find feedback tools daunting, often feeling uncomfortable with the technology or viewing the process as tedious and time-consuming. To address these barriers, workplaces and training centres need to invest in the infrastructure and support required to use, interpret and apply feedback effectively. However, what is often overlooked is the time therapists need to review and process this feedback within their already busy schedules. When time and support are intentionally built in, feedback can become a meaningful tool for reflection, learning and professional growth.

Pause and reflect...

If you were setting up a group practice and wanted to implement the use of regular feedback tools, how would you introduce this idea to your therapists? What could you say to persuade them to try it out?

Each therapist can have different views about feedback systems and processes. Some may lean towards using a standard measure while others prefer to incorporate a more free-flowing questioning stance. It could be useful to consider a different style of eliciting feedback from the style of the theoretical framework we operate within. Therapists who use more structured and manualized forms of therapy may benefit from a more free-wheeling and conversational feedback system as that will enable discussions on areas that may otherwise not be addressed by the therapy. Therapists who practice more relational or long-term work could benefit from the structure and direction that a standardized measure provides. Some clients have shared that a narrow focus on symptoms and risks does not fully capture their overall sense of how they are doing (Moltu et al., 2018). Internal change may not always manifest as a symptom reduction or a discernible improvement in functioning. We do need to think about the ways in which we define client change, healing or recovery and the kind of feedback that best informs us about this. We know that progress in therapy, and significant shifts within individuals do not always proceed along expected trajectories. Of course, the very idea of a measurable outcome itself may be antithetical to some forms of therapy, and to some therapists.

The role of therapy is often to deepen the emotional field, creating spaces for clients to engage with difficult memories and complex, even contradictory emotions. Resolving or coming to terms with oneself is not always a linear experience and clients might have months of feeling hopeless or going around in circles before they experience a breakthrough. Perhaps the breakthrough is not even possible until they truly confront their unhappiness. This unhappiness or anger is often played out in the therapeutic relationship, and we evaluate it as progress when the client feels comfortable enough with us to express negative emotions. Additionally, each client presents individual patterns of pause and change; some experiencing a dramatic moment or a turning point while it is an evolving and insidious process for others. As therapists, some of us might prefer to understand and acknowledge these patterns rather than rush to intervene. We know that grieving takes time or that ruptures (and their repairs) often strengthen the therapeutic relationship, and we need to integrate this knowledge with our response to post-session feedback.

A black-box form of therapy, where we have no idea what to expect, is not good for clients, but perhaps neither is it always useful to expect clients to conform to a strict trajectory of change. Our clients (and us) will need time for ideas and experiences to ferment and percolate, even as we keep one eye on the overall progress in therapy. In understanding client progress, some therapists might value their intuition above data from a questionnaire, but it makes sense to be open to both sets of data, integrating information to form a more complete conceptualization.

What is clear is that we need to commit time towards this critical reflection on client feedback and remember that all of us can open such conversations with clients and supervisors, even if we do not use formal feedback measures. Therapists are still the gatekeepers who decide how much session time is spent on discussing feedback, and so we need to resolve our feelings about using this methodology. As we understand the theory (and research) behind feedback and begin to seek and use it more regularly, we can realize its value, both for the client in front of us and for others in the future.

Perspectives from the Consumer/Survivor/Carer Movement

It is time to listen and respond to the chorus of voices from clients who have formed a movement. This collective voice calls on mental health professionals to critically examine psychotherapy, its role in our clients' lives and within mental healthcare systems, as well as our responsibilities as psychotherapists. This perspective implies a shift in terminology, where the terms user or consumer (in place of client/patient) refer to people who are receiving mental health services. From this vantage point, therapists view clients as consumers, people who have rights, who expect high standards of service and who do not wish to be controlled by the systems that are meant to be serving them (McLeod, 2015). The term survivor is owned by people who critique and oppose the traditional mental health paradigms as damaging based on their experiences (Sweeney, 2016). Therapist–survivors who have been through psychological distress themselves are uniquely positioned to connect with their clients' experiences and to think more deeply about the kinds of therapists and therapy that are needed. Professionals also need to privilege the voice of carers, persons who have had close encounters with the mental healthcare systems, through the experience of caring for family members. Users/survivors/carers speak from varied standpoints, depending on whether they experienced treatment and care as helpful and affirming and where they felt that the mental health system let them down or was not able to meet their needs (Daya et al., 2020).

An awareness about user/survivor movements, both locally and around the world, can help us engage with the needs of marginalized groups. Users/survivors/carers from low resource contexts face difficulties related to access, affordability of treatments and associated loss of livelihood, in addition to mental health stigma. When these factors combine with the power differentials between users and service providers and the limited opportunities for decision-making, they form monumental barriers to working towards rights and advocacy (Samudre et al., 2016). It requires persistent and committed effort to overcome these barriers, but community-led programmes do exist and thrive around the world. There is a recognition that traditional mental health systems offer pills and psychotherapy, but communities also have needs for nutritious food, employment, safe spaces or legal aid. The principles of agency, choice and inclusion are reflected in the central role of peer and therapeutic support groups drawn from within the community.

As therapists we can find ways to learn from and contribute to the user/survivor movement and advocate for meaningful change. This movement has sparked reflections on the mental health terminology and language that we use, which is often disconnected from the preferences of persons with lived and living experience of mental health distress. Some might embrace the dominant mental health language, speaking of themselves as patients, framing their distress within diagnoses such as borderline personality disorder. Others may question psychiatric labels and biomedical discourse in an effort to shift the narrative towards greater inclusivity in mental healthcare. For instance, the language of psychosocial disabilities, in place of psychiatric terminology, is seen as allowing for deeper engagement with experiences of distress and social determinants of well-being. The framework of neurodiversity is increasingly being used to celebrate the strengths of persons with different ways of processing information and engaging with the world. As a movement, it seeks to interrogate the labelling of difference and the inequalities of power that are often embedded within mental healthcare systems. As therapists, we need to be led by our clients as there are no universals in terms of what terminology is seen as affirming. While several persons and organizations advocate for the use of person-first language (e.g., a person living with schizophrenia), some question the separation of the person from something that is so central to their identities and everyday experiences. Identity-first language (e.g., an autistic person) is seen as a way to preserve the right to define themselves and embrace their uniqueness. If we dismiss this as just semantics, this reflects the limits of our awareness and responsiveness to what our clients value. Words do matter and we are advised to take a cue from our clients and frame our communication in ways that make them feel listened to and affirmed. As we engage more closely with lived experience perspective, this propels us to shift our gaze and reflect both on our own value positions and on the larger mental health systems that our clients encounter. What is our position about diagnostic criteria and categories? How much do we know about user–survivor perspectives and their experiences with psychotherapy? How do we see our role as therapists? Is it to fix problems, people or systems? Where do we see change, healing and recovery located? And are we trying to answer these questions without input from the very people we are trying to serve?

Our willingness to question the paradigms we work within, engage in dialogue and partner with persons with lived experience and then look within ourselves can help us and our profession evolve. There is much to learn about what is valued, needed or missing in therapeutic spaces from two rich veins of knowledge—survivor research and mad studies (Faulkner, 2017). Persons with lived and living experience of psychosocial distress may ask different research questions, challenge predominantly biomedical illness models and use their collective power to expand the mental health knowledge base. The interdisciplinary field of mad studies is a radical reclaiming of the word 'mad' and combines theory, education and activism to counter the dominant discourse. Leading with the word mad has both a confrontational and emancipatory intent, and reflects a resistance movement against discrimination and towards equitable and compassionate systems of care.

A Lived Experience Advocate Speaks: The Power of our Stories

Grace Gatera

My family and I survived the 1994 genocide against the Tutsi by fleeing from Rwanda to Uganda. Some volunteer doctors came to the refugee camp and diagnosed some of us children with PTSD. But then they never came back. So, it became a sort of a friend that grows with you. Everyone who knew me could say, "Oh, Grace has 'trauma'." It was this invisible thing that we attributed many things to but was okay to ignore.

Later in boarding school, I would experience depression and intense panic disorder. But I was told – you don't have malaria or cholera… you are pretending to be sick or are demon possessed. And so, because I'm a child and am told adults know better, I also believed that. If even one person told me – "Listen, you're not alone. Other people face the same challenges, or there are other refugees who are going through the same thing at this moment"—I think that would have like transformed my entire life.

When I got to university, maybe because of all the unresolved trauma from the past - I fell apart. I tried to commit suicide - twice - before I finally decided to seek help. The religion-based para counselling I was offered felt inadequate. I cannot emphasize enough how much my 'village' of relatives, friends and school staff helped me. Every time my aunt spoke to me well, every time my parents called me and said, "We love you", or every time my friend said, "You know, can we go to this together?", I felt more human. On my return to Rwanda after completing my degree (at that time it was the hardest thing I had ever done), I wanted to start over - but had a debilitating, depressive episode where I stayed in and shut myself down. It took a while to find a psychiatrist and a therapist to help me, but I was determined not to be defeated anymore.

After a break, I began working at a radio station in Rwanda that played contemporary music. While my task was to just make sure that the airwaves were always occupied, there was a lot of space to do whatever I wanted. I started a small speaking show and began talking about myself in those hours between 11p.m. and 3 a.m. – about feminism and why it saved me, about my mental health challenges and about growing up as a refugee. This was really cathartic in itself. Listeners would tune in and send messages – "I've been there, I'm a survivor myself!" My family and I started holding small retreats for other survivors like me, and these have become the highlight of my life. We played games, sang together, chatted and bonded. We saw for the first time, women sharing their survivor stories, crying from the center of their souls, shedding years and years of pain and suffering. I felt like I had finally come home and found my tribe.

At this time in 2018, a researcher from the Lancet Commission on Global Mental Health and Sustainable Development, who had heard my radio show contacted me, asking if I was interested in working with them. This took me to this Global Ministerial Conference in the UK. That's the very first time that I heard the words 'lived experience'! The biggest thing that I learned was that there were terms for *everything* that I had been through. I was not alone at all. Even the Lancet Commission was saying that mental health care had to be more focused on the rest of the global majority. And I was like, "Yes! There has to be less pain for kids who grew up like me, who grew up as a third culture."

These new opportunities opened up a new world for me - as a UNICEF Young ambassador working for young people's mental health, with Wellcome Trust and speaking at so many conferences. I have taught at Oxford and University College London. I also worked with the World Health Organization, the African Union Youth Envoy, and with Lancet Commissions on gender-based violence and depression (which was really personal), among other incredible life changing opportunities.

In all of these spaces, what we people with lived experience bring is the authenticity of our experience and the richness of expertise. Because it's firsthand, it's raw. And the thing about people who live the experience is that they can be trained to know the (mental health) language but you cannot recreate or duplicate authentic experience - so it cannot go the other way! What people with lived experience want is better services and better attention to what we are saying. We are a wide universe of people, some with lived experience that they are willing to use for expertise, and some who do not want formal roles and want their stories to remain theirs. We *all* deserve to join the field and have a say in constructing inclusive and ethical mental health services.

My work of traveling, speaking and sharing had become tiring at a point. The respect that came out of it had diminished, and it seemed like change was too slow. Sometimes, it felt like people were using our story at conferences to sort of 'other' us - to be the token 'lived experience person'. But now it feels that the role of lived experience is expanding. We have to do more, but we can only have an impactful future if experts by experience are co-producing, co-designing and co-creating funded research - when we have an immovable, unshakeable seat at the table.

What I remain passionate about is where I started. I really love sharing my story. I love connecting to other people with lived experience across the world – and that is a story in itself.

Grace Gatera is a *lived experience mental health advocate, living in Kigali, Rwanda. She is passionate about the key role of lived experience in creating a more knowledgeable and equitable mental health science.*

Completing the Circle: Client Contributions to Personal and Professional Growth

Working closely with clients as they change and grow is transformational for therapists in many ways. When psychotherapists across the world were asked to reflect on the strongest influence on their professional growth and development, it was their experiences with clients that emerged as the resounding verdict (Orlinsky et al., 2001). The everyday activity of donning the shoes of many different people can encourage the exploration of different ways of being (Kottler & Hunter, 2010). The moments when we feel stuck, have an emotionally charged session, experience a breakthrough with a client or face client dropout all offer potent opportunities for reflection and learning. Most therapists can recall at least one instance where a client's words or actions challenged assumptions or prompted a modification of therapeutic practice.

Therapists forge their professional identity through experiences with clients. This development occurs gradually, as skills and techniques are honed, feelings are attended to, missteps are reflected upon, and a realistic acceptance of the nature of change is embraced. Witnessing clients' journeys through pain, suffering, healing and growth often stimulates deep reflection within the therapist. This process not only expands professional capacities but also invites confrontation with the therapist's own self and engagement with broader questions of life and meaning (Hatcher et al., 2012). When we sit before a client who is having thoughts of self-harm, we might say that we learnt how to assess risk, how to create a safety plan and how it could be individualized. In those moments, however, we also learn to sit with distress, realize how anchoring it can be to be in the presence of another, accept that it is okay to talk openly about death and dying and experience how we can find the courage to go on even amidst great pain.

Pause and reflect…

Pause here to recollect the interactions with any one of your clients who had a significant impact on you. This could be someone who you met years ago but will never forget or someone you saw more recently.

Reflect on what you have learnt from this client—as a therapist, and as a person.

An interesting question you can ask yourself is:

In seeing my client change (or not change), have I also changed in any way?

Being a therapist requires us to think deeply about ourselves and reflect on how our feelings and experiences impact the process of therapy. Through this work, we discover and use different parts of ourselves in an ongoing process of making meaning. While some parts are challenged others may be reinforced. Our limitations and blind spots are likely to get exposed through our therapeutic interactions, and sometimes clients bring this to light quite directly. As we understand that we can be perfectly imperfect and still help our clients, this can percolate into other areas of our life as well, deepening our appreciation of what it feels like to struggle with ourselves, confront challenges or celebrate small victories. This growth may loop back into our interactions and our expectations of clients, therapists and the therapy process itself.

We work closely with clients who grapple with painful unerasable memories, loneliness, limited choices and mortality. Deliberations on such existential themes might trigger personal reflections on how we view our own life and make meaning of our existence. These glimpses of the dark side of the moon can bring an acceptance of limitations, ambiguity, uncertainty and incompleteness as a part of life while simultaneously making therapists aware of unexpected possibilities and choices (Bugental, 1991). We may notice something new or different in our lives, appreciate our blessings or become more open to new experiences. At times, when our personal struggles mirror a client's challenges, their courage and resilience can stimulate reflection and inspire us to try something different. Kottler describes this experience beautifully, "The more I confronted my clients about the ways they were inflicting misery on themselves, the more I had to look at the ways I was doing the same thing" (Kottler & Hunter, 2010, p. 10). Client stories can also bring about major transformations in our world view as we better understand the roles that love, success, humility or hard work can play in our overall satisfaction with life.

Our interactions with clients may have a strong impact on our relational selves as well. Therapists have described how they were able to value relationships that offered love and care, acknowledge their own need for support and find new ways to relate to their children and grandchildren by expressing previously suppressed parts of themselves (Hatcher et al., 2012). In seeing our clients and their struggles in relationships, we may also learn what not to do. Our constant exposure to the inner workings of the human mind can help us to feel less anger or blame in interpersonal situations as we evolve an understanding of why people do what they do. For instance, seeing the fear behind selfishness or the inadequacy that underlies control can change the way we look at selfish or controlling people in our lives. In parallel, seeing the interpersonal impact of selfishness or control can strengthen our determination to be different in our personal lives.

Clients also teach us to view the world in different ways. In inviting us into their lives, they expose us to new ideas, asking us to read about spiritual or self-care practices they may be interested in or telling us about activities, podcasts, books or resources they might have been influenced or inspired by. In our roles as therapists, we encounter individuals we might never have met otherwise, coming from diverse cultures, social backgrounds, occupations and communities. This exposure can help us shed prejudices, appreciate the value of diversity in religious beliefs or life choices and develop a nuanced and informed perspective on how we position ourselves in the world.

While no definitive map exists for integrating clinical experience and personal growth, reflecting on how clients touch our lives, who we become in their presence and what this makes possible outside the therapy room offers significant benefits. Sometimes an understanding arises through intentional reflection, while at other times, insights emerge spontaneously as a-ha moments. These learnings can be deepened and clarified through practices such as journaling, supervision and other reflective activities that encourage ongoing self-awareness and professional development.

Pause and reflect…
Reflect on your experiences with clients in your practice over time.

What are the most significant lessons you have learned about life and about what works in therapy?

Platforms where master therapists share the wisdom and life lessons they have gained from their interactions with clients could inspire many of us to reflect on our own experiences more intentionally. We certainly do not have to wait years before looking back on what we have learned from our clients. These sometimes ineffable learnings begin from the first day we sit in the therapist's chair, with some of our earliest encounters leaving powerful and lasting impacts. If more therapists spoke openly with each other about what they absorb from clients, the mutual flow of learning between therapist and client might feel more natural.

Perspectives on Training and Development

Development of Therapist Skills and Systems for Integrating Client Feedback

Encouraging comprehensive assessments that focus on clients' preferences, strengths and resources might foster a stance of learning from clients. Client feedback methods can augment supervision and track needs for additional supervisory inputs. Training programmes and practice settings can promote guidelines and systems for eliciting and incorporating client feedback, along with space for reflections and explorations about these feedback systems and processes. With trainees who are learning skills and growing into their therapist roles, it is important to think about the ways in which they would receive and respond to client feedback and address their responses in scaffolded supervisory spaces. Perhaps, therapists prefer to think of themselves as the experts in the room and are reluctant to be exposed to feedback that may not match their expectations or impressions. Effective implementation of client feedback systems outside of research projects calls for adequate attention to these attitudinal and emotional barriers.

Therapist Engagement with User–Survivor Perspectives, Movements and Advocacy

We strongly recommend exposure to user–survivor perspectives and movements as a part of the curriculum and training processes across the mental health disciplines. For these perspectives to be truly integrated into professional discourse, user-survivor-carer voices need to be embedded across the curriculum, into textbooks and resource materials and teaching–learning processes. Trainees can be encouraged to attend conferences and be part of other spaces where they can share and learn from clients as stakeholders. When trainees are introduced to best practice guidelines for user-survivor-carer involvement in mental health service design, delivery and evaluation (e.g., National Institute for Health and Care Excellence [NICE], 2019), they are exposed to a more person-centred and inclusive approach to mental healthcare.

Meaningful engagement with clients' lives and realities requires understanding their distress beyond symptoms and diagnostic labels, looking beyond the therapy room into their sociocultural and political contexts. A range of reflective, creative and experiential approaches, both within classroom and real-world community settings, can support trainees' engagement with advocacy and social action. Trainees can be sensitized to issues of social justice, power and context in their case conceptualizations and therapeutic interactions. As practitioners, a commitment to advocacy and social action involves expanding professional roles, with engagement possible either within traditional mental healthcare systems or outside them. This may include efforts to connect clients with legal, educational or economic resources, or collaborating with civil society organizations that operate within rights-based frameworks. Involvement can also extend to supporting policy changes at various levels; for example, developing sliding scale fee policies within organizations, consulting with government bodies to strengthen community-based care in underserved areas or advocating for legal and policy reforms.

Involvement of Service Users in Mental Health Education, Training and Research

At one level, engagement with service users can provide an understanding of lived experiences that are not represented in textbooks. There is potential for various levels of involvement: curriculum consultation, development of learning material, teaching and educational roles, trainee selection and assessment of training courses and modules. Inclusive models that embed the voices of service users and carers in mental health training are certainly not universal practices and can require a revisioning of training frameworks. An exemplar, *Recovery Colleges* in the UK offer free skill-based learnings courses to persons who use mental health services. What is unique is that experts by experience work as peer support workers in collaboration with persons with professional mental health training to develop and deliver these courses. While this is a laudable initiative, with the potential to scale-up across several recovery-oriented mental health services, co-created research on the cost-effectiveness, mechanisms of action and the accompanying challenges and opportunities can help strengthen this further (Van Wezel et al., 2023).

User-led or survivor research, user-controlled research and service user involvement in research are important emerging trends. There is a shift from brief involvement or consultations to one of co-production, where mental health service users may be involved in multiple ways in an equal partnership, from defining research priorities to designing and implementing the study and to the dissemination of findings (Rose & Kalathil, 2019). Training is often required to increase familiarity with participatory frameworks and iterative processes in co-designing interventions to ensure ethical and meaningful engagement for all stakeholders.

Building a democratic and participatory research process comes with multiple challenges, including deeply embedded power dynamics and structural barriers. These challenges may be accentuated in countries with hierarchical social structures and high mental health stigma and where user–survivor movements are still mobilizing. Even in contexts where the voices of service users are heard, researchers need to reflect about whether marginalized perspectives within user groups are included and valued (Rose & Kalathil, 2019). If mental health practitioners want to co-produce research with user–survivors, this first requires introspection on how democratic we are in the therapy room, the ways in which we attend to client priorities and empowerment and how much we typically engage with structural and systemic contributors to distress. Building capacity may become necessary, and guidelines from the Wellcome Trust offer valuable direction on embedding lived experience throughout all stages and domains of research, across diverse cultures and contexts (Wellcome, n.d).

Building a Stronger Research Base on Client Perspectives About Psychotherapy

We advocate a greater focus on the client in psychotherapy research so we can come closer to understanding why therapies and techniques work differently across clients, how therapeutic change occurs and the ways in which it may be obstructed. Goldfried (2019) recommends that therapists attend to a range of key client variables including their self-awareness of difficulties and possible change pathways, motivations for and expectations from therapy. These findings can be used to build empirical evidence that can inform therapeutic practice. The use of diverse research designs to examine clients' perspectives and lived experiences, including qualitative approaches and observational studies, can narrow the gap between research and practice. While there are several informative studies, there is less information on how we can integrate each perspective into our therapeutic approach. Ultimately, incorporating clients' voices into the research landscape not only enriches the understanding of psychotherapy but also ensures that treatment aligns more closely with what clients truly value.

Conclusion

Learning from clients implies seeing them as equal participants while taking responsibility for our role as co-travellers on the path of therapy—sometimes guiding and sometimes following. This perspective has already led to marked shifts in how we view therapy and how we offer services. We look forward to the next steps in this area.

References

Angus, L., & Scott Mio, J. (2011). At the "heart of the matter": Understanding the importance of emotion-focused metaphors in patient illness narratives. *Genre, 44*(3), 349–361.

Bhola, P., & Chaturvedi, S. K. (2017). Through a glass, darkly: Ethics of mental health practitioner-patient relationships in traditional societies. *International Journal of Culture and Mental Health, 10*(3), 285–297.

Bohart, A. C. (2000). The client is the most important common factor: Clients' self-healing capacities and psychotherapy. *Journal of Psychotherapy Integration, 10*, 127–149.

Brattland, H., Høiseth, J. R., Burkeland, O., Inderhaug, T. S., Binder, P. E., & Iversen, V. C. (2018). Learning from clients: A qualitative investigation of psychotherapists' reactions to negative verbal feedback. *Psychotherapy Research, 28*(4), 545–559.

Bugental, J. F. T. (1991). Lessons clients each therapists. *Journal of Humanistic Psychology, 31*(3), 28–32.

Cooper, M., & Norcross, J. C. (2016). A brief, multidimensional measure of clients' therapy preferences: The Cooper–Norcross Inventory of Preferences (C-NIP). *International Journal of Clinical and Health Psychology, 16*(1), 87–98.

Cooper, M., Di Malta, G., Knox, S., Oddli, H. W., & Swift, J. K. (2023). Patient perspectives on working with preferences in psychotherapy: A consensual qualitative research study. *Psychotherapy Research, 33*(8), 1117–1131.

Daya, I., Hamilton, B., & Roper, C. (2020). Authentic engagement: A conceptual model for welcoming diverse and challenging consumer and survivor views in mental health research, policy, and practice. *International Journal of Mental Health Nursing, 29*, 299–350.

Duncan, B. L., & Miller, S. D. (2000). The client's theory of change: Consulting the client in the integrative process. *Journal of Psychotherapy Integration, 10*(2), 169–187.

Faulkner, A. (2017). Survivor research and mad studies: The role and value of experiential knowledge in mental health research. *Disability & Society, 32*(4), 500–520.

Goldfried, M. R. (2019). Obtaining consensus in psychotherapy: What holds us back? *American Psychologist, 74*(4), 484–496.

Haber, R., Carlson, R. G., & Braga, C. (2014). Use of an anecdotal client feedback note in family therapy. *Family Process, 53*, 307–317.

Hatcher, S. L., Kipper-Smith, A., Waddell, M., Uhe, M., West, J. S., Boothe, J. H., Frye, J. M., Tighe, K., Usselman, K. L., & Gingras, P. (2012). What therapists learn from psychotherapy clients: effects on personal and professional lives. *The Qualitative Report, 17*(48), 1–21.

Kottler, J. A., & Hunter, S. V. (2010). Clients as teachers: Reciprocal influences in therapy relationships. *The Australia and New Zealand Journal of Family Therapy, 31*(1), 4–12.

Lambert, M. J. (2015). Progress feedback and the OQ system: The past and the future. *Psychotherapy, 52*(4), 381–390.

Lambert, M. J., Kahler, M., Harmon, C., Burlingame, G. M., Shimokawa, K., & White, M. M. (2013). *Administration and scoring manual: Outcome Questionnaire OQ® 45.2.* OQ Measures.

Lambert, M. J., Whipple, J. L., & Kleinstäuber, M. (2018). Collecting and delivering progress feedback: A meta-analysis of routine outcome monitoring. *Psychotherapy, 55*(4), 520–537.

McLeod, J. (2013). Developing pluralistic practice in counselling and psychotherapy: Using what the client knows. *The European Journal of Counselling Psychology, 2*(1), 51–64.

McLeod, J. (2015). Client preferences: Building bridges between therapy and everyday life. *Psychotherapy and Counselling Journal of Australia, 3*(1), Retrieved from https://pacja.org.au/2015/07/client-preferences-building-bridges-between-therapy-and-everyday-life-2/

Miller, S. D., & Duncan, B. L. (2004). *The outcome and session rating scales: Administration and scoring manual.* Institute for the Study of Therapeutic Change.

Moltu, C., Veseth, M., Stefansen, J., Nøtnes, J. C., Skjølberg, A., Binder, P., Castonguay, L. G., & Nordberg, S. S. (2018). This is what I need a clinical feedback system to do for me: A qualitative inquiry into therapists' and patients' perspectives. *Psychotherapy Research, 28*(20), 250–263.

National Institute for Health and Care Excellence (NICE). (2019). *Service user experience in adult mental health: Improving the experience of care for people using adult NHS mental health services* (NICE guideline CG136). https://www.nice.org.uk/guidance/cg136

Oanes, C. J., Borg, M., & Karlsson, B. (2015). Significant conversations or reduced relational capacity? Exploring couple and family therapists' expectations for including a client feedback procedure. *Australian and New Zealand Journal of Family Therapy, 36*(3), 342–355.

Orlinsky, D. E., Botermans, J.-F., & Rønnestad, M. H. (2001). Towards an empirically grounded model of psychotherapy training: Four thousand therapists rate influences on their development. *Australian Psychologist, 36*(2), 139–148.

Reese, R. J., Slone, N. C., & Miserocchi, K. M. (2013). Using client feedback in psychotherapy from an interpersonal process perspective. *Psychotherapy (Chicago, Ill.), 50*(3), 288–291.

Reese, R. J., Usher, E. L., Bowman, D. C., Norsworthy, L. A., Halstead, J. L., Rowlands, S. R., & Chisholm, R. R. (2009). Using client feedback in psychotherapy training: An analysis of its influence on supervision and counselor self-efficacy. *Training and Education in Professional Psychology, 3*(3), 157–168.

Rose, D., & Kalathil, J. (2019). Power, privilege and knowledge: The untenable promise of co-production in mental "health." *Frontiers in Sociology, 4*, 57.

Samudre, S., Shidhaye, R., Ahuja, S., Nanda, S., Khan, A., Evans-Lacko, S., & Hanlon, C. (2016). Service user involvement for mental health system strengthening in India: A qualitative study. *BMC Psychiatry, 16*, 269.

Sweeney, A. (2016). Why mad studies needs survivor research and survivor research needs mad studies. *Intersectionalities: A Global Journal of Social Work Analysis, Research, Polity, and Practice, 5*(3), 36–61.

Tolkein, J. R. R. (1994). *The lord of the rings*. Houghton Mifflin.

Van Wezel, M. M. C., Muusse, C., van de Mheen, D., et al. (2023). What do we not know (yet) about recovery colleges? A study protocol on their (cost-)effectiveness, mechanisms of action, fidelity and positioning. *BMC Psychiatry, 23*, 816. https://doi.org/10.1186/s12888-023-05293-8

Wagener, A. E. (2017). Metaphor in professional counseling. *The Professional Counselor, 7*(2), 144–154.

Wellcome. (n.d.). *Embedding lived experience expertise in mental health research.* https://wellcome.org/grant-funding/guidance/embedding-lived-experience-expertise-mental-health-research

Yalom, I. D., & Elkin, G. (1974). *Every day gets a little closer: A twice-told therapy.* Basic Books.

Chapter 10
Bringing Reflective Practice into Supervision

In the Grimm's fairy tale *Snow-White*, there is a magic mirror that sees all and speaks only the truth. We too, have questions about ourselves and need a mirror we can trust—one that reveals what we cannot always see on our own. When therapists feel the need to understand their work or themselves more deeply, it is their supervisor they turn to as their mirror on the wall. The supervisee deconstructs their experiences in therapy, exploring what transpired with the client while observing their own thoughts, feelings and actions. The focus of the exploration moves back and forth between existing theories and personal experience, sometimes being more analytical or critical and sometimes more intuitive and personal. Conversations we may have only had with ourselves, our half-formed thoughts and impressions, may become clearer to us in the process of thinking through these experiences with a supervisor. The presence of a supportive other enables reflection to unfold at the deepest levels. The reflective self-awareness that emerges can help us move beyond didactic knowledge and get closer to the essence of the therapeutic encounter.

In a reflective approach to supervision, the emphasis is not only on ensuring that the supervisee responds appropriately to the client, but also on supporting the development of their capacity for reflection. The supervisor models how one can think and feel their way through the therapeutic process, using reflective capacities to understand and make decisions about how to move the work forward. Through this act of shared reflection, both supervisor and supervisee encounter the inner workings of each other's minds, coming into contact with new ways of thinking, feeling, being and making meaning. Both must be willing to leave things open, as neither gains the satisfaction of complete clarity or even certainty about what to do next. This requires a certain amount of trust from both sides. The supervisor needs to trust and respect the supervisee as a developing therapist and the supervisee needs to trust that the field they have been left to play in is both boundaried and secure. Traditional methods of supervision that focus on teaching and monitoring are invaluable and form the basis of any supervisory practice…but it is in the open spaces created by reflective supervision that the supervisee can really grow and come into their own.

P. Bhola et al., *Reflective Practice in Psychotherapy and Counselling*,
https://doi.org/10.1007/978-981-96-9732-8_10

In this chapter, we highlight the role of supervision in providing the structure and support needed to facilitate reflective practice. Within this space, supervisees can identify their needs and expectations from supervision, and supervisors are invited to reflect on their own growth and development. The chapter explores the supervisee–supervisor relationship, and spotlights varied supervisory methods, tools and processes.

The Reflective Journey: Being a Supervisor and Supervisee

Being a therapist involves a high degree of responsibility. We need to appear competent in the session, regulate our own emotions and be cautious about using the right words at the right time. Sometimes though, we need a space where we can be unsure or unguarded, trusting that someone else will look out for us. This is a space that supervision may provide, with supervisors holding the frame within which we can share our strengths and vulnerabilities. In the process, we can learn how to be more effective as therapists. Supervision is also a space for reflecting on the application of theory and technique in clinical work. The supervisor and supervisee undertake the journey of supervision together, bringing a readiness to co-reflect and learn together.

Framing the Supervision Contract

The initial conversation between supervisor and supervisee typically focuses on the supervisee's goals and establishes both the supervisory contract and the nature of the relationship. The supervisor seeks to understand the supervisees' stage of professional development, nature of practice, their needs related to knowledge and skills and, of course, their expectations regarding reflective processes and methods (Orchowski et al., 2010). Initially, supervisees will want to know what reflective supervision is about and clarify their assumptions and expectations about reflective work. At this stage, setting up a supervision contract, where the goals, individual responsibilities, meeting schedules, documentation methods, boundaries, confidentiality and payment (if any) are discussed and listed, can ensure clarity (Ellis, 2017). The frame may need to be occasionally renegotiated as supervisee needs evolve.

Commitment to defined and protected time for supervision sessions is essential. This ensures that both supervisor and supervisee are able to engage fully in the process without feeling rushed or narrowly focused on the immediate tasks of upcoming therapy sessions. For those affiliated with a training institute, programme requirements for supervision can significantly influence the structure and frequency of sessions. These requirements may dictate the minimum hours of supervision needed each month, the types of documentation required (e.g., case notes, reflective logs or feedback forms) and any formal assessments that guide the supervisee's progress.

Pause and reflect...
What are you bringing to the table—as a supervisor or as a supervisee?

Consider what your counterpart might need to know about you—your stance, strengths, needs and foibles—so that you can work together effectively.

Preparation for Supervision

When we first enter supervision, there is often a mix of anticipation and anxiety. While there is eagerness to learn, it may be accompanied by concerns about receiving feedback and potential evaluation. To create a constructive environment, the supervisor and supervisee can collaboratively agree on how feedback will be shared and establish clear pathways for addressing any difficulties that arise during supervision. Some supervisees may prefer more guidance, with a clear structure and well-articulated goals, while others may be looking for a partner to explore with.

We need to thoughtfully plan the materials and the questions we wish to bring into the supervision discussion. While on-the-spot reflections have their place, using process notes or audio and video recordings carry certain advantages. Discussing process notes might help get an in-depth understanding of the therapeutic process the content of discussions and interactions as well as the therapist's internal feelings, thoughts, desires, fantasies and bodily reactions. These detailed narrative accounts are best documented soon after the session in a 'She said, I said' format (Wideman, 2019). Although maintaining process notes can be time-consuming, they bring us closer to understanding inner and relational processes, helping us become more aware of the moment-to-moment choices, actions and reactions that can enhance our reflective work.

Supervisors invite reflection by asking questions like, "What are you hoping to develop at this stage?" or "Where do you feel most uncertain in your work?" Through such dialogue, they help clarify the supervisee's current training goals and foster a sense of ownership in professional development. Supervisees who complete some preparatory reading and come in with specific questions and learning goals, stand to gain more from supervision. In terms of knowledge inputs, supervisees might have questions like, "Could you tell me how I could develop a safety plan for a client experiencing intimate partner violence?" or "What theories could I read to understand more about my client's grief reactions?" Skill-based queries may include, "Could you review my session transcript and provide feedback on how I have used Socratic dialogue to challenge this cognitive distortion?" or "What reflection could I have used here?" Discussions around challenging situations, especially those related to the client relationship or emotions triggered during the session, can deepen our understanding of the therapeutic process. Some examples of reflective questions would be, "I wanted to discuss this, because I feel termination is difficult for me"; "Can you share some ideas about how to avoid giving advice when clients keep asking?"; "Could you help me explore the anger that I am feeling towards the client's parents?" Supervisees may also articulate some of their ethical dilemmas and look to supervisors to guide them through the complex decision-making process. A supervise might share, "A client brought a gift for me, and I just could not say no!" or bring in questions such as, "Should I call a client if they have missed a session?" or "Should I continue work with a client after I leave the organization?" As supervisors, we can ensure that our supervisee's queries are heard and addressed, while prioritizing what might be important for them and their growth.

Our needs as supervisees are dynamic. At times we may require more structure and guidance, while at other moments, we benefit from encouragement to take risks or explore the unfamiliar (Bhola et al., 2017). In a reflective account, Ahluwalia (2019) shared how her supervisor failed to see beyond her façade of confidence and, as a result, offered less direction. This allowed her to remain unchallenged and emotionally protected as a trainee therapist, skimming the surface of the therapeutic relationship with her client. A subsequent supervisory relationship gently disrupted this pattern, creating space for deeper reflection on her sense of self, theoretical preferences and the emotional complexities of the therapeutic encounter. As supervisors, it is essential to stay attuned to each trainee's developmental stage and to meet them where they are. This requires an individualized approach that considers the supervisee's evolving needs, rather than relying on assumptions based on their level of training or academic background. Ongoing assessment of competencies and learning edges can help ensure that supervisory support remains aligned with the supervisee's zone of proximal development (Vygotsky, 1978).

As we grow as therapists, we learn to tolerate ambiguity and view ourselves and our sessions from more than one perspective. In response to this growth, effective supervisors begin to delve deeper into emotional experiences and their underlying explanations, posing constructive challenges or offering meta-perspectives that foster reflection and development (Ladany et al., 2013). For example, a supervisee working with a client who repeatedly avoids emotional topics may initially feel frustrated, interpreting the avoidance as resistance or failure. A supervisor, attuned to the supervisee's emotional reaction, might ask, "What does the avoidance evoke in you?" and "How do you feel about it?" This question invites the supervisee to reflect not only on the client's behaviour but also on their own emotional responses and assumptions. As the learning environment adapts to each supervisee's evolving needs, it is important to recognize that these needs can shift over time, across different domains of work or even within a single session (Borders, 2014).

When supervisor and supervisee theoretical orientations match, reflection can more easily centre on model-specific concepts. However, if they are aligned to different theoretical orientations, they can create some space for these diverse viewpoints. Reflecting together on the meanings and imperatives from each orientation, and seeing where they merge and differ, can help understand common underlying processes while experiencing the unique flavour of each orientation. The supervisor will need to be careful to present their ideas in such a way that they do not overwhelm the supervisee's conceptual framework, but rather support and expand it. The supervisee also then gets the opportunity to hold more than one perspective and reflect on their personal relationship with their orientation.

As supervisors, we can also benefit from reflecting on our own cultural background, along with that of the supervisee and client (when possible) and determine what style of supervision might be a better fit (Orchowski et al., 2010). Our social location influences our lived experiences, and being aware of aspects such as race, ethnicity, religious affiliations, class and caste can increase sensitivity to differences and power imbalances. In preparation for supervision, we can bring our locations and their possible interactions to our minds, even if we do not discuss them immediately. These are not easy conversations to have, and a deeper exploration of similarities, differences and bridges can take time to evolve. The supervisor sets the initial expectations by inviting such conversations and the supervisee can accept this invitation when they feel safe and ready.

Our early experiences in supervision deeply impact if we continue to seek supervision over time and even how we eventually supervise others. Given how crucial the supervisory experience is to therapist learning and development, we cannot overstate the need for preparation and consideration before embarking on this journey.

Pause and reflect...

Think about one of your better supervision experiences.

Describe your supervisor's approach and what they did to make it work for you.

As a supervisee, what did *you* bring to supervision that made it a positive experience?

A Safe Space for Reflection

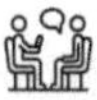

Inga had recently experienced a series of worrying dropouts and brought these concerns to Kvame, her supervisor. "Dropouts do happen, even when we try our best" Kvame said ruefully. Inga settled into the chair and felt her shoulders relax. Kvame then shared his own experience with drop out. He described a client who he felt very tuned into and who initially responded well. However, after several months of working on improving her functioning, she unexpectedly stopped coming for therapy. Inga leaned forward, sharing how she was left feeling like a bad therapist when her client dropped out. Kvame acknowledged that this was a difficult feeling and invited her to stay with the experience. They began to speak about how global self-criticism

was not useful. Instead, gently exploring specific blind spots could help us grow. Kwame shared his reflections again, "I realised I am quite sensitive about being liked ... so when my clients seem to like me, I assume that therapy is going well. This time though, it was because she liked me that my client found it hard to express how sessions were no longer meeting her needs—a nuance that I clearly missed".

Supervision is a unique space indeed. One where we are not just allowed but actively encouraged to dwell on something that is close to our hearts, yet immensely private - what happened in the session and what happened to *us* in the session. This is something we may find ourselves unable to share with either our clients or our friends. As the vignette suggests, when a supervisor responds with empathy, perhaps even sharing a story about their own difficulties as a therapist, this can help supervisees circumvent feelings of shame and become more open to reflecting on their vulnerabilities. When the inevitable vulnerabilities of supervisees intersect with a supervisory stance which is experienced as unsupportive, distant or evaluative, it can intensify fears of being judged as inadequate (both as a person and as a therapist). Such experiences further inhibit disclosures and eventually block progress in supervision. Ultimately, it is the quality of the relationship between supervisor and supervisee that lies at the heart of effective supervision. When the alliance is robust, this creates a safe space that helps supervisees access and discuss aspects of their experience that might otherwise remain hidden - subtle moments in therapy or deeper anxieties about self.

Building a supervisory alliance is not vastly different from building a therapeutic alliance and this process requires ongoing attention. If the supervisor notices a disconnect between their expectations of the supervisory process or senses a distance or disruption in the relational atmosphere, a gentle, open and direct enquiry can be helpful. For example, "This discussion didn't seem to go very well for you. Can we talk about what's happening?" This approach reflects an openness to reviewing the process, as well as a commitment to making it meaningful for the supervisee. Even a strong initial alliance can break down, and difficult moments can leave either supervisor or supervisee feeling let down or hurt. Supervisee needs often evolve over time, requiring supervisors to remain attuned to moment-to-moment shifts in the relationship. Both supervisees who seem hurried and disconnected, as well as those who only share positive stories, may prompt questions about the strength of the alliance. How we respond to these potential ruptures significantly influences the overall strength of the supervisory relationship. Supervisors who allow space for disagreement, acknowledge their own limitations and stay caring and respectful of their supervisees, are likely to do better.

The culture of supervision is embedded in institutional, professional and societal hierarchies, and these power structures can form barriers to the creation of a safe environment. Therapists first encounter supervision in the training phase, when the inequalities of knowledge and status are most prominent. This often leaves supervisees hesitant to open up, fearing that revealing their uncertainties will expose their perceived inadequacies. This sword cuts both ways, however, and supervisors can feel disempowered when they do not have the answers or insights they are expected to have. A sense of inadequacy can be triggered when a supervisee asks difficult or challenging questions, brings in a complex presentation like dissociative identity disorder or uses a theoretical lens that the supervisor is less familiar with. If they get absorbed in their own discomfort, the supervisor can miss the supervisee's underlying struggle, thereby losing the opportunity to help them work through their doubts.

We recommend a self-reflective process to help identify both the subtle and more overt expressions of our own needs for power and control. This reflection can prompt us to consider which emotions we are comfortable with our supervisees expressing—and which emotions we feel more at ease showing ourselves (e.g., "You can cry, but I would rather not…"). Supervisors who are attuned to their own interpersonal drivers (e.g., "I need to be respected") are also better equipped to recognize when these drivers are triggered during the supervision session (McMahon, 2020). While power imbalances exist globally, cultural notions of deference towards authority figures, particularly in collectivistic cultures like India, may lend the supervisory relationship a more formal tone. As supervisors, we can address this inherent hierarchy directly and strive to cultivate an environment where trainees feel safe to question perspectives, express opposing views and acknowledge their vulnerabilities (Bhola et al., 2017; Duggal et al., 2022).

When both parties acknowledge that, at its best, psychotherapy is an honest experiment, with several possible right answers and true paths, this sets the stage for deeper reflections. Supervisors can actively share their power with supervisees by inviting their input, for example, by saying, "You are the one who has actually experienced the therapy space, and you are the expert on the client… so, do you think this approach will work?" Power is also shared when supervisors acknowledge the limits of their knowledge, whether in case presentations, diagnoses or therapy modalities. Supervisors who share fleeting impressions, strong emotions and nascent thoughts, rather than offering clear-cut answers, foster an environment where supervisees feel excited to explore. This collaborative dynamic between supervisor and supervisee enables open expression of disagreement and the exchange of feedback in both directions.

A Supervisor Speaks: **Supervision Is about Creating Safety**

Maitri Chand

Supervision is not teaching, and supervision is not making a young therapist a clone of yourself. Supervision is about creating safety for therapists to become comfortable with 'not knowing' so that they may cultivate an open learning stance. This helps them to figure out who they are as therapists and helps them take steps towards what may appear scary in the therapy room as well as in their inner worlds. Early in their career, therapists feel overly concerned about helping their clients 'feel better in therapy' or ending the session on a particular note (whatever that is). Sitting with our own discomfort around client stories and emotions, as well as our own emotions in the therapy room comes from experience that the supervisor can encourage.

In my supervision work, I encourage my supervisees to explore this discomfort, especially in their own families of origin. For instance, we explore when and where in their families of origin they feel the need to 'fix' things and/or people. Or when and how they (or are expected to) help people feel better. These are challenging questions and reflecting on them in supervision is a safe way to build supervisees capacity to remain with their clients' emotional states during sessions. When supervisors express a curiosity about their supervisees, it enables supervisees to do the same for themselves, and for their clients. Whatever the tools and skills may be, I cannot emphasize enough how none of it matters if the supervisor is unable to first create a safe space. Beyond any supervision methods, a supervisor must support their supervisee's vulnerabilities and help them figure out who they want to be as therapists.

Dr Maitri Chand *is a systemic family therapist and supervisor, and Clinical Assistant Professor at Mercer University Medical School, Macon, USA. She currently has a private practice in New Delhi.*

The Supervisor's Toolkit

Reflective supervision is a process of questioning, and the questions we ask ourselves and each other can arise from many sources—from clients, peers, supervisors and supervisees. It can be a slow process, one marked by contemplation and long pauses, often with few immediate answers to our questions. Davys and Beddoe (2009, 2020) provide us a reflective learning model, beginning with identifying the event to be considered, moving on to the process of exploration, followed by experimentation in the session and ending with a shared evaluation.

Telling the Story

A supervision session usually starts with the question, "What should we talk about today?" Focusing on a key priority area, question or concern is useful, as it creates a goal and a frame for the reflections. These may be moments that evoke intense emotions in the supervisee or interactions that were surprising, confusing or felt like a breakthrough. As supervisors, we begin with helping the supervisee find their voice and share the story—in their own words and from their own perspective. The way we listen influences the story that is told. This process of retelling and reexperiencing the session in the presence of a witness is most useful when supervisors do not rush to discount, explain or soothe in response to what is shared. As the story unfolds, the supervisor notes any gaps in the narrative of the therapy process, such as the absence of the client's father or the omission of negative emotions, while also identifying the places where the supervisee lingers. In response, the reflective supervisor creates a shared experience and uses these insights as a platform for deeper exploration, encouraging the supervisee to reflect on overlooked aspects of the narrative.

Hawkins and Shohet (2012) suggest several innovative ways in which a supervisee can be invited to describe their client – perhaps asking how the client gestures, sits, or speaks, or whether they feel pulled towards or pushed away by the client. Asking a question like, "What are three things you would want me to know about your client?" can help a supervisee sift through their many impressions and focus on what they feel is most relevant. When the supervisor makes a genuine attempt to slow down their own thoughts and enter into the experience that the supervisee is sharing, images or metaphors may arise into their consciousness. In our experience, sharing such impressions helps us access unarticulated layers experience and deepens the conversation.

Pause and reflect…

The supervisor listens to her supervisee's descriptions of the therapy session with an adult client – one in which the client walked around the room, spoke of his "philosophy of life", and mentioned his incomplete college assignments in passing. Immersed in the story, the supervisor remarked, "When I close my eyes, I see your client as a young boy in shorts". The supervisee exclaimed, "That's how I experience him too! After our first session, I drew him as a little boy in khaki shorts, looking out of the window".

Bring to your mind an image or metaphor that represents one of your clients. Spend some time reflecting on this image and think about what it tells you - about your client and about how you relate with them in sessions.

Finally, ask yourself if (and how) you would take these imaginings to your supervision session…

Playing with the Story

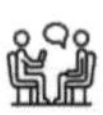

Eunsun was struggling with a new client, an investment banker who acknowledged his depression but was reluctant to discuss his feelings or the difficult relationship he felt trapped in. Although the client followed her suggestions to engage in mastery and pleasure activities, he remained task-focused and seldom brought up his concerns. He reported that his mood had not improved. Eunsun brought this to supervision, seeking guidance on how to get unstuck and move the therapy forward.

The supervisor began by asking Eunsun a series of reflective questions, as outlined by Senediak (2014), to explore her experience in the session. These questions were designed to help Eunsun gain insight into her experience and identify changes to consider for the next session. The supervisor first asked her to reflect on her thoughts and expectations about the interaction, then inquired, "What is the emotional atmosphere in the room as you are speaking with him?" This prompted Eunsun to recognize the emotional flatness and low energy in the session. She had assumed that the client was not very depressed, as he seemed functional at work, but soon realized he was mechanical and detached in all aspects of his life.

Next, the supervisor asked, "Have you had an experience with a similar client before?" This question led Eunsun to notice the ways in which this client differed from others she had worked with. As their discussion deepened, the supervisor prompted Eunsun to reflect on her own approach, asking, "Through what lens can you best relate to this person?" This invitation led Eunsun to step back and consider the client's unique experiences and background. The supervisor then followed up with, "How would this shift your approach in the session?" encouraging Eunsun to think about how these new insights could influence her interactions and adjust her approach moving forward.

When the supervisor directed her attention to her personal style, Eunsun realized that her chirpy, high-energy approach—which worked well with younger clients—might feel overwhelming for this particular client. Reflecting on the client's words, she recalled how he described his father as impatient with weakness and unwilling to accept 'excuses' for failure. Viewing the situation through the lens of gender and connecting it with the client's past experiences, she understood how difficult it must be for him to be vulnerable with her and how terrifying his depression might actually be. Together, they explored more subtle and sensitive ways to engage the client, such as slowing down her pace, adjusting her expectations, and focusing on experiences and conversations rather than directly addressing feelings.

This exploration stage exemplifies the active role of the supervisor in scaffolding the supervisee's development. The supervisor provides affirmation, reassurance, and support, teaches theory and skills, and suggests therapeutic approaches. Most importantly, the supervisor opens the door to reflective discoveries, helping the supervisee navigate complex emotional dynamics. The timing of these reflective explorations is crucial. If the supervisee—or the supervisor—is feeling too distressed, angry, or defensive, they need to pause and address these immediate emotional needs before proceeding. The supervisor alternates between zooming in to reflect on the personal impacts and meaning of the issue for the supervisee and zooming out to consider any influences from professional, organizational, or sociopolitical contexts that may be at play.

The supervisor can choose from a variety of methods to help supervisees reflect on difficult moments in therapy, connect with their emotions, and understand how their personal experiences shape the therapeutic process. When these explorations focus closely on the micro-processes of the session, they foster a deeper level of both interpersonal and intrapersonal awareness. Methods like *Interpersonal Process Recall* (IPR; Kagan, 1976), where segments of recorded therapy sessions are reviewed together, can be quite time-intensive but highly effective. During this process, the supervisee is encouraged to listen carefully and enter a reflective space, connecting with their covert thoughts and feelings both before and during the interaction.

The exploration often begins with asking questions to examine the supervisee's experiences. "What bodily sensations or images were evoked during the session?" or "What were you feeling and thinking about the client or the therapeutic process at that moment?" A deeper level of reflection involves unpacking the expectations and perceptions that both the therapist and the client may have had of each other. The supervisor may ask questions like, "What do you think your client wanted from you?" or "Do you think your client was aware of what you were feeling during that moment?" These questions invite the supervisee to consider how their perceptions of the interaction might differ from those of the client. Some insights emerge only when we give time and space to consider smaller moments and meanings within the session. For example, asking, "Was there anything you wanted to say to your client but didn't?" can uncover new layers of the interaction.

Even if we are unable to record sessions, the discovery-oriented, process-focused stance of the IPR approach can still be valuable in helping supervisees deepen their reflective practice. A recent extension of the IPR method, proposed by Ivers et al. (2017), introduces a series of questions designed to enhance multicultural awareness. These questions address issues of cultural differences between supervisor and supervisee and any cultural assumptions and biases held by the supervisee, and bring a focus to the cultural factors in the client's story. For example, the supervisor might ask about the supervisee's reactions to aspects of the client's social location, such as their accent, religious beliefs or skin colour. Additionally, the supervisor may explore perceptions of the client's comfort in discussing experiences of injustice or discrimination. By considering these factors, we can piece together and integrate aspects of the client's story, ultimately fostering a more sensitive and inclusive practice.

For example, a supervisor might ask, "It seems like you're feeling deeply about working with X. Could you share what you're experiencing?" This gives the supervisee an opportunity to express their emotional responses, such as feeling frustrated when the client was late again or anxious after the client disclosed using an addictive substance. Both the supervisor and supervisee can then explore these emotional reactions together, naming and understanding them in the context of the therapeutic work. They might identify emotions like anger, sadness, impatience, excitement, or confusion and explore how these feelings could be influencing the therapeutic relationship (Heller & Gilkerson, 2009). These reflective conversations offer the supervisee the chance to explore the sources and implications of their emotions, some of which could be tied to personal vulnerabilities or past experiences. For example, the supervisee's reaction to the client's addiction might be connected to struggles with addiction within their own family of origin. Such conversations help to unpack the emotional landscape and provide a deeper understanding of how personal histories can inform therapeutic practice.

Building on this foundation, some frameworks for reflective conversations are rooted in specific theoretical models. One example is the *reflective communication and questions method* (Gray & Smith, 2009), which draws from solution-focused and narrative models to frame exploratory questions. For instance, a supervisor might ask the miracle question, "Imagine for a moment that in your next session with your client all of the current problems and conflicts you are having disappear. You know, the session of your dreams. Tell me, what would that look like?" (Gray & Smith, 2009, p. 164). Other narrative therapy-based questions could help identify the source of any disabling narratives in the supervisee's social and cultural landscape while keeping the focus on supervisee strengths. Another interesting method is the *prismatic dialogue approach* which deepens engagement with different perspectives within the supervision session. We all know the importance of stepping into our client's shoes, but when we are in the midst of a session, it can be hard to truly sense what the client is feeling or how we are coming across to them. In this exercise, the therapist plays the client, while the supervisor plays the therapist, asking relational and circular questions to uncover underlying relationship patterns. Once the exercise ends, the supervisor checks, "How do you think this might help your next conversation with your client?" (Bird, 2006).

Pause and reflect...

Try the *prismatic dialogue approach* in your supervision session.

Reflect on your experience as a supervisor: What was it like to step into your supervisee's shoes? Did it help you understand what kind of input or support they might need from you?

Reflect on your experience as a supervisee: How was it to step into your client's shoes without also needing to think about being a therapist?

Reflect together: Did it open any new aspects of the experience for both of you?

Supervisors are in a unique position to help the supervisee gain insight into how their personalities, past experiences, and beliefs can influence therapeutic interactions. Therapists' difficult personal experiences and histories have often been viewed as red flags, blind spots, or obstacles, especially when they resonate with what unfolds in therapy. Because of this, supervisees may hesitate to acknowledge or bring their vulnerabilities directly into the conversation. While the supervisee's life experiences can be potential obstacles in the therapy process, they can also be a strength, lending a sensitivity that another therapist might not have. As supervisors, we can validate their experiences and facilitate exploration through resource-focused questions such as, "How do your life experiences help you to be more compassionate toward your clients? How do they allow you to understand your clients on a deeper level? How can you use your previous life experiences to inform your work?" (Timm & Blow, 1999, p. 334). When we see our personal lives as neither good nor bad, but as experiences that make us who we are, we can be more balanced in how we use them in therapy. And having a good supervisor is key to this process.

Moving Forward

The supervisee next moves to the stage of experimentation and application of possible actions and solutions in the therapeutic process. This is positioned as something to try with the client and not as a definitive path. When the supervisor and supervisee decide to move forward with a plan, for instance, to try the empty chair technique with a client, they also need to consider if the supervisee has the necessary support and resources. The supervisor might share some reading material, involve the supervisee in a role-play and discuss any apprehensions about how this will be received by the client or if it will work. In this stage, we put our reflections to test, applying them in the real-world situation, aware that every move we make is based not on a fact or a certainty but on a hypothesis to be verified.

Revisiting the Story

This last phase is an opportunity to review what has been learnt through these reflections and allow space for new questions to emerge in supervision. A supervisee might begin thinking about their work with certain types of clients or contexts, their development as a therapist, an ethical conundrum or wonder about the role and value of therapy. Together, the supervisor and supervisee can plan when to explore these questions and address these learning needs. A supervisee who notices that they relate differently to clients across the gender spectrum may anticipate that this issue is likely to come up again. The supervisor can help them proactively explore the way they feel about themselves and their own gender and examine the gendered messages they have received. Together they can unpack how these beliefs and feelings might manifest in session contexts and plan how to address them. This model of reflective supervision privileges supervisee experience over supervisor expertise, and sees reflective processes as having the potential to transform therapists. The evaluation and feedback stage completes the reflective loop, though, in truth, the process is never complete. Rather, we may move back and forth through stages, asking new questions and arriving at new answers.

Reflecting Together: Supervision in Group Formats

As we begin to test our wings after training, creating a group with our peers can offer a space for continued supervision, and a sense of being in the same boat. Peer supervision can be a particularly useful resource for both novice therapists and experienced therapists who work independently and have limited access to professional networks. A space with less prominent power differentials can be freeing but, like all other groups, a cohesive and sustainable framework is helpful. These groups are not necessarily leaderless and may have varied formats for leaders, moderators or observers, and can also involve rotating roles. Peer supervision groups can vary significantly in how they define their scope and focus. Some groups emphasize personal development, creating space for members to reflect on their emotional responses, therapist identity and the impact of clinical work on their well-being. Others may concentrate on case conceptualization, offering opportunities to discuss clinical material, explore therapeutic dilemmas and deepen understanding of client dynamics. Some groups are oriented toward skill-building, using activities such as structured feedback, role-plays, or technique-focused discussions to strengthen therapeutic competencies. Additionally, groups may choose to align with a specific theoretical orientation—such as psychodynamic, cognitive-behavioural or humanistic approaches—or adopt an integrative or pluralistic stance that accommodates multiple perspectives..

A Supervisor/Supervisee Speaks: A Work in Reflection

Hargun Ahluwalia

For the longest time, as a therapist I have thought of myself as a work in progress. Progress, understood as onwards and forward movement, has meant learning new techniques and modalities in psychotherapy— like addingg storeys to a skyscraper or pages to a resume. More recently during the lockdowns in the pandemic, I wondered if onwards and forward was the way to be.

The social realities of the pandemic began to creep up on me. The news of thousands of deaths, lost jobs, the migrant worker crisis and the systemic challenges, which I had deftly drowned out, began to get louder. I felt shame at my ignorance and privilege and wondered if other psychologists thought about and felt for the world outside of academia. I brought these ideas into my online peer supervision group and realized that most of my peers felt deeply uncomfortable bringing their personal feelings into this intellectual space. I remember doing with their discomfort what I did with my shame—tried to understand it, first silently and by discussing together. The group evolved into a smaller one, where there was some comfort in looking into our histories and acknowledging difficult emotions. We talked about the world around us by understanding how it made us feel. After the brutal gang rape of a young girl belonging to the Dalit community, a few of us cried and some of us reflected on our emotional distance. We asked, "Had we always been deaf to the horrors around us?" "What purpose does our ignorance serve for us?" "Do we feel safe this way?".

In the safety of this reflective group, we could experience unsafe feelings. We supported each other's uncomfortable journeys through gentle questioning and sometimes by just letting the question be. I carried these questions outside of the group and into therapy sessions with my clients, "Do I distance myself from my clients' social realities?" "Am I really empathizing if I'm trying to remain safe by not allowing myself to feel discomfort?" Reflecting on my emotions and reactions made me learn more about who I am, what I value and what I need. In turn, I became more attuned to my clients and better able to guide them to discover parts of themselves. Peer supervision has become a profoundly life-changing experience. I have learnt that progress isn't about moving onwards and forwards but inwards and maybe even backwards, where I look at my past. I'm not as interested in building storeys as I am in examining the foundation. In this space, I can look inwards without judgement, be vulnerable in front of others, allow myself to be taken care of and learn from others.

Dr. Hargun Ahluwalia *is a senior clinical psychologist and a board approved supervisor at a Psychological Trauma Recovery Service in Melbourne, working with adults with cPTSD and PTSD.*

Group formats leverage the advantages of multiple voices to nurture reflexivity and support the shared process of meaning-making. Group supervision, where one supervisor works with several supervisees at the same time, is a commonly used format among both trainees and practicing professionals. In this setting, the supervisor holds overall responsibility for helping each supervisee meet their individual learning goals. They also maintain a safe and reflective space in which therapists can share difficult experiences or explore their struggles with clients. However, group dynamics can be challenging. When supervisees are met with a rapid succession of critical or probing questions or are not given adequate room to think and process, they may feel defensive, shamed, or angry. The facilitator needs to see to it that questions, comments and feedback come at a pace and style that the supervisee can handle, in order to stimulate reflection rather than shut it down. Using a more tentative and open-ended style of inquiry—such as "What struck me when I heard her talk about the incident…," "This brought up my own experience with…," or "I wonder what might happen if they traded roles for a day or two…"—can open up possibilities for all group members (Paré et al., 2004, p. 122). The supervisor can model this gentle and reflective style, encouraging group members to consider how they are asking questions and what this says about their position. Asking group members to talk about how they felt during a line of questioning can encourage greater awareness of emotional dynamics. Noticing and drawing attention to one member's discomfort, or setting aside time to discuss each person's preferred interaction style and confidence level, can also help the group become more sensitive and attuned to one another.

In the *group reflective case discussion model,* one supervisee is invited to share a therapeutic experience and observe the groups members' responses. After a round of clarifying questions, participants offer their reflections and draw connections between the case and their own work. The focus then shifts to exploring relevant theoretical frameworks and potential ethical concerns. At that point, the presenter re-enters the discussion, and together the group identifies key themes, lessons learned, and strategies applicable to similar situations. The supervisor plays a less active role but keeps the discussion focused and ends by consolidating the reflective learnings. The process of exploring ideas and perspectives rather than offering solutions or searching for the one truth minimises judgement and increases the therapist's repertoire.

The *interacting–reflecting training exercise* (Rober, 2010) uses a similar format with an interesting blend of experiential work in small groups. Metaphorical images are used to describe the client, the supervisee and the therapy process (e.g., a train leaving a station, a tree with strong roots, a flock of seagulls in flight, walking through a fog, peeling an onion). Room is created for supervisees to experiment and take risks with their reflections, delving into inner conversations that are not easily acknowledged or expressed in sessions. The exercise often includes a role-reversal component, where participants alternate between being the interactor (the one engaged in a therapeutic conversation) and the reflector (the one observing and reflecting on the interaction). The blend of metaphor and action components encourages supervisees to weave between different levels of reflection.

Edward de Bono's (1999) *Six Thinking Hats technique* offers an innovative approach for group supervision, ideal for a collaborative exploration of therapy situations (Li et al., 2008). In this method, the multiple voices are given some shape and coherence, so that they can blend constructively. Each group member takes turns 'wearing' a different hat, starting perhaps with the White Hat, which prompts the question, "What do we know?" With the Red Hat, group members shift to expressing their feelings and intuition, without having to provide reasons or justifications. The Black Hat poses critical questions about potential problems and what does not fit, asking "What can be hazardous?". Wearing the Yellow Hat brings a more optimistic outlook, encouraging the group to explore possibilities "What could happen?" This reminds members to focus on what is feasible, beneficial and wished for. Next, the Green Hat encourages group members to think creatively and out of the box, asking "What have we not considered so far?". The supervision session ends with everyone wearing the Blue Hat to create space for reflections and blending all the ideas generated, moving towards asking "What is our conclusion?" This dynamic approach brings structure and creativity to group supervision, ensuring that multiple perspectives are fully explored and integrated.

Pause and reflect…

Try the *Six Thinking Hats* method, and reflect on your experiences:

Did you wear some of the hats more often than others?

Did you find yourself going off track and forgetting which hat you were wearing?

Did any of the hats dominate the group session?

Along with using the group space to gain insight into our therapy work, we also have the opportunity to reflect on the group process itself. Participants may note times of belonging and separateness within the group, exploring why this might be so. The awareness of emotional reactions to specific group members, or of habitual roles and positions within the group lends insights about our interpersonal patterns.Ultimately, the value of all these models lies in accessing a polyphony of voices to guide and enrich future therapeutic practice.

Reflecting on the Supervision Process

As a system already integral to a psychotherapist's work, supervision naturally lends itself to fostering reflection. Each supervisory framework brings its own flavour and focus, and we tend to gravitate toward those that suit our preferences, workload and available time. To deepen or shift our reflective practice, we can experiment with unfamiliar approaches or mix diverse methods and modalities. It is important, however, to consider how each method aligns with our supervisory goals and whether it truly furthers the learning and growth we envision. Before introducing a new approach, a collaborative discussion of expectations, learning objectives and desired growth pathways helps both supervisor and supervisee feel empowered. Insights gained from discussing one client often inform how we work with others, and we may experience retrospective insights when revisiting past sessions with fresh eyes. When both supervisor and supervisee commit fully to reflection, the supervisory space becomes deeply enriching and mutually satisfying.

Relational reflexivity encourages practices that allow both parties to reflect on how supervisory conversation and interactions are experienced (Burnham, 2005). The supervisor could initiate questions such as, "Is this going okay for you?" "Is this what you want us to discuss first?" and "Does my style of listening work for you?" Regular discussions about the learnings from each session can ensure that the supervisee becomes comfortable with reflection and will not be thrown by a sudden deep question. As supervisors, we may also reflect aloud on how the process of supervision is going for us, again modelling the process of reflection for supervisees (Curtis et al., 2016). As supervisor and supervisee reflect together, it can balance the power differential in the relationship, teaching supervisees how they can do the same with clients. Introspection can also help supervisors recognize if they are avoiding reflective work by throwing questions back at supervisees or frequently referring them to theory and textbooks.

Building Our Internal Supervisor and Internalized Supervisor

As we engage with our supervisors, we develop an internalized supervisor—an internal representation of their presence and guidance, experienced in visual, auditory, or felt forms (Watkins, 2018). It is possible that we incorporate both positive and negative voices of our supervisor, eventually leading to a 'good' or 'bad' internalized supervisor. If supervision experiences have not been reflective enough and exclude personal reactions and histories, this can impede the development of confident, reflective inner voices (Mammen, 2020). When we imagine a compassionate supervisor, it develops the capacity to soothe ourselves and be less self-critical (Bell et al., 2017). It is the supervisor's approach, presence, supportive statements and guidance that get represented and become resources to be used later while working with a client. Holding the supervisor in mind helps us handle difficult moments, further our work with our clients and grow as therapists.

While the internal representation of the supervisor plays a crucial role in our early professional development, Casement (1985) proposed the idea of an internal supervisor. This could be imagined as a mental space to reflect, explore and monitor our work from a supervisory perspective (Bell et al., 2017). It involves spontaneous reflection, where we can look at our own work and what is happening between us and our client—something that stands apart from the internalized supervisor. This internal supervisor has its origins even before we receive any formal supervision. As we progress, an island of intellectual contemplation; "a mental space within which the internal supervisor can operate" (Casement, 1985, p. 28)—develops and what eventually becomes possible is the dialogue between the internal and external supervisors. Both the internalized supervisor and the internal supervisor support development as reflective practitioners, so that dialogue and perspective taking become part of our everyday practice.

Pause and reflect...

We invite you to engage in a visualization exercise.

Picture how your internalized supervisor looks.

Do they seem calm and confident or worried and unsure?

Do they sound more critical, compassionate or perhaps dispassionate?

End your reflections by considering whether the two of you speak often enough.

Room to Grow: Developing as a Supervisor

As therapists, we may enter a supervisory role because it feels exciting and is a natural progression in our careers and/or a job requirement. Quite often, we may be expected to step into the role of a supervisor soon after training to become a therapist. Finding our own feet as professionals and having to guide others at the same time can leave us feeling unprepared and even like an imposter. Doing supervision, or undertaking the tasks of supervision, can be differentiated from being a supervisor or assuming the identity of a supervisor (Burnham, 2012). We may *do* supervision for years, before we can say with confidence that we *are* supervisors. Being a supervisor requires more than therapeutic and reflective skills. We also need to draw on our love for teaching and our sense of responsibility towards the profession.

We recommend the use of the pantheoretical *seven-eyed model* (Hawkins & Shohet, 2012) to teach and learn reflective supervision processes. Each of the seven eyes suggests an area of focus and detailed exploration during the supervisory process. The first eye in this model is a focus on the *client*, making space for them in the supervision room and experiencing them as deeply as possible. The second eye reviews the *interventions*, looking at what was done and what was not done and seeking to understand how these choices were made. The third eye looks at the *supervisee-client relationship*, helping the supervisee get in touch with their feelings about and towards the client and noticing the relational dance between them. This naturally moves to the fourth eye where the *supervisee self* is brought to the front. The supervisor pays attention to how the client is impacting the supervisee, explores the supervisee's emotional and relational patterns and attends to their needs for self-care, resources and support. The focus shifts from the therapy room to the supervision room, with the fifth eye looking at the interactions within the *supervisor-supervisee* relationship, leaving room for the possibility that some patterns might mirror those in the therapy room. This is also the time for the supervisor to reflect on their feelings and preferences, perhaps wondering if they relate more easily with certain supervisees—the one who is more independent? The one who obviously values their opinion? Or perhaps the one with whom they feel emotionally connected? Using the sixth eye, the *supervisor* focuses on their own here-and-now experiences which serve as potential messages about what is happening in the therapy and supervision rooms. The seventh eye expands the field to encompass the *wider context*, the professional systems and sociocultural economic-political contexts in which client, supervisee and supervisor are embedded. Here the supervisor takes care to understand how the therapeutic work is impacted by these systemic connect expectations and experiences with the larger system to the therapeutic work. As we integrate this framework into our supervisory practice, we hone our skills in choosing which aspect of the process to focus on, shift between different perspectives and integrating all that we observe.

Pause and reflect...

Use the *seven eyed model* to reflect on your approach to supervision:

Which eye/s do you look through most often in your supervision sessions?

Which eye is usually (tends to stay) closed during supervision sessions?

Is there an eye you are uncertain about looking through?

The Balancing Act

There are several balancing acts we may need to engage in as we straddle both the therapy room and the supervision room. We need to put ourselves into the shoes of our supervisee and their client(s) while simultaneously remaining firmly in our own. We need to be in touch with the self of the therapist that lies within each supervisee but also be careful not to slip into casting them as clients (Borders, 1993). We need to support our supervisees as well as guide or course correct them when required. This equilibrium takes time to evolve, and supervisors may find themselves being pulled to one or the other side in different situations. A supervisor who recalls stressful supervisory experiences and is determined to create a warm and supportive space for their own supervisees, might be reluctant to offer a challenge, even when it is required. A supervisor needs to judge the optimum balance between providing scaffolding or direction and allowing space for the supervisee to reflect and explore a therapeutic impasse. Supervisee needs may vary, depending on their developmental level, emotional distress, the complications in client presentation and a host of other factors. In this context, the wisdom to know the difference often comes with reflecting on our own experiences.

As supervisors, we carry varied responsibilities—to clients, to our supervisees, the training institution and to the profession. It is not uncommon for supervisors to feel pulled between the needs of the client and the needs of our supervisee. For instance, a client may need an intensity of connection and care that our supervisee feels overwhelmed by. This is really a time for the supervisor to hold both the client and the supervisee in their mind. Supervisors may provide more direct support than usual, helping supervisees connect differently with their clients by modelling the empathy and relatedness the supervisee struggles to experience. When it seems difficult to reconcile the needs of the client, the standard of care expected by the organization, and the supervisee's current capacities, this calls for deeper reflection. When we are in touch with our supervisee's lives, emotional worlds, challenges and current capacities, we better positioned to identify when self-care must take priority. Supervisory time can then be devoted to helping the supervisee express personal emotions and dilemmas rather than focusing exclusively on the client. Supervisors may model strategies for strengthening boundaries, managing workload and work–life balance, or building emotional support systems. If a supervisee appears persistently overwhelmed, discussing and recommending personal therapy becomes an appropriate intervention.

As supervisors develop, there is growing comfort with looking within and become increasingly adept at noticing subtle interactional cues during supervision. Although therapy and supervision happen in different rooms, the interactional processes between supervisee and supervisor sometimes mirror what is happening in the relationship between client and supervisee. This analogous or parallel process (Ekstein & Wallerstein, 1958), that emerges in the client-supervisee-supervisor triangle, is often quite elusive. A supervisee may not realize that they are replicating their client difficulties in their interactions with their supervisor. Just as the client feels stuck, hopeless and passive, the supervisee may experience frustration with the pace of supervision. If the supervisor remains oblivious about the supervisee's lack of engagement, they may in turn re-enact the supervisee-client dynamic in the supervisory relationship. Supervisors who are alert to currents in their supervisory relationship and within themselves, can use their understanding of to speculate on what might be happening between supervisee and client. When the emergent parallel process is explored in a gentle, curious and collaborative way, its value as a communicative bridge between the two rooms can be realized. As the supervisor meta-communicates about what might be going on in the supervisor-supervisee interaction, this also models how to address relationship dynamics with clients. Newer possibilities for working with the client may begin to open (Calvert et al., 2016).

The meanings we ascribe to such parallels must be tempered by the possible influence of our subjectivities on the links that we make between the two rooms. It is also possible that feelings that emerge within the supervisee-supervisor dyad must be addressed within *this* relationship, before speculating about possible unconscious communications of the client's difficulties. While discussions on such relational dynamics can be illuminating and even strengthen therapeutic work, we also recommend pausing to think about possible ramifications for the supervisee, their interactions with the client and their professional growth. Supervisors can look for a window to introduce these hypotheses in a tentative manner, depending on their supervisee's developmental level and capacities, while always staying grounded in the implications for therapeutic work. It takes consistent practice in reflection and reflexivity for a supervisor to hold so many threads of awareness together.

While it is hard work to be a supervisor, it is also an extremely rewarding experience. As we reflect with supervisees on their therapy experiences, we may come to see newer perspectives and ways of approaching therapy. Working through another therapist's struggles can also bring our own blind spots and strengths to the forefront. As supervisors, maintaining supervision notes can help us track the overall development of the supervisee, as well as review our own progress. We need to continually assess our comfort level with asking reflective questions during supervision and commit to developing this skill throughout our professional journeys. Ultimately, becoming a supervisor is one of the quickest paths to growth as a therapist, and being an effective supervisor is a meaningful way to contribute to the profession.

Supervision can sometimes feel like a very tall order, prompting us to question whether we have the skills and abilities required. As supervisors, we do not need to be perfect. Being 'good enough' while being willing to learn, *is* actually good enough (Hawkins & Shohet, 2012). We can acknowledge that we do not know everything and also accept that we do not need to know everything in order to be effective supervisors.

Pause and reflect…
How would you like to foster your own development as a supervisor?

As a supervisor, what are your learning goals for this year?

A Supervisor Speaks Integrating the Social Justice Lens in Supervision

Chetna Duggal

Our training program for supervisors has been designed to include structured lectures and skill learning sessions along with reflective spaces where supervisors bring in challenges and dilemmas they experience while working with their supervisees one on one and in groups. An illustrative example[1] would be as follows: A supervisor shares their dilemma about how directive they should be with their supervisee, who expresses helplessness about being unable to help a young client who is feeling alienated in school and missing classes. In the supported supervision sessions, the supervisor begins with presenting the *marker* (what they and/or their supervisee identified as the issue/concerns) followed by reflections on how they made meaning of the marker using supervision models and theory. This is followed by sharing specific questions that they would like input on. While bringing challenges and dilemmas requires courage, this presents a great opportunity for learning.

With a deep commitment to centre the value of social justice in supervision practice, there is an intentional focus in these sessions to reflect on therapist (supervisee) and supervisor positionality and the power dynamics in the therapist-client and the supervisor-supervisee relationship. Since the group is already oriented to the social justice lens through theoretical ideas/models and reflective exercises in the lectures, there is usually a shared language and comfort within the group that makes this conversation possible. Going back to the example, the group may actively think about the social location of the client and use an intersectional lens to understand the marginalisation and alienation that this young client may be feeling based on identity markers such as gender, class, caste, ability. There could also be reflective dialogue on the role of systems or contextual discourses that may not allow this young person to speak their mind thereby contributing to their isolation. As the group reflects together, the supervisor-in-training may at times connect to biases or blind spots within themselves or their supervisees. They may recognise how in some ways they can be a part of systems that has power over this young person. Having a diverse group, which brings together supervisors from various contexts, cultures and countries, with different social identities or positionalities, also ensures that there are multiple voices and perspectives in the room. Even on occasions when the discussion has been dominated by clinical or theoretical lenses, there has always been someone who is able to point the group towards the unheard or unseen.

In supported supervision sessions, the reflective work and the act of seeing often brings to the forefront questions about the practice of doing. Wondering how we empower and advocate for our supervisees and clients and what would it mean to work towards social justice, the group is able to envision a practice that is informed by values that are held dear. Some of the broader questions we ask ourselves could include: What do we say to this young person, what might empower them to speak their mind, how could we advocate with the school leadership with them, or what might need to change within the system for them to belong? Going granular - thinking of possible steps to take, the words to use to start this conversation within the therapy room and outside, or how our emotional tone could convey our value stance - makes the work real and possible. When I think of what this feels like, it is like being on a swing, going up to explore the possibilties of our ideas, and coming down to see how we can bring them alive in our practice.

What has been interesting to see is how reflection-on-action during supported supervision sessions gets internalized and is then transformed to reflection-in-action by the supervisor-in-training. There is tremendous power in being witnessed and being seen, and in the group shining light on the supervisor's strengths and pointing to sparkling moments. Most importantly there is power in the group being able to hold hope when the supervisors-in-training doubt their supervisory competence. Over time what is practiced in the reflective space with peer feedback and facilitator support gets incorporated into the supervisory style, and is beautifully integrated into the supervisory identity. What is experienced by the supervisor as empowering in the reflective space, does not just stay with them alone. We imagine that it is recreated in the supervisory relationship with other therapists, and in turn with many clients.

Dr. Chetna Duggal *is a psychotherapist, trainer and supervisor. She heads Rahbar, a field action project to promote training, supervision and professional development for mental health practitioners in India and anchors a post graduate diploma on Supervision for Mental Health Practice.*

Perspectives on Training and Development

Frameworks and Training for Supervisor Development

We advocate the use of competency frameworks to focus attention to support supervisor development in psychotherapy training. Best practice guidelines for supervisors could include the necessary technical, relational and ethical supervisory skills, along with an intentional focus on reflective processes (Border, 2014). The success of implementing reflective supervision components in training programmes depends on circumventing barriers due to competing academic and clinical demands and on support from leadership and key stakeholders.

Initial and ongoing training opportunities in the form of courses and workshops in generic supervision competencies, or specific methods such as use of interpersonal process recall or genograms, are critical to support supervisors' growth. For an understanding of what supervision looks like in different theoretical orientations, we recommend the American Psychological Association video series that showcase ten approaches, in addition to competency-based frameworks. This spans multicultural/

feminist, accelerated experiential, emotion-focused, systems, critical events, integrated developmental, cognitive behavioural, integrative, relational–dynamic and experiential perspectives.

Inclusive approaches, such as the *Clinical Supervision Research Collaborative*—a global, cross-disciplinary online community of supervisors—play a crucial role in fostering supervisor development. This initiative provides opportunities for supervisors, across experience levels, disciplines and geographical locations, to engage with diverse supervision practices, access key learning resources and build research networks. Such spaces that nurture supervisors are vital to the process of supervisor development, offering both valuable resources and a platform to connect with peers.

Supervision for Trauma-Informed Practice

One of the most important transformations in supervisory practice is the emerging focus on trauma-informed care (Borders et al, 2023). As members of the healing professions, we have always encountered clients with complex histories of trauma, and the rise in violent conflicts and war have contributed to the continued legacy of trauma across the world. The role of supervisors in providing a safe space for supervisees to learn to work with trauma, while buffering them from potential vicarious traumatization, is increasingly recognized as critical. Trauma-informed supervision goes beyond educating supervisees about trauma, its embodied experience and varied impacts and its treatment. As supervisors hold space for supervisees to become aware of their own trauma histories, their responses to clients' trauma stories, and assumptions about forgetting, remembering and healing, their own memories may be evoked in ways that may be difficult and helpful.

In practice, trauma-informed supervision guides supervisees to titrate interventions carefully, ensuring that clients are supported without being retraumatized. At the same time, supervisors must monitor supervisees' emotional well-being and self-care needs, which can include tracking caseloads of clients with significant trauma histories. We regard trauma-informed supervision as an essential competency domain and strongly recommend Courtois's (2018) reflective account as a key resource for deepening this practice.

Developing an Ethos of Supervision for Lifelong Learning and Development

As supervision is not always mandated and regulated, seeking it depends more on a supervisee's inclinations or on the resources of time, money and available supervision opportunities. We note significant cross-cultural variations in access to psychotherapy supervision. For instance, while only 17 per cent of a sample of psychotherapists in

India reported receiving formal supervision after training (Kumaria et al., 2018), the rates are far higher in several other countries, even among more experienced practitioners (Orlinsky & Rønnestad, 2005). Institutional support in terms of time, training and support can strengthen psychotherapy supervision in training contexts. We also recommend that professional associations create resource networks for ongoing supervision and emphasize this as a priority for continuing development. We see a growth in peer supervision groups and tele-supervision and anticipate that such opportunities will be strengthened and promoted, particularly in resource-constrained contexts.

Conclusion

The supervision process belongs equally to the supervisee and supervisor, and requires commitment and investment from both for it to succeed. In reflective supervision, both stand to learn from each interaction, mutually stimulating personal and professional growth as they reflect together on the experience of being a therapist.

References

Ahluwalia, H. (2019). A work-in-progress: A supervisee's reflections. *Psychotherapy Bulletin, 54*(1), 56–62.

Bell, T., Dixon, A., & Kolts, R. (2017). Developing a compassionate internal supervisor: Compassion-focused therapy for trainee therapists. *Clinical Psychology & Psychotherapy, 24*(3), 632–648.

Bhola, P., Raguram, A., Dugyala, M., & Ravishankar, A. (2017). Learning in the crucible of supervision: Experiences of trainee psychotherapists in India. *The Clinical Supervisor, 36*(2), 182–202.

Bird, J. (2006). *Constructing the narrative in supervision.* Edge Press.

Borders, L. D. (1993). Learning to think like a supervisor. *The Clinical Supervisor, 10*(2), 135–148.

Borders, L. D. (2014). Best practices in clinical supervision: Another step in delineating effective supervision practice. *American Journal of Psychotherapy, 68*(2), 151–162.

Borders, L. D., Lowman, M. M., Eicher, P. A., & Phifer, J. K. (2023). Trauma-informed supervision of trainees: Practices of supervisors trained in both trauma and clinical supervision. *Traumatology, 29*(2), 125–136.

Burnham, J. (2005). Relational reflexivity: a tool for socially constructing therapeutic relationships. In C. Flaskas, B. Mason, & A. Perlesz (Eds.), *The space between: Experience, context and process in the therapeutic relationship* (pp. 1–19). Karnac.

Burnham, J. (2012). Are you sitting too comfortably? Using the praxis of positioning to move between the activities of therapy-supervision and the identities of therapist-supervisor. *Clinical Child Psychology and Psychiatry, 17*(2), 171–180.

Calvert, F. L., Crowe, T. P., & Grenyer, B. F. S. (2016). Dialogical reflexivity in supervision: An experiential learning process for enhancing reflective and relational competencies. *The Clinical Supervisor, 35*(1), 1–21.

Casement, P. (1985). *On learning from the patient.* Tavistock.

Courtois, C. A. (2018). Trauma-informed supervision and consultation: Personal reflections. *The Clinical Supervisor, 37*(1), 38–63.

Curtis, D. F., Elkins, S. R., Duran, P., & Venta, A. C. (2016). Promoting a climate of reflective practice and clinician self-efficacy in vertical supervision. *Training and Education in Professional Psychology, 10*(3), 133–140.

Davys, A. M., & Beddoe, L. (2009). The reflective learning model: Supervision of social work students. *Social Work Education, 28*(8), 919–933.

Davys, A., & Beddoe, L. (2020). *Best practice in professional supervision: A guide for the helping professions.* Jessica Kingsley Publishers.

Duggal, C., Dua, B., & Kothari, A. (2022). Holding space for those who heal: Reflections from the Rahbar Supportive Supervision Programme during the Covid 19 pandemic. *The Clinical Supervisor, 41*(2), 127–148.

De Bono, E. (1999). *Six thinking hats.* Little, Brown and Company.

Ekstein, R., & Wallerstein, R. S. (1958). Supervisor and student-therapist and patient-the parallel process. In R. Ekstein & R. S. Wallerstein (Eds.), *The teaching and learning of psychotherapy* (pp. 177–196). Basic Books.

Ellis, M. V. (2017). Clinical supervision contract & consent statement and supervisee rights and responsibilities. *The Clinical Supervisor, 36*(1), 145–159.

Gray, S. W., & Smith, M. S. (2009). The influence of diversity in clinical supervision: A framework for reflective conversations and questioning. *The Clinical Supervisor, 28*(2), 155–179.

Hawkins, P., & Shohet, R. (2012). *Supervision in the helping professions* (4th ed.). McGraw-Hill.

Heller, S. S., & Gilkerson, L. (2009). *Practical guide to reflective consultation.* ZERO TO THREE.

Ivers, N. N., Rogers, J. L., Borders, D. L., & Turner, A. (2017). Using interpersonal process recall in clinical supervision to enhance supervisees' multicultural awareness. *The Clinical Supervisor, 36*(2), 282–303.

Kagan, N. I. (1976). *Interpersonal process recall: A method of influencing human interaction.* Kagan, Michigan State University.

Kumaria, S., Bhola, P., & Orlinsky, D. E. (2018). Influences that count: Professional development of psychotherapists and counsellors in India. *Asia Pacific Journal of Counselling and Psychotherapy, 9*, 86–106.

Ladany, N., Mori, Y., & Mehr, K. E. (2013). Effective and ineffective supervision. *The Counseling Psychologist, 41*(1), 28–47.

Li, C.-S., Lin, Y.-F., Nelson, J., & Eckstein, D. (2008). Hats off to problem-solving with couples. *The Family Journal, 16*(3), 254–257.

Mammen, M. A. (2020). Attachment dynamics in the supervisory relationship: Becoming your own good supervisor. *Journal of Psychotherapy Integration, 30*(1), 93–101.

McMahon, A. (2020). Five reflective touchstones to foster supervisor humility. *The Clinical Supervisor, 39*(2), 158–177.

Orchowski, L., Evangelista, N. M., & Probst, D. R. (2010). Enhancing supervisee reflectivity in clinical supervision: A case study illustration. *Psychotherapy: Theory, Research, Practice, Training, 47*(1), 51–67.

Orlinsky, D. E., & Ronnestad, M. H. (2005). *How psychotherapists develop: A study of therapeutic work and professional growth.* American Psychological Association.

Paré, D., Audet, C., Bailey, J., Caputo, A., Hatch, K., & Wong-Wylie, G. (2004). Courageous practice: Tales from reflective supervision. *Canadian Journal of Counselling, 38*(2), 118–130.

Rober, P. (2010). The interacting reflecting training exercise: Addressing the therapist's inner conversation in family therapy training. *Journal of Marital and Family Therapy., 36*, 158–170.

Senediak, C. (2014). Integrating reflective practice in family therapy supervision. *Australia and New Zealand Journal of Family Therapy, 34*(4), 338–351.

Timm, T. M., & Blow, A. J. (1999). Self-of-the-therapist work: A balance between removing restraints and identifying resources. *Contemporary Family Therapy, 21*, 331–351.

Vygotsky, L. S. (1978). *Mind in society: The development of higher psychological processes.* Harvard University Press.

Watkins, C. E., Jr. (2018). The supervisee's internal supervisor representations: Their role in stimulating psychotherapist development. *International Journal of Psychotherapy, 22*(3), 63–73.
Wideman, D. (2019). Working with process notes. In S. G. De Golia & K. M. Corcoran (Eds.), *Supervision in psychiatric practice* (pp. 63–68). American Psychiatric Association Publishing.

Chapter 11
Being in Personal Therapy

Visitors to the National Gallery in London, walking past the iconic painting *The Ambassadors* by Hans Holbein, are suddenly confronted with the image of a skull on the canvas. The painting depicts two men dressed in ceremonial outfits, along with meticulously detailed objects including globes, dials to tell time, textiles, books, musical instruments and religious symbols. An indeterminate oblong shape at the bottom centre of the canvas transforms into a skull *only* when viewed from a particular angle. The Renaissance artist used a technique called *anamorphosis*, where an image viewed from a different angle or position, or through a special device, makes something visible which was concealed or could not previously be seen.

Just as changing the vantage point makes it possible to see something new, therapists who have experienced being in the client's role in personal therapy may be able to access a unique and layered understanding of the therapy process that is not possible from the therapist's chair alone. As we reflect on what it feels like to be a client, being vulnerable or needing support, we may connect with a new aspect of ourselves. We are all part therapist and part client, and different parts may be dominant at different times. The process of reworking this figure and ground and looking at both ourselves and the therapy experience from both perspectives can really help to develop our professional sensitivity (Berman, 2005). As we become more aware of our personal self and therapist self, we may notice overlaps and discontinuities. We can feel more congruent if we acknowledge that these dualities co-exist within all of us and allow both identities to mutually inform and enrich each other rather than remaining disconnected and isolated, or competing for dominance within us. In keeping with this perspective, we use the term *therapist-client* to denote therapists in personal therapy.

The earliest form of training in psychotherapy involved mandatory and regular analysis for the practitioner, based on the belief that only a therapist aware of their own unconscious could help a client become aware of theirs (Freud, 1915/1958). While personal therapy continues to be intrinsic to psychoanalytic and psychodynamic orientations, its influence has percolated to practitioners of varied persuasions

P. Bhola et al., *Reflective Practice in Psychotherapy and Counselling*,
https://doi.org/10.1007/978-981-96-9732-8_11

(Orlinsky et al., 2011). Engagement with personal therapy continues to be a strong tradition, almost a rite of passage for therapists. Some may initiate this as a mandatory training requirement, or as is more often the case, seek this space for themselves—to heal, learn and grow.

As therapists, each of us may have questions about the need for personal therapy or how best to use this space. In this chapter, we explore how and why personal therapy is accessed, break down how it influences our personal and professional development and address other pertinent questions about the personal therapy experience. We end by examining the challenges and rewards of being a personal therapist.

Why Seek Personal Therapy?

In her candid memoir, *Maybe You Should Talk to Someone,* therapist Lori Gottlieb (2019) invites us into the therapy room to meet her both as a therapist and as a patient. She chronicles her transformative personal therapy experience, which began after the end of a relationship and lasted longer than planned. Her journey is juxtaposed against the stories of four of her patients—a woman diagnosed with terminal cancer; an abrasive, self-focused Hollywood producer; a woman struggling with alcoholism and relationship difficulties; and an older woman searching for meaning. As therapists who are contemplating or undergoing personal therapy or looking back on our experiences, there is much we can learn from and relate to in this narrative. Gottlieb draws our attention to the fact that, although therapists do attend therapy, there is a tension between the desire to be an invulnerable helper and the acceptance that one is human and needs a space for self-reflection, growth and change. We witness Gottlieb's difficulties in getting started, choosing a therapist and gradually immersing herself in the therapeutic process and her journey of self-discovery. In this process, she connects her reflections and process of self-discovery in both roles and rooms.

Personal therapy has traditionally been seen as a professional requirement, and as the most direct route for working on the self of the therapist. We can be motivated to start therapy by our experiences with clients, wondering: Why was I feeling the way I did with *this* client? Our emotions and memories are often triggered by specific session experiences and even when we take this to supervision and consultation, the need for deeper reflection or resolution can remain. Emotional and interpersonal patterns that we notice over time can also act as stimuli. For instance, in response to experiences of stagnation in our work, we might ask ourselves: Is this all I have to offer clients? Is this as far as therapy goes? Is there something more I need to understand about myself, or about people, that can help me go further?

Of course, it is also true that most therapists seek therapy for the same reasons that anyone does—looking for support in dealing with early experiences, trauma, long-standing patterns, current stressors or even psychiatric disturbances. Like our clients, we may encounter moments when we realize that, despite coping well, our internal resources are becoming overwhelmed. At other times, we may feel drawn to grow further, by developing healthier relationships, acquiring new skills or striving toward greater personal congruence. These are all relevant reasons to seek personal therapy.

Regardless of our initial motivations for approaching therapy, like Gottlieb, we may find that reflecting on the resonance and dissonance between the personal and the professional can deepen this experience. As we become more aware of ourselves, address our life issues and become happier as people, our therapist selves also develop. We learn to draw better boundaries, be more attuned to client experiences and have more patience and generosity to offer our clients. Research supporting the pivotal role of the therapist in therapy outcomes implies that any method of improving therapist functioning is likely to be relevant and useful for clients (Moe & Thimm, 2021). Why then are all therapists not in personal therapy? Our emotions of shame at needing help, doubts about the helpfulness of therapy, worries about confidentiality and fears of giving power to a therapist are possible barriers to seeking help. The anonymity and freedom that our clients experience may not be available to us since we are part of the same profession. There might be concerns about how a trainer or colleague might judge us if our inner struggles are revealed. The culture of training institutes and the professional milieu also tends to shape perspectives on personal therapy. If training institutions, teachers and colleagues do not consider personal therapy as important but rather perceive it as a sign of weakness or inadequacy, therapists are less likely to seek help. Of course, the same is true if therapists themselves do not see it as valuable or an essential requirement for being good practitioners. Even when these emotional barriers have been overcome, there can be lingering hesitation about the time and financial commitment that therapy calls for.

When we look at the footprint of personal therapy, mapped across six countries in North America, Europe and Australasia, an overwhelming majority (almost 87%) of psychotherapists reported engaging in personal therapy at least once (Orlinsky et al., 2011). Overall, the investment was rated as one of the most salient contributors to professional growth and development, supporting and deepening the lessons from their experiences with clients. There are wide variations in therapy access and engagement across countries and contexts, and our knowledge about the global landscape is still limited. We do know that practitioners in majority-world contexts like India ranked the experience of personal therapy as last on a list of 10 potential positive influences on their professional development (Kumaria et al., 2018). Perhaps, this was due to a range of contextual constraints, such as high caseloads, fewer trained professionals and the large mental health services gap (Bhola et al., 2017). Trainees may be unable to afford therapy and even if they can, finding an available personal therapist who can offer subsidized rates is challenging. The mental health community may be small enough that dual relationships are difficult to avoid, and concerns about confidentiality and stigma may be more pronounced. The increasing availability of online therapy over the last few years is a welcome development, as it addresses both emotional and practical barriers. It vastly increases the pool of available therapists, makes therapy more accessible and offers privacy in seeking help. While it may not always be more affordable, this significantly reduces the time commitment involved.

Finally, we do recognize that therapy is ultimately a personal choice. There is no need to reify therapy or see it as the only pathway for personal and professional growth. It is also true that not all therapists feel like they *need* therapy. They may be coping well, have enough social support or might prefer to draw from supervision, reading or professional interactions for professional development. Psychotherapy is not the only way to address a personal or psychological needs, and some therapists may prefer alternate routes. Each experience we have—a lecture, a workshop or a chat with a friend—is valid and useful in its own way. Much depends on how we engage with and make meaning of our life experiences. It can sometimes feel like we already know too much about therapy and therapists to really be able to find new value from being in personal therapy. We may prefer to develop another side of ourselves, looking to spirituality, creativity, adventure or just healthy relationships to help us heal or cope. Or we just may not be ready to open that door yet.

Pause and reflect...

Take a moment to consider what you might gain from personal therapy or what might keep you from trying it.

If you are not in personal therapy, do you wonder if there might be anything you are missing out on?

Experiments with Clienthood

The focus has gradually shifted from whether personal therapy benefits therapist-clients to how it benefits us. The process of reflecting on personal therapy experiences and integrating the learning into professional repertoires is a key pathway to gaining from personal therapy. For those who decide to take the plunge and seek personal therapy, there are many possible rewards.

***A Therapist Speaks*: Therapist on the Couch**

Nupur Dhingra Paiva

I have been a client in psychotherapy in different ways (individual and group; twice-per-week depth therapy, weekly therapy and intensive dynamic therapy consultations) with different therapists over an 18-year period. The most powerful, memorable and effective were when I was invited to be an active participant, instead of on the couch or as an anxious–silent group member.

While on the couch, I wanted to see my therapist's reaction to what was shared, to look at her face and perhaps to keep an eye on her. I have always been tuned in to how others respond to me, but it took years to realize how this was a core part of my character structure.

In group therapy, I was overwhelmed by anxiety, wanting to become invisible and disappear. Simultaneously, I wanted the group leader to be a benevolent, giving, leading presence. I was again keeping an eye on her, to see how she reacted to me. Clearly, I was placing myself in a needy, passive, helpless child position to this powerful figure, and I constantly needed her validation. This is ironic because helplessness in others, especially women, has always been a source of irritation when it enters the room in my patients. Yet here I was, doing exactly the same. So, it becomes easy to see how it was a disavowed part of myself which I could see and reject in others but not see in myself. When my therapist reacted positively, I would be emboldened to continue. When she reacted with impatience or dismissiveness to my contribution, it would sting, leaving me wounded and enraged. I wanted her permission and encouragement—I wanted her approval the way I wanted my father's approval.

This personal therapy journey made a big impact on my interactions with my patients, most of whom are adolescents with emotional and relationship difficulties. I am very aware of the tone of my voice ever since I heard myself speak on a video-recorded session; I was horrified to find how strict and clipped I sounded—not empathic or gentle at all. I am now more aware of the relationship patterns that the patient invites me to fit into: Do I become active when my patient is passive and helpless? Do I do the hard work when my patient is detached and disinterested? Whose therapy is it—mine or the patient's? So, who needs to be doing the hard work? How do I respond when there is veiled aggression, sarcasm or devaluation? These are a few tricky aspects of the quality of the relationship which only became evident to me by having been a patient repeatedly.

Ms. Nupur Dhingra Paiva *is a child and adolescent psychotherapist, and the author of Love and Rage: The Inner Worlds of Children. She uses Intensive Short Term Dynamic Psychotherapy in her work with adults. She previously worked at the Tavistock and Portman NHS Foundation Trust, London, and currently practices in India.*

Getting in Touch with the Self

Personal therapy is first and foremost a way of taking care of ourselves in a reflective space. Being a therapist does not guarantee psychological health or a supportive environment. Many of us choose to be in therapy because we need it as individuals, whether it is to cope more effectively, address personal challenges, enhance self-awareness, foster self-acceptance or achieve greater satisfaction in life. Above all, personal therapy is a vital form of self-care for therapists—a space to feel at home, put down our burdens and let somebody else carry the load for an hour. It may not be possible or necessary for every personal therapy experience to immediately feedback into professional development. It is a happy coincidence that the focus on personal selves often adds to therapist development rather than taking away from it.

The finest gift from this dedicated hour to reflecting and talking about ourselves every week is an increase in self-awareness. This is one of the fundamental purposes of personal therapy and is frequently reported as its primary benefit by therapists (Willemsen et al., 2023). Therapist-clients who gain awareness of their inner world can leverage this understanding to respond more effectively to their clients' emotions (Noble & Rizq, 2020). For example, a therapist in personal therapy might become more aware of their difficulty tolerating uncertainty and recognize how their pressing need for closure might lead to a push for premature solutions. This increased self-awareness can influence how they respond to a client who is struggling with doubt. As the therapist learns to tolerate and accept their own uncertainty, they may also develop the capacity to tolerate, and even value, similar emotions in their client. For the therapist, staying in touch with discomfort can also support the ability to differentiate between their own feelings and reactions and those of the client. The better therapists know and understand themselves, both personally and professionally, the better equipped they are to maintain boundaries and distinguish the client's experience from their own.

Building Our Reflective Capacity

Therapy spaces engender a habit of reflection, encouraging deeper thought about oneself and one's relationship with the world. The felt security in the therapeutic relationship can enhance the capacity to reflect and mentalize (Rizq, 2011). As therapists, it is almost inevitable that our personal reflections will inform clinical work but is the intentional effort to integrate experiences from these two spaces that enriches and consolidates our learnings.

Wigg et al. (2011) derived a model to outline how personal therapy impacts the development of reflective practice. They describe a generative process across four areas of reflection: beginning with *personal reflections.* These centre on the self, working to enhance self-awareness and acceptance, along with understanding the ways in which personal aspects enter the therapy room. As these connections are made, *professional reflections* on the role and identity of the therapist are strengthened, beliefs about the value of therapy are reinforced, and therapeutic skills and competence are honed. New aspects of the self may continue to emerge over time, both in everyday life and within personal therapy. While we may never know ourselves completely, the process of searching and engaging in personal therapy over a period of time and examining our changing motivations and needs can build *extended reflection.* Finally, there are *meta reflections* which involve an intentional process of assimilation and integration of our experiences and reflections, marked by greater ease in bringing our authentic selves into our therapeutic work.

It can be valuable to allow personal therapy experiences the time and space to settle. When these experiences are crowded by client work, academic demands or supervision, their impact may be diminished. We may revisit therapy experiences at different times, making new meanings as we evolve as individuals and therapists. For instance, a therapist may first notice a need for recognition in a specific context at a particular point in time, later connecting this to other experiences and reflecting on how it influences interactions with clients. This need may manifest in feelings of hurt or withdrawal when clients do not fully engage, or in a tendency to work harder to feel valued by them. As the therapist explores these dynamics, they become more aware of what happens when they acknowledge their strong need for recognition. Through self-reflection, they might discern where this need serves them and where it does not. This self-awareness deepens the therapist's understanding of their own emotional landscape, allowing for more precise attunement to clients' journeys and identifying what might be most supportive in each moment. Over time, the therapist develops a personal narrative or theory around the need for recognition, which can then be integrated into their clinical practice, deepening their therapeutic approach. This represents the deepest layer of reflection, one that bridges the personal and the professional, unfolds across time and illuminates how each domain of reflection interacts with the other.

Deepening Our Connection with Clients

Sitting on the client's chair brings an awareness of a range of subtle thoughts and feelings that may remain inaccessible within the therapist role. Experiencing what it is like to be spoken to as a client may stimulate us to think more carefully about how we speak to our own clients. For instance, did we find it comforting or alienating to hear our intimate experiences described as symptoms? If we received a mental health diagnosis, did it feel accurate or reductive? Such moments invite reflection on the ways in which a therapist's choice of language influence a client's sense of being seen, understood or defined within the therapeutic encounter.

The experience of being a client can also make us aware of the courage it takes to seek help, the vulnerability when sharing parts that we feel ashamed of, the occasional reluctance to enter sessions and the sense of eager impatience while awaiting the next chance to speak. As we sit in this chair, our experiences can concomitantly lead to a reduction of any feelings of omnipotence. Our familiarity with the client's world can deepen both the experience and expression of empathy. We will be better placed when we have a lived experience of being a client and are not just curious tourists in their world.

Pause and reflect...

If you were in personal therapy, would you disclose it to your client?

What would indicate to you that this disclosure might be helpful, or best avoided?

Several tangible and intangible experiences can occur in the corridor between the therapy room with one's personal therapist and the therapy room with one's client. The area of greatest impact and perhaps the most significant contribution of personal therapy to professional development seems to be in terms of building relational depth and interpersonal competencies (Rake & Paley, 2017). As we learn to open up and allow ourselves to develop intimacy with our personal therapists, we grow to accept ourselves better. This in turn creates the conditions for a more flexible relationship with intimacy, enabling us to experiment with different levels of closeness and distance. The experience of personal growth can translate into the ability to meet clients where they are, and increased comfort with clients who push us away as well as with those who need us to be very close. Noticing what helped us connect with our own therapist and the relational strategies they used can clarify how we might build stronger alliances with our own clients.

Learning Through Experience

Therapy can feel like a closed box. No matter how much theory has been read or how many videos have been watched, it remains challenging to fully imagine what it feels like inside the therapy room. The importance of showing unconditional positive regard to clients may be understood, but the ways in which this can be expressed and felt are continually unfolding. We may not realize how much the expression on a therapist's face can communicate, until the moment comes when we closely observe our therapist while sharing our own story. In essence, personal therapy is a great opportunity to learn how to be a therapist. It helps with zooming in on the minutiae of the therapeutic experience, of course, but it can also bring theories to life. This experiential part of personal therapy is likely to have the deepest impact on our learning.

On the same day, you may *be* a client who is finding it hard to manage their emotions, and you may also *have* a client who is finding it hard to manage their emotions. As you reflect on what your therapist did that helped you change your emotional state, you may try the same with your client. Or as you notice how when your therapist draws your attention to more constructive emotions it enables you to let go of more destructive ones, this can help you experience emotion-focused therapy in action. As we keep looking at different aspects of both experiences, we may not only learn how to manage our own emotions better, but also fine tune how we can help our clients manage theirs.

The personal therapist is thus an important role model for us as therapists. This is not just in the context of teaching us what to do, but also in the context of teaching us what not to do. Having a therapist who is usually late may inspire us to always be on time for our clients. Having a therapist who does not maintain boundaries can make us more conscious of times when our personal material is spilling over into the session. Of course, all therapists make mistakes, and this is also an important lesson. When a personal therapist makes a mistake, acknowledges it, takes responsibility and works to repair any harm, it offers an opportunity to recognize and accept the inevitability of mistakes in therapy (Bellows, 2007). Perhaps most importantly, this could help reconfigure our expectations from the therapy process and come closer to embracing the idea of being a good-enough therapist.

Pause and reflect

Take a moment and ask yourself if there was anything your personal therapist did that made you feel: 'Yes, I want to be like that as a therapist'. Or 'No, I don't want to do that as a therapist.'?

Have your experiences in personal therapy influenced you to adopt or avoid any behaviours with your own clients?

The power of insight, the strength that comes from being truly accepted or the thrill of feeling equipped with a strategy for self-help can leave a lasting impact. As personal issues are worked through, faith in clients' ability to address their own challenges grows, along with the courage to challenge or push clients when necessary. Speaking to clients about therapy, and how and why it works, becomes rooted in experience rather than just theoretical knowledge, lending more emotional depth and impact.

Growing into Our Own Style

Experiencing personal therapy reveals the unique style of each therapist. While some may model themselves after their personal therapists, others may use this experience to become the kind of therapist they wish they had. These insights provide an opportunity to reflect on a style or stance that aligns with one's personality, resonate with particular aspects of orientation or technique and identify language that feels both natural and effective. While the connection with a personal therapist is important, so is the process of individuation—allowing the expression of the 'self' in ways that are spontaneous and authentic. This transition from idealization or blind imitation to the creation of an individual identity fosters growth as a therapist (Wiseman & Shefler, 2001). As personal therapy experiences are processed, intentional reflection on strengths, vulnerabilities, values and even unique aspects like a sense of humour supports the process of becoming one's own kind of therapist. This journey can also lead to the development of personal techniques and theories, as seen in the case of Pinsof, who created integrated problem-solving therapy. He described his own experiences as a patient as one of the most profound influences on model development, "It is a model that I can sell, because I have bought it. I know it from the inside as well as the outside" (Pinsof, 2005, p. 146). Of course, such integration requires observing how theory and technique are applied, experiencing their impact and using this experience to refine and deepen one's understanding of theory.

Every Silver Lining Has a Cloud

Of course, not every experience in therapy is one of affirmation and growth. Personal therapy can be a mixed bag, especially when it is mandatory or introduced in the training phase. A glimpse into this intensely private space, we reveals testimonies to the transformative power and value of personal therapy, along with several divergent voices. Trainees undergoing mandated therapy have also described a gamut of negative responses; a lack of readiness, a sense of disconnection from the process or just ticking a box to anger and resentment and feeling like there was a gun to the head (Rizq & Target, 2010; Von Haenisch, 2011). There is so much to learn during therapy training—about connecting with our clients' needs, developing skills and growing into our therapist identity and findings time to process difficult emotions evoked in personal therapy can indeed be challenging. Immersion in personal exploration can particularly overwhelming when trainees are vulnerable with difficult relational histories and memories. While most research centres on trainees, the possible negative effects of personal therapy could be experienced at any point in the professional trajectory. We may seek to emulate our personal therapist, how they relate with clients, their choice and timing of interventions, their language, stance and philosophies of change. It can be disconcerting, even painful, if we realize that much of this needs to be unlearnt later along the professional journey. Sometimes, negative experiences strengthen the conviction to take a different path and carry the potential to shape an individual into the kind of therapist they aspire to be (Råbu et al, 2019).

It may be assumed that investment in personal therapy will yield dividends in terms of improved client outcomes, but definitive conclusions are difficult to draw from extant research. Questions about how the timing or duration of personal therapy engagement impacts client welfare remain, yet answers tend to be drawn more from the shared reflections of therapists than from methodologically sound quantitative studies. Those of us in personal therapy need to take the time to reflect on what we are learning and how we are growing (or not). When therapist-clients delve into their experiences more actively, attempting to connect the dots between the personal self and therapist self, there is much more to gain from the experience.

A Therapist Speaks: **The Habit of Honesty and the Limits of Technique**

Nancy McWilliams

I began my analysis at age 23, and I saw my analyst, a warm man with a reputation as a classical Freudian, three times a week on the couch for four and a half years. The most enduring outcome of my personal analysis, which preceded my formal clinical training, was the discipline of trying to engage honestly with my internal life. There is a humility that comes with unflinching immersion in the depths of one's own mind, and with that humility comes a greater openness to learning from others about what one tends to get wrong. Perhaps most critical to my maturation, I internalized my analyst's voice—the voice of someone who could acknowledge having made a clinical error.

A turning point in my analysis happened after I cancelled my appointment twice in a row due to physical distress after a minor medical procedure. This was highly unusual for me—I was trying to be an exemplary patient. My analyst asked if there was any psychological dynamic behind my having been in unexpected pain or having missed my appointments. I reacted with devastation based on a powerful transference. My father had sometimes been abruptly critical, and what I projected onto my analyst was the accusation, "You are not a good-enough patient. If you really cared about this analysis, you would have pushed through the pain. Maybe the pain isn't even real! You were in a state of resistance to the treatment, and you didn't even know it!" So, in response to his query, I went into a long, angry diatribe: how much it felt like unfair, harsh paternal criticism; how hard I had tried to be a good daughter to my father; and how painful it had always been when I seemed suddenly not to meet his standards. My analyst listened quietly for a long time, bearing silent witness to my rage and my anguished memories, and then asked, rather mildly, "Didn't your father ever make a mistake?".

The implicit admission that *he* had made a mistake, that he should not have asked the question, or should have listened longer before exploring the possibilities of somatization or resistance, was deeply touching to me. As I write about it now, it seems a fairly ordinary human interaction, hardly the stuff of enduring gratitude. But knowing that he had deviated from the then-prevailing psychoanalytic party line about non-disclosure and experiencing how gracefully he both acknowledged the limits of his own understanding and confronted my idealization of my father, it had a profound impact. It was clear to him, but not yet to me, that my internal sense of never being good enough reflected a fantasy that if only I had been the perfect child, my father, whose judgment I wanted to believe was beyond question, would never have been upset with me.

I now believe that learning technical approaches such as trying to confer emotional validation, or mirror feelings, or give cognitive reframes to patients' problematic beliefs, are not sufficient to become an effective clinician. Therapists have to be able, as my analyst was, to admit to the limits of their capacities for empathy and be nondefensively honest about their misunderstandings and failures. I learned to accept criticism from my patients not because I was taught to do so but because my analyst accepted it from me. At the heart of the analytic attitude is a commitment to a level of honesty that is exceedingly demanding. This radical honesty may be even more fundamental than empathy and deserves more attention in our psychotherapy training programs.

I remember a patient, early in my practice, who repeatedly attacked me for not understanding her. The referring psychiatrist spoke of her as a "borderline from hell," and indeed, from our first meeting on, she engaged in long, angry rants about my inability to make her feel better. I struggled valiantly to overcome her negativity with my best efforts at empathy. I wanted to show her I understood that behind her angry tirades was terrible anguish. But all my efforts to mirror her internal devastation and show her my understanding failed—in fact, they seemed to exacerbate her pain. She became more and more infuriated with my impotence, often leaving an appointment early, slamming my door in exasperation as she exited. I came to dread her sessions.

After weeks of fruitless efforts, as she once again insisted, "No, you DON'T understand!" it dawned on me that she was right. I knew cognitively how much she was suffering, but emotionally, I could not fully join her experience. This was a painful truth to admit, an assault on my narcissistic need to see myself as able to connect emotionally with any human experience. But just as a witness to a person in physical pain cannot quite imagine what the sufferer feels (and doesn't want to), I had no visceral sense of my patient's anguish (and would have resisted feeling it if I had). After reflecting on this insight for a few moments, I said, "I have to admit that you are right. I *don't* understand what it's like to be you. And I *can't*. I've never been as depressed as you are, and I hope to God I never am, because from my perspective, it looks like hell on earth."

For the first time, she felt a genuine connection with me. Paradoxically, she experienced my admission that I could *not* feel empathy as empathic. This shift led to her willingness to describe her internal world ("racing thoughts," "restless energy," "inability to sleep") well enough that I realized that the diagnosis with which she had been sent to me was wrong. She actually had a bipolar illness in which her mania expressed itself as rage. This was the turning point in our work, which in retrospect she sees as lifesaving. Once she was consistently taking a mood stabilizer, her rage relented, and therapeutic collaboration became possible, enabling several years of productive treatment. It is now four decades since her termination, and she is still doing well. Some months after she enlightened me about the limits of my empathy, I ran into the physician who had been prescribing her medication. "What a lovely woman!" he exclaimed. "It must be a pleasure to work with her!".

In my own experience as a patient, I learned that there is a radical humility in the attitude of a genuinely helpful therapist. Theodor Reik, whose work originally inspired me, framed this virtue as moral courage. As a therapist, I am neither a knowing authority nor a flawless empath. I am an *employee* of my patients. Just as my analyst was open to learning from me how to do his job, I try to approach my work as the apprentice of the individuals who hire me. Only with their instruction and correction can I learn how to be of genuine help to them.

Nancy McWilliams *is Visiting Professor Emerita at Rutgers Graduate School of Applied & Professional Psychology and has a private practice in USA. A former president of the Society for Psychoanalysis and Psychoanalytic Psychotherapy of the American Psychological Association, she is a member of the Austen Riggs Center Board of Trustees. She is author of four textbooks (on psychoanalytic diagnosis, case formulation, therapy, and supervision) and is co-editor of the Psychodynamic Diagnostic Manual.*

Our Journey of Personal Therapy

Psychotherapy can take many forms, and no one knows this better than a therapist-client. Taking the time to reflect on options and preferences, perhaps even trying out a few different approaches, can help identify the therapy that works best for us.

Pause and reflect

If you are in personal therapy, reflect on what contributed to your decision.

Think about the influences on your choice of therapist and the form of therapy.

Who is the Best Therapist for Me?

Once we decide to take the plunge and seek personal therapy, the first steps involve making the critical decision of who to see. As therapists, we may be especially discerning when choosing our own therapist, aware of how significantly the quality of the therapist can influence the therapeutic process. While some therapists may find senior professionals or colleagues more accessible, others may prefer to seek therapists outside their professional circle to preserve boundaries and ensure confidentiality (Norcross, 2005). Much like any client, therapists seek someone they feel safe with, whose competence they trust, and a form of treatment they believe is likely to help. Of course, it is the match between personal therapist and therapist-client that matters the most. With the growing online presence of therapists, it also common to explore professional websites, social media content and client testimonials to gain a sense of their therapeutic approach, style, values and professional alignments.

It could well happen that it does not work out with the first therapist we try. Perhaps there is no relational fit, or the therapeutic orientation of one's personal therapist may not align with the needs of the moment. As we develop professionally and gain insight into how different therapies work in practice, we may use this knowledge to make more informed choices when seeking a personal therapist. It can be an interesting exercise to reflect on what draws us towards a particular therapist.

Pause and reflect…

What would you like or expect from your relationship with your personal therapist?

What might you find intimidating about your personal therapist?

What would you experience as reassuring about your personal therapist?

Staying Home or Going Out?

Another decision the therapist-client may face is whether to seek therapy within their own theoretical orientation or explore a different one. Some may feel they can deepen their understanding by working with a therapist who shares their orientation, while others might be drawn to a modality they are curious about or interested in integrating into their own practice.

Notably, while psychoanalytic and psychodynamic therapists tend to stay closer to home in choosing therapists from their own orientation, practitioners from other approaches have shown more varied preferences (Norcross, 2005). In fact, cognitive-behavioural therapists have been known for seeking personal therapy outside their orientation (Laireiter & Willutzki, 2005). Choosing a therapist from a different orientation can be an interesting experience, providing the opportunity to have our personal material examined through the language and philosophy of another school of thought. Allowing ourselves to enter into our experiences rather than intellectualizing or labelling them creates more space for change and growth—and seeing a therapist from a different orientation can stimulate such change, shaking us out of familiar and repeated thinking tracks. It is then easier to let go of our therapist selves, just be clients and allow ourselves to receive.

A positive personal experience with another orientation can also impact the way we view our own. Trainees from a cognitive-behavioural orientation described a tension between the manualized protocols they were learning as students and the more relational therapies they were experiencing as clients (Noble & Rizq, 2020). At this early stage, it may be too soon for them to learn how to integrate practices from two different orientations, and the experience of therapy in their own orientation may feel less confusing and help in crystallizing theoretical concepts (Laireiter & Willutzki, 2005). However, later in one's professional development, exposure to other orientations of therapy can broaden or deepen our skills and competence. Perhaps a more experienced dynamic therapist will be able to use their experience of feminist therapy to enliven their own sessions, noticing when stepping forward to meet the client can significantly change client experience. A more experienced therapist who works from a cognitive-behavioural perspective may feel they have already absorbed much of what this approach offers, and may now seek to learn something new, both about therapy and about themselves. Ultimately, the choice of therapeutic orientation depends on the reasons for seeking personal therapy and the role the therapist envisions it playing in both their personal life and professional development. Is it a tool to learn techniques? A means of understanding the therapeutic alliance? A pathway to explore less explored parts of the self? Or a hope of healing fractured relationships? Each therapeutic orientation offers a unique perspective on human suffering and may be able to meet our needs in different ways. As we move through different phases of life, the challenges we face change, and so may the type of therapy that best supports us. While seeing a therapist from our own orientation can enhance professional development, our personal selves might also enjoy the freedom to experiment.

Are We There Yet?

There is no one right time to seek personal therapy and no one recommended duration of therapy. For some, personal therapy may be a brief, mandated requirement during training or something that seems expected. For others, it becomes an essential pillar of support they cannot imagine doing without. There is a sense that therapists accumulate a lot of emotional detritus every day, making personal therapy an important space to support both their clients and themselves. Some research suggests that therapists prefer long-term therapy and are encouraged to pursue it by their own therapists (Norcross et al., 2001). However, this is not to say that only long-duration therapies are helpful. Hoyt (2011) speaks about how a single session of hypnotherapy helped him prepare for a surgery he required.

A long duration of therapy does not necessarily mean seeing the same therapist, week after week for years. Rather, therapy may extend over time as our needs evolve, involving work on different issues, exploring various therapists and modalities, and integrating varied insights about psychotherapy and ourselves. Several factors beyond duration likely influence the impact and value of personal therapy. Ultimately, the significance of therapy's length may be less important than each therapist's thoughtful reflection on the reasons behind their preferences regarding duration.

Pause and reflect…

If you were in personal therapy, what would you feel about wanting to take a break?

Would you find it hard to tell yourself (and your therapist) that you are done or that therapy is not working for you?

When would you consider your personal therapy complete?

Helping the Helper: Being a Personal Therapist

Having explored the experience of being a therapist-client, we now turn our gaze towards the other chair, seeking to understand the nuances and demands of being a personal therapist.

Nasir, a seasoned therapist in his 40 s, was asked to be a personal therapist for the first time. While he was initially flattered and felt recognized by his professional community, he wondered how to proceed. Would personal therapy be different from regular therapy? How would he prioritize and balance the twin goals of personal and professional development? Would a therapist-client be easier or harder to work with than a regular client? Would he feel more relaxed talking to a colleague who understood his language, or would he feel more tense at being open to evaluation by a peer? What would he do if he ran into the therapist-client outside the session? He felt the need to focus his reflections and to consult someone with experience as a personal therapist.

If you were in Nasir's shoes, what would you have wanted to know?

In many ways, therapy is therapy, and the required skills, processes and foci remain largely consistent. However, when another therapist occupies the client's chair, it introduces subtle influences that can permeate the therapeutic process, whether consciously recognized or not. The personal therapist therefore encounters unique challenges in creating a workable dynamic with their therapist-clients. Many of these challenges can come from therapist-clients and their discomfort or unfamiliarity with being clients. But these struggles can also arise from within the personal therapist themselves, who may feel judged for not being good enough or uncertain about what to prioritize in sessions.

A meaningful starting point is to explore what being a personal therapist truly means to us. Is it incidental that some of our clients are therapists? Do we wish to make it a larger part of our professional identity and actively position ourselves to see therapist-clients? Do we see therapist-clients (especially those in mandated personal therapy) as not having a real need or issue, unlike our other clients? This choice can be influenced both by our theoretical orientation as well as the value we place on self-awareness and personal therapy. For those intrigued by the possibilities inherent in being personal therapists, it is valuable to establish some guiding principles that can support us as we navigate this complex role.

Easing Therapist-Clients into the Other Chair

When they first enter the therapy room, therapist-clients can bring different expectations and vulnerabilities with them. Some may feel eager to finally have their personal therapy experience, others may fear judgement from colleagues, while many, often trainees undergoing mandatory therapy, may feel pressured into the role and uncertain about whether they truly need it. As personal therapists, we often start by exploring what personal therapy means to our therapist-clients and addressing any apprehensions about the process. In particular, we need to recognise that our clients may feel especially vulnerable and unsure, struggling to follow in a room where they usually lead. Even when we are confident of its value, the shift from taking care of to being taken care of is rarely an easy one. Openly exploring what it might feel like to be in the other chair and addressing their questions and concerns by discussing our approach or plan can foster a more balanced partnership.

We ourselves might feel intimidated by having this 'expert' client who speaks our jargon, enquires knowledgably about our approach or declares clearly what they want and do not want from sessions. If a therapist-client tells their personal therapist that, "Mindfulness meditation doesn't really work for me, I need something more from you", this appearance of confidence can unsettle us, making us question our typical methods or approaches. Absorbed in this self-examination of our own training and skills, we may miss asking the client why mindfulness doesn't work for them or fail to explore what could work better and why. Therapist-clients use jargon or put on their professional hats for various reasons. Perhaps they feel nervous and exposed, striving to establish their own sense of self; or maybe they seek a more equal relationship. It is also possible that they hesitate to take off their professional hats because this is such unfamiliar territory. The use of a shared language can also be a way of drawing us closer and sharing inner worlds. A therapist-client who uses the term dysregulated to describe their emotional state could be conveying, "I know you will understand what I mean when I say I feel dysregulated and it is a relief to not have to explain quite how out of control or desperate I can feel sometimes". This could of course, also be a way of keeping distance and intellectualizing issues, a therapist-client may find it easier to say dysregulated than to allow themselves to experience and express that dysregulation in the moment. A reflective openness to possible meanings, coupled with genuine interest in the client's underlying experience, is essential in creating a healthy therapeutic alliance. We would not ask any other client to leave their profession or professional language at the door. Instead, we honour the strengths and knowledge they bring into the session. As personal therapists, perhaps we need to reflect on what it is that makes us uncomfortable with the therapist who lives within our therapist-client.

Attending to the Personal and Professional

Each client takes a different journey to the therapy room, carrying their own hopes and goals for who they wish to become or how they hope to change their lives. In personal therapy too, the focus arises primarily from the client's needs and experiences, and it is important that we take the time to understand what these goals are. Therapist-clients may dismiss some of their own goals as too insignificant and worry about revelations that are too painful. They might wonder, "How can I as a therapist actually need help with parenting? How can I reveal my extra marital relationship or share that I am dependent on substances?".

We may need to offer explicit permission to bring both smaller and larger goals into the therapy space, and to reassure them that heightened functioning is not expected because of their profession. Asking the question, Why now? can help them connect with the immediate experiences that led them to seek therapy, while also giving us the opportunity to validate their needs, whatever they might be. As personal therapists, we try to respect and treat therapist-clients like fellow professionals, without ever forgetting that they are also vulnerable human beings. This balancing act requires ongoing sensitivity to the therapist-client's evolving needs, allowing all parts of their experience to enter the session. Our capacity to welcome both their functional and struggling aspects can support them in accepting all parts of themselves.

Personal therapists may also hold professional development as a conscious goal, drawing on various approaches to explore the interplay between the personal and the professional. For instance, we might invite reflection on what motivated the therapist-client to enter the field, what being a therapist means to them and how this shapes their clinical work. We can also explore what sustains them in the role, what they find meaningful, and where they encounter challenges. A therapist-client who tends to avoid conflict, whether in personal or professional contexts, can examine this pattern from both perspectives, perhaps using their therapeutic skills to build personal insight or drawing on personal breakthroughs to strengthen their professional capacities.

Therapist-clients might value the opportunity to discuss their professional choices and build congruence between their personal and professional selves. Sometimes, therapist-clients may wish to discuss their work-related difficulties, describing a difficult or painful session with their own clients. They may even want to discuss a positive experience, where they found hope or direction from witnessing how their clients resolved their issues. When therapist-clients bring up professional issues, we strive to stay away from a supervisory position, instead, keeping focus on the inner life and needs of the client in front of us. Even when they talk about their work, we need to keep in mind that they are really talking about themselves and help them also to make the same connection. Sharing reflections such as, "You are telling me about this client who made you very angry, I wonder if this is similar to the anger you feel with your partner when they challenge your ideas", could be useful. In this way, we can use their professional experiences as a pathway into understanding their personal values, concerns or difficulties.

What Makes the Therapist-Client Unique?

Having a client who is also an expert on therapy can be both deeply satisfying and uniquely challenging. We may feel friendlier and warmer towards our therapist-clients and experience sessions as livelier and more natural. Personal therapists report that they enjoy sessions more and are more likely to discuss research or matters relevant to the profession with their therapist-clients as compared to other clients, creating a feeling of intellectual closeness (Norcross et al., 2001). A pre-existing knowledge of therapy can work as a shortcut, as therapist-clients often require less psychoeducation, and their intellectual knowledge of concepts makes the shift to the emotional level much easier. There can also be a sense of shared camaraderie and experience, with both therapist and client being aware of the highs and lows of a therapist's work life.

However, seeing a therapist-client can bring out a different part of our professional self, as the approval of an expert will always carry more weight than the approval of a lay person. There could be a stronger desire to be appreciated or acknowledged by the client, accompanied by a heightened sense of scrutiny. We may find ourselves being more on time, maintaining more detailed notes or monitoring our moment to moment responses more critically. If our therapist-client tells us that they do not feel accepted or that they wonder if therapy is going anywhere, it can be hard not to feel defensive. The imposter feeling that lurks within most therapists could quickly get activated.

Therapist-clients may also have different expectations from therapy as compared to lay people. They might be hoping for a magical transformative therapy experience and feel let down or be critical when this does not happen. When combined with an insider's awareness of its underbelly such as the recognition that we don't always like our clients, or that we are sometimes just guessing and hoping something will help, this can leave therapist-clients feeling ambivalent about both the process and the therapist. Perhaps it is experiences like these that have led many personal therapists to describe therapist-clients as more challenging or critical (Geller et al., 2005).

As personal therapists, we may need to be extra sensitive to boundaries and how they may be interpreted by our therapist-clients. Therapist-clients might push us to treat therapy like it is nothing more than a conversation between colleagues, wanting to contact us after hours or seeking career advice. While we might occasionally choose to shift between the therapeutic frame and regular life, it is not useful to do so at the behest of the therapist-client, as this can make therapy feel like less of a safe and certain space (Probst, 2015). When the personal therapist is firm about maintaining boundaries and treating the therapist-client like any other client, this can be experienced by therapist-clients as a rejection of their professional selves. On the other hand, it might easier for them to truly let go within this frame, trusting the personal therapist to be the professional in the room and freeing them to just be clients. Personal therapists will need to reflect on what these choices will mean to particular therapist-clients and navigate accordingly.

Finally, we can keep in mind that the likelihood of extra session contact is far greater with therapist-clients than with other clients, as we often share professional spaces. We can try keeping such contact to a minimum, but where this is unavoidable, we need to explicitly negotiate around client preferences. For instance, we might directly ask, "What would you like to do if we run into each other at a conference?" Reflecting together on the meaning of these experiences can also be useful.

Both theoretical and research literature do not really address the issue of the kind of support personal therapists might need. We assume they are experts and know what they are doing, but of course, this is not always true. Personal therapists may even need more supervisory support, especially to address potential feelings of professional ineptitude. The space to reflect on the session process, including power struggles with therapist-clients and feelings of vulnerability or jealousy that may arise, can be invaluable for personal therapists. Equally important is the ability to separate our own projections about how we think the therapist-client sees us from what is actually unfolding in the interaction. Conversations on how to support and strengthen the work of personal therapists are limited, and we see this as an important area of growth for our profession.

Too Much Information: Dealing with Disclosures

Sharing a common professional world means that therapist-clients may sometimes speak about colleagues and contacts, leaving the personal therapist privy to information that can feel difficult to hold. Such disclosures may evoke curiosity, fascination or discomfort. Feelings of protectiveness or defensiveness can also emerge, especially when someone the therapist-client criticizes is personally known and valued. It becomes important to consider how personal relationships with colleagues can be maintained without allowing confidential information to influence those interactions. Anticipating the possibility of such disclosures allows space to reflect on how best to respond. At the same time, clients must feel safe to speak openly about their feelings and difficulties with people in their lives. This places the responsibility on the therapist to manage any internal conflict that arises. Offering an explicit assurance of confidentiality may help therapist-clients feel reassured that these conversations are both safe and welcome.

Therapists may also feel disturbed when therapist-clients bring up information about ethical violations they have engaged in, either deliberately or unintentionally. These disclosures can range from seemingly minor lapses, such as receiving an expensive gift from a client or conducting a session in a non-professional setting, to more serious breaches that challenge the core values of the profession. As personal therapists, uncertainty can arise about whether such ethical breaches should be brought to the therapist-client's attention while considering the impact on the therapeutic alliance. If a significant ethical breach is uncovered, there may also be an obligation to consider reporting, which adds layers of complexity and tension. These are complex issues with no simple answers. Consulting with trusted peers and reflecting on the possible outcomes of different choices can help balance obligations to the therapist-client, their clients and the profession. One approach is to discuss the ethical breach openly with therapist-clients, exploring why they made that choice and whether they are aware of the ethical principles involved. For instance, helping them recognize that it is an inability to say no that led to accepting an expensive gift, can open pathways for developing stronger ethical competencies. However, this ideal outcome may not always be achievable. Some therapist-clients might be too vulnerable or defensive to critically examine their behaviour at a given time. In these cases, suggesting a temporary sabbatical from clinical work can provide necessary space for healing and reflection, reducing risks to clients and the therapist-client alike. If resistance persists and the therapist-client refuses to acknowledge unethical behaviour, the personal therapist must grapple with their own conflicting ethical duties in balancing respect for confidentiality with the imperative to protect clients and uphold professional standards.

In conclusion, while there are several unique aspects to seeing therapist-clients, we would recommend Laura Brown's advice to remember that "…the therapist-client is a client, first, last, and in between" (Brown, 2005, p. 280).

Perspectives on Training and Development

Debates About Mandatory Personal Therapy During Training

A compelling argument for making therapy obligatory is the initiation of a strong foundation for self-exploration and reflective work. However, personal therapy is not necessarily intrinsic to psychotherapy training worldwide, and there are significant variations across countries, mental health disciplines and training programmes. For instance, while training programmes in Germany have stringent requirements for licensure (Bundes Psychotherapeuten Kammer, 2022), the presence and nature of requirements and specifications vary widely across courses in the UK, while the Rehabilitation Council of India (2016) does not mention personal therapy in its guidelines for clinical psychology training in the country. In countries where there are fewer resources for personal therapy, it may be up to each educational institution to decide if they wish to make this mandatory, suggest it as an option and provide some institutional support in the form of designated time and a list of possible therapists, or ignore it altogether.

While personal therapy during training can be a valued experience, concerns about potential negative effects for some trainees and infringements on their autonomy are being expressed more openly and stridently. The economic and time costs of personal therapy reduce access, and this can deter some persons from joining certain training courses or even from choosing psychotherapy as a profession. We recommend that while available options for personal therapy can be discussed, the elements of choice are important—to seek therapy, decline, or even defer the decision. As trainers and supervisors, we need to reflect on our position on personal therapy for trainees and consider whether and when we would recommend it.

Best practice guidelines can be helpful for training contexts that encourage, recommend or continue to mandate personal therapy. These can support trainees in making informed choices, engage safely with the process and learn to use personal therapy in a meaningful way. Training courses need to have clarity about the aims and rationale for this form of experiential learning and share this with trainees in advance (Moller et al., 2009; Murphy et al., 2018). Space for dialogue, choice regarding the therapist, therapeutic orientation, duration and frequency of sessions or even discontinuation of therapy are advocated (Malikiosi-Loizos, 2013). Information about therapists who provide care at reduced fees may be particularly important for trainees, especially trainees who may have limited economic resources. If personal therapy is not mandated and is being suggested or recommended, then outlining the approach and protocol for that might be important. Trainers may need to reflect on their reasons for recommending personal therapy for a particular trainee and peer-consultation may be helpful to ensure that personal biases are considered.

An authentic engagement with personal therapy and assimilation of its potential benefits can be fostered by reflective processes to help trainees integrate their therapy experiences and convert these learning into more effective work with clients.

Attunement to the trainees' experience and commitment to their safety and well-being are paramount with clear pathways for support and redressal for any difficulties with the personal therapist or other negative experiences (Edwards, 2018). What these recommendations translate into is that teachers, trainers and supervisors need to consciously guide students on their personal therapy journeys. This can include practical recommendations of how to find a therapist and perhaps even how to manage the spillover from personal therapy in to work with clients. It may be as simple as scheduling personal therapy sessions so that they are not followed by difficult client work, or it could be a more complex process of understanding how to park some of the more overwhelming personal therapy experiences so that they do not enter sessions with clients until they are more processed. Supervisors can make it a habit to enquire about personal therapy experiences and how they are currently impacting the therapist-client's identity and clinical work. At one end of the spectrum, the student-therapist-client might be left feeling very inadequate as they note the vast difference between their level of competence and their therapist's level. At the other end, the therapist-client may feel no benefit from personal therapy leaving them questioning their choice of profession or orientation. These are both valid responses and trainees could benefit from having an open space to explore and integrate their personal therapy experiences with their professional development.

Multiple Pathways to Personal Development

There is an emergence of training recommendations which call for introducing trainees to a range of reflective and experiential activities rather than personal therapy alone (e.g., European Association of Psychotherapy, 2023). Sometimes in our zeal to speak of the benefits, we may discount how some therapists who have never been in personal therapy have deep enduring relationships and good outcomes with their clients, while others may remain less effective as therapists despite their personal therapy experience (McWilliams, 2004). Experiential groups, supervision spaces or a commitment to self-reflection, perhaps through activities such as journaling can also provide scaffolding to develop self-awareness and promote personal growth. Personal practice frameworks, which are shorter and perhaps more contained than personal therapy, are gaining research and theoretical support. Each of these spaces offers different reflective possibilities that we might find useful as therapists. Supervision is perhaps one of the first spaces for trainees to bring in their selves, emotions, memories and experiences and explore the connections with therapeutic work. Therapeutic elements may percolate into supervisory spaces and while we cannot fence the personal entirely, we recommend that the integrity and safety of supervision spaces be protected. For supervisors, this calls for reflection on the supervisory process with each trainee and on their own emotional responses, perhaps guiding supervisees towards personal therapy when this seems to be needed.

Conclusion

Entering personal therapy calls for the courage to be able to meet parts of ourselves that we may otherwise avoid. But this is a space that can reward our courage with reflective opportunities for personal and professional transformation. It is when we are compelled by our own reasons and choose to engage deeply with this form of personal exploration that personal therapy may be most valuable. It plays a unique role in the lives of therapists because the only way to truly experience what it is like to be a psychotherapy client is to *be* a psychotherapy client.

References

Bellows, K. F. (2007). Psychotherapists' personal psychotherapy and its perceived influence on clinical practice. *Bulletin of the Menninger Clinic, 71*(3), 204–226.

Berman, E. (2005). On analysing colleagues (trainees included). In J. D. Geller, J. C. Norcross, & D. Orlinsky (Eds.), *The psychotherapist's own psychotherapy: Patient and clinician perspectives* (pp. 235–253). Oxford University Press.

Bhola, P., Raguram, A., Dugyala, M., & Ravishankar, A. (2017). Learning in the crucible of supervision: Experiences of trainee psychotherapists in India. *The Clinical Supervisor, 36*, 182–202.

Brown, L. S. (2005). Feminist therapy with therapists. Egalitarian and more. In J. D. Geller, J. C. Norcross, & D. Orlinsky (Eds.), *The psychotherapist's own psychotherapy: Patient and clinician perspectives* (pp. 265–281). Oxford University Press.

Bundes Psychotherapeuten Kammer (2022). Muster-Weiterbildungsordnung: Psychotherapet*innen. https://www.dptv.de/fileadmin/Redaktion/Bilder_und_Dokumente/Psychotherapie/Junge_PT/Muster_Weiterbildungsordnung_Nov_2022.pdf

Edwards, J. (2018). Counseling and psychology student experiences of personal therapy: A critical interpretive synthesis. *Frontiers in Psychology, 9*, 1732. https://doi.org/10.3389/fpsyg.2018.01732

European Association of Psychotherapy. (2023). *The European Certificate of Psychotherapy*. ECP Official document. Version 8.0. voted AGM Vienna March 2023. Retrieved from https://www.europsyche.org/ecp/ecp-standards/

Freud, S. (1915/1958). The unconscious. In J. Strachey, J. (Ed.), *The standard edition of the complete psychological works of Sigmund Freud* (pp. 159–215). Hogarth Press.

Geller, J. D., Norcross, J. C., & Orlinsky, D. (2005). Research on conducting psychotherapy with mental health professionals. In J. D. Geller, J. C. Norcross, & D. Orlinsky (Eds.), *The psychotherapist's own psychotherapy: Patient and clinician perspectives* (pp. 345–364). Oxford University Press.

Gottlieb, L. (2019). *Maybe you should talk to someone: A therapist, her therapist and our lives revealed*. Scribe Publications.

Hoyt, M. F. (2011). Psychology and my gallbladder: An insider's account. *Journal of Clinical Psychology: in Session, 67*(8), 766–775.

Kumaria, S., Bhola, P., & Orlinsky, D. E. (2018). Influences that count: Professional development of psychotherapists and counsellors in India. *Asia Pacific Journal of Counselling and Psychotherapy, 9*(1), 86–106.

Laireiter, A.-R., & Willutzki, U. (2005). Personal therapy in cognitive-behavioural therapy: Tradition and current practice. In J. D. Geller, J. C. Norcross, & D. Orlinsky (Eds.), *The psychotherapist's own psychotherapy: Patient and clinician perspectives* (pp. 41–51). Oxford University Press.

Malikiosi-Loizos, M. (2013). Personal therapy for future therapists: Reflections on a still debated issue. *The European Journal of Counselling Psychology, 2*, 33–50.

McWilliams, N. (2004). *Psychoanalytic psychotherapy: A practitioner's guide*. Guilford Press.

Moe, F. D., & Thimm, J. (2021). Personal therapy and the personal therapist. *Nordic Psychology, 73*(1), 3–28.

Moller, N. P., Timms, J., & Alilovic, K. (2009). Risky business or safety net? Trainee perceptions of personal therapy: A qualitative thematic analysis. *European Journal of Psychotherapy and Counselling, 11*(4), 369–384.

Murphy, D., Irfan, N., Barnett, H., Castledine, E., & Enescu, L. (2018). A systematic review and meta-synthesis of qualitative research into mandatory personal psychotherapy during training. *Counselling and Psychotherapy Research, 18*, 199–214.

Noble, A., & Rizq, R. (2020). It's led me astray': How cognitive behavioural therapists experience personal therapy in clinical practice. *Counselling and Psychotherapy Research, 20*, 29–38.

Norcross, J. C. (2005). The psychotherapists own psychotherapy: Educating and developing psychologists. *American Psychologist, 60*(8), 840–850.

Norcross, J. C., Geller, J. D., & Kurzawa, E. K. (2001). Conducting psychotherapy with psychotherapists II. Clinical practices and collegial advice. *Journal of Psychotherapy Practice and Research, 10*, 37–45.

Orlinsky, D. E., Schofield, M. J., Schroder, T., & Kazantzis, N. (2011). Utilization of personal therapy by psychotherapists: A practice-friendly review and a new study. *Journal of Clinical Psychology, 67*(8), 828–842.

Pinsof, W. M. (2005). A shamanic tapestry: My experiences with individual, marital and family therapy. In J. D. Geller, J. C. Norcross, & D. Orlinsky (Eds.), *The psychotherapist's own psychotherapy: Patient and clinician perspectives* (pp. 145–161). Oxford University Press.

Probst, B. (2015). The search for identity when clinicians become clients. *Clinical Social Work Journal, 43*(4), 337–347.

Råbu, M., McLeod, J., Haavind, H., Bernhardt, I. S., Nissen-Lie, H., & Moltu, C. (2019). How psychotherapists make use of their experiences from being a client: Lessons from a collective autoethnography. *Counselling Psychology Quarterly, 34*(1), 109–128.

Rake, C., & Paley, G. (2017). Personal therapy for psychotherapists: The impact on therapeutic practice. A qualitative study using interpretative phenomenological analysis. *Psychodynamic Practice, 15*(3), 275–294.

Rehabilitation Council of India. (2016). M.Phil. (Clinical Psychology): Guidelines and syllabus. Retrieved from www.rehabcouncil.nic.in

Rizq, R. (2011). Personal therapy in psychotherapeutic training: Current research and future directions. *Journal of Contemporary Psychotherapy, 41*, 175–185.

Rizq, R., & Target, M. (2010). "We had a constant battle". The role of attachment status in counselling psychologists' experiences of personal therapy: Some results from a mixed-methods study. *Counselling Psychology Quarterly, 23*(4), 343–369.

Von Haenisch, C. (2011). How did compulsory personal therapy during counselling training influence personal and professional development? *Counselling and Psychotherapy Research, 11*(2), 148–155.

Wigg, R., Cushway, D., & Neal, A. (2011). Personal therapy for therapists and trainees: A theory of reflective practice from a review of literature. *Reflective Practice, 12*(3), 347–359.

Willemsen, J., de Condé, H., Kaluzeviciute-Moreton, G., Guogaite, G., Polipo, N. F., & Zech, E. (2023). A qualitative meta-analysis examining the impact of personal therapy on clinical work and personal and professional development. *Counselling and Psychotherapy Research, 24*, 853–869.

Wiseman, H., & Shefler, G. (2001). Experienced psychoanalytically oriented therapists' narrative accounts of their personal therapy: Impacts on professional and personal development. *Psychotherapy, 38*(2), 129–141.

Chapter 12
Investing in Self-Care Through Reflective Practice

As therapists, we share our self and use our feelings, experiences and strengths to foster connection with our clients. This investment in the relational process often brings deep satisfaction, rewards and meaning to our lives. However, therapeutic work is not easy and is often marked by unexpected challenges and uncertain endings. Therapeutic work involves emotional labour (Hochschild, 2003), where we are encouraged to show empathy and consciously mask and regulate our own difficult and intrusive emotions. We also experience the pressure to do the right thing and be vigilant about client welfare. These continued responsibilities can take a toll on our well-being. Being a psychotherapist involves going through a repeated cycle of caring, which includes the phases of engaging with clients (empathic attachment), caring for and working with them (active involvement) and then separating from clients at the end of each session (felt separation). The fourth phase in this cycle of care is the time to pause for reflection, restoration and re-creation of the self (Skovholt & Trotter-Mathison, 2016).

Pause…

The Pause is a practice initiated by a nurse, after the experience of losing a patient to cardiac arrest. The nurse requested the team to pause and honour the life of the individual, before continuing with their routine. This collective pause encourages empathy during critical moments and allows space for an acceptance of difficult feelings (Ducar & Cunningham, 2018).

After a difficult session, psychotherapists can also feel the need to ground themselves.

and reflect…

When is the last time you needed a pause?

P. Bhola et al., *Reflective Practice in Psychotherapy and Counselling*,
https://doi.org/10.1007/978-981-96-9732-8_12

When did you last ignore your need for a pause?

The societal construction of therapists as "poster people for healthy emotions" (Van der Merwe, 2019, p. 38), and as role models equipped with all the answers, can be restrictive. In conforming to this image, therapists might portray themselves as impervious to stress and vulnerability, leading to feelings of shame when they need support. This became sharply evident during the COVID-19 pandemic, where therapists responded to the increased mental health needs of clients and front-line workers. Many quickly adapted to remote work, providing support from behind their screens—often while feeling tired, anxious and exhausted. Self-care is tyically framed as an ethical imperative, essential to ensure that personal challenges did not interfere with professional responsibilities. These experiences reinforced the need to view self-care not merely as a way to cope with stress, but as a means to foster growth, resilience and generativity. This perspective encourages therapists to see self-care as an integral to both personal and professional life, as something that enhances well-being, supports life goals and deepens the transformative potential of their work. Rather than a set of discrete tasks, self-care becomes a commitment to fostering positive emotions, cultivating meaningful relationships and embracing values that resonate on a deep level. When therapists take ownership of this process, self-care practices naturally integrate into their daily routines, much like writing session notes or consulting with supervisors.

Self-care is both an attitude and a practice. It allows us to sit with our feelings, embrace vulnerability and enhance our capacity for reflection and dialogue, ultimately improving our effectiveness at work. In this chapter, we explore how self-care and resilience-building can be more valued and visible aspects of our professional lives. Attitudes toward self-care are critically examined through the lens of systemic pressures for productivity and individuals' resistance to these demands. We spotlight self-care needs and practices within the contexts of challenging work contexts (e.g., palliative care), difficult experiences (e.g., client suicide), personal life transitions (e.g., parenthood) and organizational practices (e.g., leave policies). Additionally, we introduce diverse strategies to build a personalized toolkit for nourishment, sustainability and finding meaning in work.

The Right to Rest

Neoliberal notions about rest often frame it as a luxury rather than a necessity, prioritizing productivity and economic output over well-being. In this context, busyness is seen as something that defines worth, leading to a belief that time spent resting must be justified by future productivity. For therapists, who hold the emotional and psychological well-being of their clients as a priority, the dynamics of leisure and rest can be particularly complex and fraught with challenges. Cancelling a session, for instance, can trigger guilt over letting a client down and anxiety about their well-being. Clients may respond with disappointment or even resentment, and the collaborative process can be undermined if the sense of trust falters. Even a well-deserved vacation or a break can feel fraught—something therapists hesitate to take outright, as if they must ask for permission. This internal conflict is compounded by the pervasive expectation for therapists to remain available and responsive to clients via email, text, or tele therapy, even during periods of intended rest. On an individual level, therapists must confront their own beliefs about productivity and self-worth, while on a structural level, the demands of their profession often make it difficult to prioritize self-care without incurring professional or financial consequences.

Pause and reflect...

Women at Leisure, is an Instagram-based photo project that captures women in moments of rest, joy and self-care, challenging societal norms that deny them unstructured time. The creator, Surabhi Yadav frames leisure as a feminist issue and as an act of resistance, emphasizing how access to guilt-free time is informed by intersections of gender, class, caste and geography (Yadav, 2023).

In what ways do you think societal expectations influence your engagement in self-care practices?

How do your intersecting identities influence the guilt or ease you feel when taking time for yourself?

Factors such as race, gender, socio-economic status, ability and cultural background weave a complex pattern of privilege and disadvantage and determine who is entitled to self-care and who can genuinely access it. For example, women often experience guilt when prioritizing their own needs, influenced by cultural narratives that glorify self-sacrifice and caregiving. This guilt can be particularly pronounced for women in the caring professions, such as nursing, teaching and therapy, where the expectations to prioritize the well-being of others in their personal life is reinforced by similar expectations in their professional life. With men, the imperative to provide and be successful can leave them valuing achievement over satisfaction or care. Similarly, individuals with disabilities often face intersecting social, economic and physical barriers that can severely restrict their ability to engage in meaningful self-care, further illustrating how access is unequally distributed. Movements like the Nap Ministry offer a counter-narrative to capitalist ideals, framing rest as a form of resistance against the relentless pressure to be productive (Hersey, 2022). By challenging the dominant culture that equates busyness with worth, these movements advocate for rest as a necessary component of personal and societal health.

Critical reflections on self-care attitudes can help therapists recognize when they feel compelled to work despite being depleted. The problem is compounded when organizations and institutions expect therapists to draw on their own resources without questioning the systemic status quo (Stiles & Fox, 2019). Even when organizations prioritize employee well-being, their systems and processes can become overwhelmed due to limited funds and resources. Nonetheless, there is a limit to how much responsibility can be placed on individual therapists to fill these gaps. By emphasizing individual responsibility, we risk overlooking the need for societal and institutional change that is essential for creating supportive environments conducive to well-being. A balanced approach would frame self-care as a shared responsibility between individuals and systems, and as both a personal and collective commitment. We strongly advocate for self-care to be recognized as a systemic concern, integrated into institutional and organizational structures from the onset of professional training. It is essential to develop policies and practices that dismantle obstacles, ensuring self-care is acknowledged as a fundamental human right—accessible to all, regardless of their circumstances.

The Matrix: Clients, Therapists and the System

Becoming aware of the interplay of stresses that emerge from therapeutic interactions with clients, the person of the therapist as well as organizational and structural contexts, can guide us towards better self-care. A good experience in one area (e.g., a great session with a client) can buffer us from stress in another area (e.g., a difficult experience with a department head). Of course, negative experiences can also be cumulative in their impact and experiencing stress in more than one area can really stretch our resources.

Caring for Clients While Caring for Self

Our clients' stories and emotions often linger on with us long after the session has ended, entering discussions with supervisors or peers, colouring our day and even infiltrating our dreams. While these ideas and impressions can trigger deeper reflections, they can also be experienced as intrusive, not allowing us enough respite from our professional lives.

Pause and reflect…

Can you remember a client who 'followed you home' in your mind?

Think about why this might have happened.

Consider whether there are certain clients or issues that you find harder to leave behind.

Reflect on any recurring difficulty in disconnecting from your clients and your work.

More than the number of hours spent at work, it is the emotional toll of those hours that deeply impacts therapists. Bearing witness to stories of trauma, displacement and loss while meeting clients with complex needs or personality vulnerabilities can exacerbate stress levels and deplete personal resources (Yang & Hayes, 2020). In settings like palliative care, close encounters with death and dying or interactions with grieving families can draw out our own existential questions. When therapists work in settings such as de-addiction centres or inpatient facilities, repeated exposure to a slower and often fragmented pattern of change can contribute to emotional fatigue. The experience of feeling the client's pain can lead to indirect trauma (Knight, 2013), an umbrella term that encompasses manifestations of secondary traumatic stress (Figley, 2002), vicarious traumatization (McCann & Pearlman, 1990) and compassion fatigue (Figley, 2002). Therapists who work with many clients with trauma histories may be vulnerable to anxiety, hypervigilance, numbing and re-experiencing of their client's trauma—all experiences that are analogous to post-traumatic stress disorder. Cumulative exposure to stories of trauma can also lead to potentially permanent and pervasive changes in the cognitive schemas and the self of therapists (McCann & Pearlman, 1990; Pearlman & Mac Ian, 1995). When clients' worlds are marked by a lack of trust, safety or control, therapists may begin to feel a similar absence in their own lives. Such experiences can contribute to compassion fatigue, particularly when it becomes difficult to access our most fundamental tool—empathy for clients. In these moments, it is essential for therapists to make intentional efforts to address their self-care needs, while maintaining a sense of purpose and satisfaction in their work. Drawing a line between work and personal life is often challenging. Developing a reflexive awareness of why we make certain choices can help us critically explore our patterns and discover where change is needed.

A Therapist Speaks: The Power of Care - For Self and the Other

Hiba Siddiqui

A few years ago, our team was treating an elderly lady with a terminal cancer diagnosis. With both children residing overseas, she was being cared for by her 83-year-old husband, her primary and only carer. He was stoic when I first met him – evidently reluctant to speak to a younger psycho-oncologist. But after a few conversations, we were able to strike a rapport. He would speak about his fears of losing his wife and had kept a framed photograph of their 50th wedding anniversary by her bedside in the ward. He would ensure that his wife's nail paint was changed every two days, even though she was in an unconscious state. He told me that she had always been particular about her nails.

I too had been a caregiver to someone with cancer at a time when I understood little of this world. So, it wasn't surprising for me when this couple's story felt very close to home. During our conversations through caregiver counselling, his dedication to her well-being felt familiar and so did the grief of eventually losing her. I vividly remember the difficulty of facing him when we were informed of her loss. The fear of shedding even a single tear in front of him was crippling. I struggled, believing that the rulebook said I shouldn't be overwhelmed by my own emotions while caring for someone else. But I also knew that trust and rapport form a large component of therapy and that they stem from my intrinsic ability to empathise. This awareness helped me let go of any guilt about my emotions in the moment, allowing me to humanize my practice.

Working in a private tertiary care hospital, it is common to find oneself navigating such complex situations and facing the dilemmas that arise from them. These often come from forming deep connections with patients and caregivers in their long and arduous journey of experiencing cancer. A parent, helpless for their child, unable to stop the deterioration; a patient with no social support struggling to pull through the harsh side effects of the treatment; or a person, unable to sustain the financial burden of the disease, resorting to withdrawing treatment—what can I possibly say in situations like these to make them feel better? Many times, the pressure is draining, leading me to break down in my own personal spaces.

Experiencing varied intensities of emotional upheaval in this professional space can safely be equated to a roller coaster ride for me. Numbness and apathy also make their occasional visits, and for someone whose daily life revolves around the mechanics of emotional connections, this can be tricky. In so many ways, my patients become a part of me, a part that is often lost and grieved for. Self-reflection and dialogue with team members and peers allow me to process my sessions, find peace with troubling conversations, deconstruct complex emotions and gain a fresh perspective on my own therapeutic trajectory. Being an expressive person myself, I often reach out to those who can hold space for me and allow me to articulate my emotions. It's important to have people to talk to, whether it's family, friends, or coworkers. It helps me feel less alone and keeps me connected. My own weekly psychotherapy sessions help me ascertain my grieving process and make sense of it. I now recognize the importance of self-care in a profession predominantly centered around the wellbeing of others.

It is true that the relational intricacies between the care provider and person in care can be difficult to navigate. But it is also true that it's possible to build a bridge between the two by exchanging personal stories of loss, pain and grief, along with sharing moments of love, laughter and joy. Yes, the care provider is susceptible to emotional fatigue. That is why it is a part of our journey to know when to withdraw as an individual, only to return to the system as a professional to support more lives.

Hiba Siddiqui *is currently working as a Senior Psycho-oncologist and is engaged in doctoral research on cancer survivorship and sexual health communication in India. She also engages with the community through awareness initiatives and has established support groups for patients, survivors and carers.*

Self-Care in the Face of Client Suicide

All therapists hope never to experience the pain of losing a client to suicide. While we recognize that not all clients get better in the ways we hope for or imagine, the finality of suicide can affect us deeply, both as persons and as practitioners. Many therapists begin recounting the experience of losing a client by describing how they first received the news and recalling their initial discussion with a supervisor or colleague. A minimal or dismissive response, or worse, a critical or blaming one had long-term effects on their ability to process this experience (Knox et al., 2006). Intense feelings of shame, guilt, anger and loss can jostle with self-doubt about therapeutic skills and fears of being judged incompetent or unfit for our chosen profession. Mourning for the client, dreading facing their family and worrying about legal or institutional repercussions only intensify the emotional turmoil (Sandford et al., 2020). This journey is not one we can walk alone, and the support of friends, family, colleagues, supervisors and institutions is essential.

Grief can ebb and flow, leaving therapists vulnerable over extended periods. To cope, some may attempt to block these feelings by distancing themselves from clients or immersing in busy work. On the other hand, anxiety about the possibility of losing another client can lead to hyper-vigilance, often resulting in frequent risk assessments and preemptive referrals for medication or admission (Sandford et al., 2020). While this heightened sensitivity and caution can enhance risk assessment skills, discussions with supervisors are valuable for distinguishing between effective evaluations and overly defensive approaches (New Zealand Psychologists Board, 2017). Emotional struggles may also manifest as unconscious pressure on clients to get better, stemming from therapists' need for reassurance regarding their effectiveness. These patterns often take time to resolve, and a gradual approach can be beneficial - beginning with addressing immediate feelings of grief, guilt and concerns about competence, and eventually examining how these emotions may influence therapeutic style. While addressing these emotions at a comfortable pace is important, actively engaging with them is essential for growth and resilience.

Sharing this experience with other therapists, and hearing or reading about therapist experiences with client suicide can drive this point home. Supervision provides a supportive space for processing grief, articulating feelings and exploring questions about what could have been done differently, helping to create a meaningful narrative of the experience (Whisenhunt et al., 2017). Supervisors can create a healing space when they share the burden of loss and responsibility with their supervisees. They can emphasize their joint involvement in the conceptualization and decision-making regarding the client or share their own past experiences related to client suicide. Part of their responsibility is to gauge the supervisee's need for additional support or personal therapy, their readiness for work and the appropriate case load for the immediate future. In the process of providing support, supervisors may find it challenging to hold it together and create space to process their own difficult emotions. They could be impacted by their own loss history and experiences with client suicide and bear the additional burden of worrying that they have failed their supervisees. At these trying times, both supervisors and supervisees need to feel safe under the umbrella of the organization's support. When training centres and organizations actively support therapists and provide necessary time and resources, it attenuates the negative and enduring effects of client suicide. Preemptive discussions about the possibility of client suicide during training, along with an acknowledgement of the impacts of secondary trauma, and the importance of self-care can help therapists prepare for and traverse this difficult terrain (Sanders et al., 2008). Practitioners working outside academic and organizational settings, particularly those in private practice need to establish support networks for conversations, capacity building and consultation.

Learning to care for ourselves and embrace life in the face of its uncertainties and vicissitudes is a vital lesson for therapists. In processing the loss of a client to suicide, it is crucial to reflect on questions of individual responsibility and choice regarding life and death (Sanders et al., 2008). The interactions among various risk factors, the limited efficacy of available tools and the reality that clients may conceal their suicidal ideation and plans make predicting and preventing suicide quite challenging (Kessler et al., 2020). It is important to remember that a therapist does not have complete control of their client's choices and actions. What is expected of therapists is to do the best we can.

The Personal Lives of Therapists

Our personal qualities and experiences can be positive contributors to our craft, but they can also manifest as vulnerabilities. For instance, attention to detail may enhance our work but can also lead to rigidity. An inflated sense of responsibility for our clients' outcomes can lead us to do too much in sessions, overlooking how 'the more the therapist does, the less there is for the client to do' (Kottler, 2010, p. 193). It can be useful to remind ourselves that perfectionistic therapists are not perfect. In fact, exacting standards have been linked with poorer client outcomes (Presley et al., 2017). There is the danger that early maladaptive schemas such as unrelenting standards and self-sacrifice can make therapists more susceptible to burnout (Simpson et al., 2019). Even a well-functioning therapist can be temporarily laid low by stressors like the loss of a loved one, relationship challenges, financial or health difficulties and a range of life events. Being preoccupied with urgent personal issues can leave less room for clients' difficulties and reduces the capacity to maintain the therapeutic alliance. While some stressors are temporary and not entirely unexpected, others, such as caring for a child with a chronic illness, necessitate ongoing adjustments. Pregnancy marks a transitional stage towards a new identity as a mother and the creation of a new bond. Many women therapists report experiencing strong pulls between impending motherhood and their professional identity as therapists. This dual focus can create tension in the therapeutic relationship. Clients may feel resentment about sharing the therapist's attention, while therapists might experience mixed emotions—sometimes resenting clients for taking them away from their baby and, at other times, resenting the baby for taking them away from work (Way et al., 2019). Although women make up a large portion of the therapeutic workforce, there is limited guidance and support for managing the substantial feelings of anxiety and guilt that therapists may experience during pregnancy, maternity leave and childrearing.

Both past and present experiences of stress and trauma can leave therapists more attuned to their emotions and, at times, more vulnerable. When a client's experiences resonates with personal pain, it can evoke retraumatization, with the resurfacing of difficult memories and emotions. It is reassuring to remember that although everyone has difficult personality traits, burdens and even trauma, these do not have to hinder their effectiveness as therapists. Awareness and acceptance of personal challenges signal the need for better self-care and encourage exploration of different ways to heal and grow. We could find it challenging to acknowledge that personal difficulties, suffering and failure can occur—just like for anyone else. There are moments when it seems impossible to keep the therapist self-separate and intact. Acquainting ourselves with therapist narratives of personal adversity and coping (e.g.,Lubner & Luca, 2019; Murray-Swank, 2019) can help us acknowledge and respond to our struggles. It helps when supervisors act as role models for self-care, demonstrating that neither they nor we are above psychological stress. Therapists often speak of a reluctance to ask for help from their colleagues, fearing their judgement or evaluation—a fear that is not completely unfounded. Sensitivity to a colleague's distress enables timely emotional and practical support, potentially preventing their difficulties from escalating further. Such actions can create a generation of therapists who accept the intersections between personal and professional lives and are not so reluctant to help and be helped.

In challenging personal times, work can offer a comforting refuge—a place to feel capable, valued and needed. However, it is essential to pause and consider the balance between the capacity to work and the need for time to heal. Adams (2014), in discussing bereavement, highlights that grieving, engaging in rituals of loss and finding inner strength require time. Using therapeutic work as a means of coping can shift the focus toward the therapist's needs, potentially placing unintentional pressure on clients to provide emotional gratification. Difficulty being fully present in sessions or struggling to connect with clients may indicate a need for personal healing. Using a trusted friend, colleague or supervisor as a sounding board to discuss thoughts about taking time off or returning to work can be invaluable. Upon returning to work, therapists may find that their experiences have transformed them, adding depth to their practice. Waldman (2003) illustrates how her bond with her baby enabled her to tap into the positive mirroring and loving gaze that her client needed. Painful experiences can leave individuals feeling exposed and raw, often breaking down usual defences and coping methods. This vulnerability can create opportunities for enhanced self-care and even the exploration of newer therapeutic approaches. In this context, Murray-Swank (2019) shares how he started to integrate more self-compassion *and experiential methods into his therapeutic approach, acknowledging their importance during his own challenging times. Difficult experiences can create a sense of shared humanity with the client, reducing the feeling that therapist and client are from "different worlds" (Adams, 2014, p. 107). When we transform ourselves, we experience changes in the way we relate with our clients. For how can a new therapist have the same old relationship?

Building Communities of Care at Work

The work context is often a double-edged sword, contributing significantly to well-being but also being the source of much stress. Therapists may find little time to recuperate between sessions, tasks or responsibilities, leading to the accumulation of smaller stressors. Work culture often demands constant activity, discouraging rest until tasks are completed. People in roles with less decision-making authority may have limited control over their workload and schedules, while those in positions with greater responsibility often face continuous demands on their time and attention. Employees in organizations may experience less autonomy and control over the quantity and type of work compared to those in private practice, increasing the risk of burnout (McCormack et al., 2018). Most organizations provide opportunities to take on multiple rewarding roles, including trainer, teacher, researcher or administrative team member. Therapists can either focus on refining their skills to cultivate a strong focal identity or explore diverse roles to discover what they find most fulfilling.

Organizations employing therapists must be sensitive to the significant impact of work-related stresses. The broader context of the organization—including hierarchies, operational rules and values, resources and facilities—contributes to a reciprocal contract between employees and employers. If this contract feels unfair or imbalanced, job satisfaction may be threatened (Maslach et al., 2001). Therapists can feel a sense of misalignment with the organization's frameworks and policies, such as when they desire to focus on therapy conflicts with expectations to prioritize research. Rigid policies that allow little room for negotiation and compromise can lead to feelings of disconnection and uncertainty about belonging.

Since a significant portion of the day is spent at work, the interpersonal atmosphere becomes one of the primary environments experienced. Unsupportive bosses, difficult colleagues and a culture of conflict and rivalry can lead to burnout. Within the community, some members hold more power than others, and founders and leaders play a crucial role in fostering a safe, inclusive and supportive work environment that offers mentoring and growth opportunities. Creating reflective and inclusive spaces, promoting a culture of empathy and implementing supportive policies can contribute to a joyful and enriching workplace.

***Interview*: Organizational Self-care Frameworks—The RAHI model**

Anuja Gupta and Ashwini Ailawadi

In this excerpt from an interview with ***Anuja Gupta*** *and* ***Ashwini Ailawadi****, we learn about the self-care practices and systems at the pioneering non-profit RAHI (Recovering and Healing from Incest) Foundation, India's first incest/child sexual abuse response organization set up in 1996.*

Gupta and Ailawadi emphasize that being in touch with one's emotions and being willing to reflect on and deal with personal issues are the very cornerstones of work with issues of trauma. This deep engagement can be potentially triggering or may bring up various vulnerabilities. This is true for everyone: those on personal healing journeys, those involved in support, advocacy and rights-based initiatives, communication and outreach through awareness and capacity-building programs and even administrative work.

At the recruitment stage for volunteers and staff, there is an assessment of coping abilities and support structures. Gupta remarks, "At RAHI, there is a very high quotient of it being *personal*. We have systems to take care, but it is also important for people to have some external support structures. In our experience, if they have both, they have done well, else it is difficult to sustain in this work." An employee welfare scheme provides low-cost psychotherapy services for staff members, which is co-paid by RAHI. There are processes to build a culture of sharing about stories of abuse, with guidelines to support safe sharing in small group team meetings. The founders speak of the dangers of a them and us split in the team and emphasize that reflective work and support are required by all members—survivors of abuse as well as those who are impacted by working closely with trauma or are struggling with other vulnerabilities. Close mentorship is provided to survivors, with a special focus on those who need to work with unresolved childhood trauma. Ailawadi speaks of engaging with personal definitions of strength and weakness, as these can impact survivors' journeys of healing and self-care. Social action is seen as an important tool for self-care and growth among survivors through the Firebird Project. Before a survivor engages in the sharing of personal testimony, "We constantly judge if it is going to enhance their recovery," says Gupta.

Apart from self-care practices of "meditation, doing fun things, not having very strict working methodologies", and drawing boundaries to protect personal time, Gupta emphasises the sustenance and meaning drawn from witnessing recovery and transformations. "One of our peer educators recently said that she is going to have a child and wants to name it Rahi. Something we are doing right … this is why we still do what we do."

Anuja Gupta *is the Founder and Executive Director at RAHI Foundation and is an Educator, Trainer and Therapist in the area of incest/child sexual abuse. She was awarded the Ashoka Innovators for Public Fellowship and is a past Fellow of the MacArthur Population Innovations Program.*

Ashwini Ailawadi *is the Co-founder and Creative Director at RAHI, India, and is involved in conceptualising and shaping RAHI's training and advocacy programs and media communications.*

Our colleagues, both within and outside an organization, form a part of our professional community, A mutually supportive and enriching community benefits not just the individual therapist, but the profession as a whole. When we have a whole community that takes care of us, that we can lean on when we need, the imperative for individual self-care reduces and can be replaced by a notion of community care. This is even more significant in low resource contexts, where therapists are often overworked and underpaid by organizations that are themselves struggling to survive. Here, the usual advocated avenues for self-care and professional development like peer supervision and personal therapy are scarce, leaving little room to tailor work lives to individual needs. During the COVID pandemic, it became clear that the survival of the human community depends on collective effort and solidarity.

Mental health quickly became part of popular discourse and while the role of mental health practitioners was valued and even glorified, their own needs for psychosocial support became evident only as the pandemic progressed. In India, initiatives such as listening circles, applied theatre methodologies, helplines and support groups created spaces for solace and solidarity (Bhola et al., 2022). A sense of community emerged as therapists across the world found new ways to meet, seeking more supervision, peer engagement and professional interactions in both online and offline spaces. As the world moves forward from the pandemic, many of these initiatives seem evanescent, even as the demands on the mental health community endure. There is a pressing need to develop cascading and sustainable programs that ensure scaffolded self-care becomes an integral part of a psychotherapist's journey, embedded within training programs, peer supervision, and professional organizations. We envision a system where we trust that the community will care for us, and we can be free to care for the community. We wonder what such a supportive community might look like for psychotherapists.

Working Towards Well-Being

Often, the stress we experience is manageable, and the joys and rewards of work nourish and sustain us. At other times, we can find ourselves exhausted and ineffective, feeling cynical about our role or the enterprise of therapy itself. Periodically reviewing our self-care status can help us catch these patterns early and plan a response while we still have the energy to execute it. Research indicates that emotional and physical exhaustion are the aspects of burnout most often seen with psychotherapists (Simpson et al., 2019). Psychotherapists can also reflect on whether they are experiencing meaning burnout, which occurs when work no longer holds meaning and feels routine, boring or valueless; or caring burnout, which occurs when the ability to care gets eroded, leaving them disconnected from clients and their concerns (Skovholt & Trotter-Mathison, 2016).

When we recognize that we are struggling, it's common to feel disappointed or frustrated with ourselves about our circumstances. An attitude of self-compassion where we acknowledge our own humanity and treat our troubles with the same care we offer to clients or friends, is a better approach (Neff, 2011). A self-compassionate stance can be liberating, helping us to see troubles as a part of life and caring for ourselves as a natural and valid response. Individualized self-care practices include a combination of proactive and preventive steps that help buffer stress as well as emergency responses to mitigate acute stress or imminent burnout. Of course, the cycle is recursive, so beginning a yoga and meditation class as a response to current experiences of compassion fatigue can mitigate the likelihood of recurrence. Basic lifestyle changes like attending to sleep, nutrition or exercise are always a good place to begin. Developing a social media policy that regulates contact with current and former clients and defines a time frame for response can mitigate some of these encroachments on our privacy. Of course, what is even more important is the ability to mentally switch off from online work-related communication during weekends or vacations and create time and space for our own needs.

In this section, we use vignettes to highlight common constellations of challenges that are particularly relevant for therapists: poor work-life balance, a sense of incompetence at work, difficulty with recognizing and responding to emotions and loneliness or isolation. We offer suggestions that can help a therapist better understand and take care of their self. The goal here is not to guard against negative experiences but to allow the self to be touched or shaped by them without being overwhelmed. This creates space for softening and growing to encompass and integrate the painful realities of our client's lives, as we expand the capacities of our personal and professional selves.

Too Much to Handle

Helga is a recently qualified psychiatrist who is feeling very rushed and tired. She wants more time to pursue her own research, which excites her, but her clinical load is extremely high. This is her first job, so she spends much of her time reading up and planning her work. Her training certainly did not prepare her for everything she needs to deal with. She feels frustrated and depleted, regrets having to drop her yoga class and spends more and more time dreaming of a holiday in the hills.

The quantum and range of work responsibilities that are common to the lives of most mental health professionals can be overwhelming. Like Helga, we can feel like we just do not have the energy to pursue all our different interests, and our desire for excellence can be a very relentless driver. Self-care activities are often the easiest to drop when we feel pressured for time, adding to experiences of depletion in the long run. The way we view our professional role and its contribution to our sense of self also influences how much we give to our jobs, and how we feel about ourselves for doing so. For instance, women often experience the pressure to be completely caring at work while also feeling guilty about not being able to attend to the needs of their families. As therapists who are sometimes so involved in the care of others that we do not take care of ourselves, it is useful to consider how we can build a web of care that holds both ends.

Work–life balance and me time are often heard terms but are among the hardest things to achieve. To find the time to do the things that matter to us as individuals, we might need to negotiate time away from work or family. Of course, work *and* family are typically high priority, and it can seem overwhelming if either is threatened. How are we to then find time for the self? Not all therapists have the privilege of choice. Some may be unable to afford a lighter workload or self-care activities like joining a gym or taking a holiday. Instead, self-care may need to be reimagined within the context of real limitations, focusing on what is achievable. Making the decision to take that morning walk, alter sleep routines or turn off phone notifications in the evening are all intentional steps that can help manage milder manifestations of stress. It is crucial to assess when capacities are too stretched to handle additional work and to have the courage to say no when needed. A good starting point is to closely examine how caseloads are planned and how days are organized, ensuring there are breaks between therapy sessions to recharge for the next interaction (Kottler, 2010). Therapists like Helga can reach out to their organizations for support, advocating for necessary changes that facilitate healthier work practices.

Reflecting on whether it is financial pressures, workplace expectations or a personal work ethic drive us to work long hours can also provide valuable insights. Incorporating variety and diversity into our tasks can be a refreshing way to both energize and restore ourselves. As psychotherapists, our work life is very peopled, and seeking a degree of solitude may allow for contemplation and regulation of emotions. Incorporating practices such as brief visualization or mindfulness exercises, along with changing our physical environment, can lead to lasting benefits by allowing us to retreat inward and recharge. When everything feels like a chore, it can signal the need to look for motivation and lightness within us. Since psychotherapy is 'serious business', it is easy to forget that aspects of life can be fun or temporary. No one can, or should, be an intense professional at all times—and laughing, giggling and allowing ourselves to be silly is also hugely restorative.

A Therapist Speaks: The Secret Room

Deepti Guruprasad

Engaging in a creative activity can help therapists get in touch with their emotions and express their inner wisdom. Maintaining an attitude of openness and playfulness while creating is important, as such exercises are designed for personal reflection rather than social comparison or public display. This art experiential, *The Secret Room,* is designed to help therapists escape to a peaceful, quiet space, one that is their own and can be accessed at any time (adapted from Haeyen, 2018).

Materials: Art paper, paints, pastels, markers, coloured paper, magazines, scissors and glue.

Instructions: Imagine a secret room and see what it looks like. It is a room in which you relax, to which you retreat when you feel over- worked or drained. The door is closed to everything that might tire you out. The room is calm, pleasant and lovely. Make an image of this room using any materials of your choice.

Ask yourself these questions:

How did you design your secret room?

What elements were important in it? What makes it comforting?

How often do you need this room? Was there a time when you needed it more?

In your daily life, is there a place in your surroundings where you can feel this way?

If so, how often do you use it?

Ms Deepti Guruprasad, *is a clinical psychologist and registered art therapist with a decade of clinical experience across diverse racial and socioeconomic settings in the United States. She has recently moved back to India and follows a strengths-based* *integrative approach in therapy while emphasizing the mind–body relationship in healing.*

Feeling Too Much or Feeling Too Little?

Meera is a sensitive social worker who works closely with young clients in a drug rehabilitation centre. Many come from disturbed homes, and she can feel their pain and empathize with their need for escape. She works hard to reach her clients, constantly thinking of new ways to keep them engaged. Recently, a favourite teenage client started using substances again and left the centre. Meera is extremely disappointed with herself. She feels anger rising towards clients who are slow to progress and finds herself disconnecting from the more difficult ones. "What's the point in caring?" she thinks. "Anyway, I can't make a difference".

Meera feels the need to remain positive for her clients, providing the hope and belief that is so lacking in their lives. This can lead her to minimize her own feelings of doubt or resentment. Therapists are expected to perform in an emotionally regulated and caring manner in both professional and personal spheres. From the beginning of our training, there is a tacit understanding that we do not discuss unwanted emotions about our clients. Anger, frustration, hopelessness or contempt, especially when directed towards the client, can become unspeakable even in the privacy of our own minds. Denial, however, has the same detrimental effect on therapists as it does on clients, and these difficult emotions can manifest in unexpected ways, often influencing how therapists interact with other clients or even how they treat themselves. When these emotions are acknowledged as legitimate and valid reactions to therapeutic work and expressed in informal sharing with colleagues, or in supervision and personal therapy, this offers significant relief. Psychotherapy models provide various avenues for acknowledging and processing emotions without becoming too overwhelmed. Mindfulness meditation, acceptance-based techniques, grounding exercises or distress tolerance methods are as useful for therapists as they are for clients, though they do require a regular commitment to be most effective.

Our resilience as therapists is closely tied to how we make meaning of our experiences. Meaning can emerge from a multitude of sources for each of us, whether it's the belief in making a difference in a client's life, the respect that the profession commands, or the conviction of being a good person and aligned with one's spiritual values. Furthermore, witnessing the resilience and growth of clients can inspire personal growth in return. Resilient therapists feel a sense of alignment between their beliefs and practices, remain strongly connected in both personal and professional spheres and continue to be curious, self-reflective and self-aware (Hou & Skovholt, 2020). When feeling disconnected and disillusioned with work, it can be helpful to remember what initially inspired a career in the field or to reconnect with the core values that brought meaning to the work (Posluns & Gall, 2020). Additionally, the negative emotional atmosphere that often arises in therapy rooms can be counterbalanced by cultivating positive emotional spaces in other areas of life. When things are not going so well at work, it might be helpful to think of what could be restorative—perhaps spending time with family or seeking solitude in the mountains.

A Therapist Speaks: **Pan'nin Zaar Khudayas Waninn**

(Seeking Help from the Almighty[1])

Asiya Niyaz

People call Kashmir the Valley of Saints, engulfed with shrines where they seek spirituality and peace. During my clinical practice, I have witnessed many of the clients using religious means of coping, such as reciting the Holy Quranic verses to ward off difficulties in their lives and seeking help through prayers. Since we share a collective unconscious, I also regularly visit the holy shrines or offer prayers alone at home to find solace and cope with the stress and challenges of my work. By this way, I am able to connect with myself and the clients.

Years ago, at the start of my career, I was really struggling to build a therapeutic alliance with a man who spoke about his extra-marital relationship. There was this moral dilemma because I felt it was wrong that he was deceiving his wife, but there was also this deep guilt within me—he was my patient, trying to get some help. And then I thought, "Who am I to judge him? This matter is between him and his God. Maybe Allah has made me a reason to help him currently. The biggest judge is up above, and he will see. After all, there are gray areas within me as well, and that does not make anyone less of a human being." So that's how I dealt with it.

In our profession, we constantly hear about people's agonies, tragedies, and struggles, and there is this constant wear and tear within us. For me, it is particularly overwhelming when I see patients who are grieving a loss or have life circumstances that cannot be changed. As a clinical psychologist, it seems that the only thing that can be enhanced is coping. And sometimes that may not be possible as well. In situations like these—when I need help, when I am in a dilemma, when I am stressed, when I am depressed, when nothing seems to be possible—I always turn to the Almighty, pour my heart out, and seek his guidance. Alhamdulillah, he has always helped me. This is how I have handled my emotions ever since I was a teenager. It is not just the rituals but the deep sense of connection that matters. This connection is the revival of whatever is lost; it gives me strength and a different perspective and makes me feel rejuvenated. At these times, I remember a verse in the Quran that says, Allah does not burden a soul beyond its capacity.

Ms. Asiya Niyaz *is a consultant clinical psychologist at the Institute of Mental Health and Neurosciences, Srinagar, Kashmir, and has previously worked with Médecins Sans Frontières (Doctors without Borders).*

[1] Translated from the Kashmiri language.

The Lonely Road

George is a thoughtful intellectual therapist who recently moved back to his hometown to take care of his ailing mother. He works in a busy community mental health centre, and his dedication to work leaves little time for friends or family. George becomes aware that he is not doing very well but feels helpless in the face of his own unhappiness. He finds it hard to share his experiences with his new colleagues who he fears may not understand him. He wants to get married, but where to find the right person? Although he spends his days engaged in intensely intimate conversations with clients, his evenings stretch out emptily in front of him.

Like many other therapists, George finds it easier to connect with his clients than he does with people in his personal life. The bonds we make in the therapy room can contrast with a pattern of withdrawal from social connections (Råbu et al., 2016), and we need reflection to understand this phenomenon better. Perhaps George lacks the interpersonal skills to strike up or nurture new relationships, only feeling confident of himself within the structure of the therapy relationship. Even with the necessary skills, immersing in the lives and emotions of clients can leave therapists feeling raw and vulnerable, impacting their personal and social relationships. It can also result in diminished interpersonal energy, making it challenging to extend care or concern to others. This issue becomes more pronounced when the therapist role is assumed even in personal interactions and relationships. The therapist is the provider of care and not the receiver, the therapist sticks to relatively serious and meaningful conversations, and the therapist is in charge. Personal and social interactions, however, are replenishing and pleasurable when we allow ourselves to *receive* care, to be less than perfect, vulnerable or needy and to have lighter conversations that are about nothing in particular. Furthermore, as keepers of secrets, therapists often become accustomed to compartmentalizing experiences and emotions, which can hinder their ability to share struggles or even everyday occurrences with friends and family. Reflections on the lack of flexibility and openness in revealing different aspects of oneself to the world may reveal fears about the consequences of breaking internalized codes of emotional suppression and secrecy. This heightened sensitivity to negative behaviours and exposure to human frailty can also lead therapists to become anxious or demanding partners and parents, and even cynical or mistrustful of others (Hatcher et al., 2012). The capacity for empathy can function as a double-edged sword—while therapists are attuned to others' needs, they may quietly long for that same understanding from those around them. When loved ones overlook the subtle signals of our need for support, not receiving the care we offer so freely to others can feel especially painful. Preemptively deciding that personal experiences are too complex to be really shared can lead therapists to invest less in personal relationships. When this becomes a consistent pattern, it also denies the joy of connection. Of course, many therapists successfully leverage the skills and insights about human relationships gained through their work to understand and communicate better with those around them. Complete self-care practice includes understanding how we can nurture our personal relationships, perhaps through articulating our relational needs, or learning how to take our therapist hat off when speaking to friends and family. Therapists are often seen as "experts at one-way caring" (Skovholt & Trotter-Mathison, 2016, p. 162), overlooking their own struggles as long as they continue to function effectively.

Sometimes, we might need to be our own therapists.

A Therapist-Poet Speaks: Khudkalami (Self-Talk[2])

Muzammil Karim

Khudkalami	*Self-talk*
Dil ko ye samjhana hai	I must counsel my heart
Apna khayaal bhi rakhna hai	To take care of myself too
Ghum ka lamba daur chale	When sadness stays for long
Dard ke qisse aur mile	And pain weaves more stories
Mann to rooth jaata hai	Mind spirals into sulking
Dil bhi toot jata hai	Heart finds itself broken
Thak haar ke ye zehen	Tired and exhausted my mind
Soonch mai kahin kho jaata hai	Gets lost in endless worries
Pyaar se ghum sehlaana hai	Love is the cure for sadness
Dil ko ye samjhana hai	I must counsel my heart
Apna khayaal bhi rakhna hai	To take care of myself too
Kabhi hansi kho jaati hai	Laughter is lost at times
Neend kabhi marr jaati hai	At times even sleep perishes
Koi khalal pad jaata hai	Dissonance cuts through the soul
Mann bhaari ho jaata hai	Heaviness weighs on the mind
Dil ke khaali kamron mein	Within the empty rooms of the heart
Ghum barf sa jam jaata hai	Sadness freezes like snow
Umeed ko dhoop banana hai	Hope must bring new sunlight
Dil ko ye samjhana hai	I must counsel my heart
Apna khayaal bhi rakhna hai	To take care of myself too

Muzammil Karim *is a clinical psychologist and couple therapist, practising in Delhi and Srinagar. Born and brought up in the beautiful valley of Kashmir, he likes to read and write poetry and has a keen interest in the understanding of human behaviour from psychological as well as socio-cultural perspectives.*

All of us need a web of relationships to carry us through life and meet our needs to be seen, acknowledged and valued by those around us. This could include someone to call when we are having a difficult time at work or someone to celebrate our success with. While some friends meet our intimacy needs, others offer us resources, information and company in our activities. Think about who you could call if you were feeling lonely or who might help figure how to file your taxes. If you felt the need to strengthen your support system, where would you make a start? As psychotherapists, we actually have tremendous resources at our disposal in the form of friends, colleagues and classmates. Fellow professionals not only truly get our experience but also possess the skills to alleviate feelings of isolation. We can build networks by

[2] Translated from the Urdu language.

prioritizing and investing in healthy, nurturing relationships, reconnecting with old friends and family and cultivating new connections whenever possible. By letting go of dysfunctional relationships, we create space for new and enriching interactions - perhaps someone with a very different background from us, who can offer fresh perspectives and nurture new aspects of our personalities.

What Am I Doing Here?

Neel has begun doubting his competence as a counsellor after three clients dropped out of therapy. He is feeling the need to update his skills and wonders if peer supervision will offer answers for his questions. He finds himself questioning his therapeutic decisions and being more unsure with clients. His days start to feel heavier, and he feels a reluctance to get out of bed and start work every morning. "Have I committed to the wrong profession?" he wonders.

As with Neel, there are times that therapists experience self-doubt. Our clients may only get slightly better, or better just for a period of time. Even when we do our best, rarely do clients say that they are completely fine with all issues resolved. At times when the client's dissatisfaction with us becomes more visible through their dropping out or missing sessions, we can feel our doubts rising to the surface. Again, like Neel, we can be reluctant to seek help for this, fearing judgement from supervisors or colleagues, even going so far as the make global judgements of our own fitness for the profession.

As therapists, we can feel that all aspects of the client's trajectory lie within our hands, and it is solely our competence that determines the success of a therapy. A cognitive and emotional shift is crucial here, and we need to remember that clients are not always ready or motivated for change, and we can only work within these constrained possibilities. We need to have realistic expectations of what therapy, and what we as therapists, can do for each client. Even when we help a client accept their childhood experiences, we cannot really change their past. There is a limit to how much therapy can change life's circumstances—and no matter how hard we and our clients try, some concerns remain. When we look up from an overly close examination of our own responsibility, we may notice that systemic factors like the number of sessions a client can afford or their biological vulnerabilities also impact outcome. Therapists also need the wisdom to understand what can and cannot be changed—whether in relation to their own competence or to their client's lives.

It is only when we give voice to our doubts about our professional abilities and decisions and can sit more comfortably with not knowing, that we create growth pathways in our therapeutic work. Being more accepting of ourselves as human beings, gives us a more secure platform from which we can examine our professional performance, facilitating problem-solving and course correction as therapists. We can also bolster our sense of competence by remaining in touch with our positive experiences as therapists. Savouring these moments—immersing ourselves in the experience, anticipating or reminiscing about them and sharing them with others—provides a meaningful counterpoint during times of low mood or discouragement.

It is not just about feeling better but also about doing better; and an acceptance of our limitations often motivates us to improve our competencies. We can proactively track and build our skills with reference to professional competency frameworks (e.g., British Association of Counselling & Psychotherapy, 2020). Competency frameworks help us determine where we are and where we would like to go, and it can be very reassuring to have a map that guides our self-improvement plan. We enhance our competencies through reflecting on what we learn through academic activities, workshops and conferences, and translating this learning into specific and tangible changes in practice. This places us in the driver's seat instead of passively waiting for time and experience to build our expertise. The process of deliberate practice involves setting incremental and personalized learning objectives that are just beyond our current abilities, with time allocated to repeatedly rehearse and refine specific skills (Rousmaniere, 2024). Keeping a learning log that tracks what we did and could have done, using therapy recordings and asking for and responding to client feedback are all strategies that predict better client outcomes (Chow et al., 2015).

We do not need to engage in this journey alone but can reach out to a supervisor who can walk with us and offer a space for regular reflection and course correction. As therapists, we can never know enough to competently deal with every situation we face, and it helps us to acknowledge that learning is a continuous process. Perhaps what is most important is that we learn how to learn, a skill that can stimulate growth and mitigate stagnation and burnout.

Pause and reflect...

Sometimes our self-care plan is more a set of dreams or intentions rather than an actual plan.

Reflect and outline your matrix of self-care needs.

Commit to any one change you would like to make in your self-care practices and identify the steps that will help translate your ideas into action.

A Therapist Speaks: Sanctuary

Pallavi Banerjee

Often, the initial work in therapy involves the patient just getting in touch with their intuition to recognise the need for rest, before continuing with the grind of deeper work. Unfortunately, we therapists may be as divorced from self-care as our patients.

I am a psychotherapist who works from her home-based office. Previously, I have been in stressful jobs, managing both my clinical practice and full-time teaching assignments. This stress gradually showed up in therapy sessions - minor signs like feeling bored in the session or feeling impatient with a resistant client. Nothing out of the ordinary, right? We all have these feelings as part of the countertransference baggage that is a given in our work. But burnout is insidious, and that is what makes it a silent enemy.

What alarmed me was the fuller presence that I would bring to the sessions, when rejuvenated after vacations - the mental suppleness I would feel, my curiosity, and a plethora of other deep feeling states that would tune me in to my patient. This, along with other life circumstances, motivated me to slow down in life and take a serious practice of Study-Meditation-Contemplation in Buddhism, my own analysis and the practice of psychotherapy, as the primary functions in my life. The mind states I accessed during silent meditation retreats in the hills, and later through my systematic training in Buddhist meditation practices under guidance of a qualified Teacher, gave me the taste of a different life. Then there was no going back to the fast 'ten thousand to-do-lists' kind of life.

Along with my work as a psychodynamically informed psychotherapist, I also provide supervision to younger psychotherapists. Though I work from home, I take on patients for therapy only if slots are available during pre-decided work hours. That way, there is a uniform routine. As part of professional care, I take supervision from seniors in the field and peers. Meditating, participating in the study and prayers in the Buddhist Centre, occasionally going for retreats, attending seminars and talks - mainly related to psychoanalytic psychotherapy, reading books, reflective conversations with friends and family or spending a quiet evening listening to music, watching a film or listening to a Spiritual talk, helps me work through mental fatigue.

My choices in the last few years have led towards making me more fully present in sessions with my patients, making each day of work something to look forward to. The more I slowed down and made room for reflective practices, the more my intuitions guided me to move in these directions.

Dr. Pallavi Banerjee *is a psychotherapist, who has undergone psychoanalysis for 10 years and has been training in study and meditation practices within the Tibetan Buddhist framework. She is an Associate Member of Indian Psychoanalytical Society and a Trustee of Atish Dipankar Dhyan Kendra, a Centre for Meditation and Study of Buddhist Psychology and Philosophy. She tries to bring reflective practices from both psychoanalytic-existential framework and Buddhism to her work as a psychotherapist.*

Perspectives on Training and Development

Integrating Self-Care Within Training Contexts

Self-care can be fostered through the creation of formal learning opportunities for trainees to reflect on and identify signs of personal distress, burnout, compassion fatigue and vicarious trauma. Lessons from positive psychology, such as recognizing and honing strengths, aligning work with our values and investing in strong relationships, can enrich the self-care curriculum. The self-compassion and mindfulness strategies that are advocated for clients could be helpful for therapists as well. Self-care can be approached from various angles, using a combination of didactic and more experiential and exploratory methods: assigned readings, guided discussions and self-reflection exercises (Thériault et al., 2015). Engaging with the narratives of other therapists who have faced similar challenges, such as losses due to suicide, can help trainees and supervisors feel less isolated and provide guidance on the journey toward healing. We recommend exploring the resources available from the website of the *Coalition of Clinician Survivors* (https://www.cliniciansurvivor.org/) which offer information, support and guidance for clinicians who have experienced loss or trauma. Periodic tracking of experiences of stress and resilience *in* both personal and professional domains, through completion of measures like *The Practitioner Professional Resiliency and Self-Care Inventory* (Skovholt & Trotter-Mathison, 2016) can help trainees recognize their strengths, challenges and opportunities.

A range of self-care opportunities within the campus/workplace, for example, mindfulness meditation, fitness activities or acceptance and commitment therapy techniques can broaden the repertoire of trainees and employees. When we help trainees devise concrete individualized self-care plans, this can support their well-being, enhance the quality of care provided to clients and set the foundation for restorative practices throughout their professional pathways. Trainees can imbibe enduring lessons from teachers and supervisors who model effective work–life balance and self-care. Any implicit and explicit messaging that positions overwhelming stress as a rite of passage for entry into the (invulnerable) psychotherapist's role needs to be interrogated and addressed within the organization. Self-care initiatives do not have to stand apart from training in other professional skills. Frameworks such as the Person-of-the-Therapist (POTT) model, which focus on self-awareness and acceptance of vulnerabilities, can foster self-care among clinicians (Kissil & Niño, 2017). The evaluation of self-care initiatives can indicate which self-care approaches work, whether they lead to change and where the impacts are felt. However, there is no substitute for participatory dialogue and ongoing evaluation, where trainees are asked what is working well and what changes could further strengthen individual and organizational self-care cultures.

Organizational Policies and Structures that Facilitate Self-Care

Organizations that invest in strengthening supervision frameworks and in training for reflective supervision can build an important layer of support for trainee well-being. Supervision plays a vital role in normalizing early experiences of uncertainty and anxiety and in the development of self-care competencies during and beyond psychotherapy training. A commitment to student and faculty welfare requires that all organizational policies and practices be regularly reviewed to examine their impact on self-care and well-being. This includes a critical review of academic demands and schedules, workload, supervision time, workplace interactions and communication, time off from work/vacations/sabbaticals and processes for grievance redressal. An assessment of felt needs and a feedback system can help organizations make more substantive and effective changes. Trainees and employees need to feel that taking designated time-off or advocating for needed changes is encouraged and valued in the organization. Training institutions and organizations can share their best practices and innovative approaches for professional development and well-being and facilitate the development of effective models for resilient workplaces.

Responding to Therapist Mental Health Vulnerabilities and Impairment

Distress and vulnerabilities are universal human experiences, and the therapist community is not immune to mental health difficulties. Initiatives such as peer buddy systems, mentoring and ongoing student wellness initiatives can help build networks of support within training programmes. Organizational provisions for mental health accommodations and services, leave rules, health insurance and employee assistance programmes are all part of the web of support for trainees and employees who may be experiencing emotional distress, personal crisis or professional burnout. There are some special considerations to keep in mind when therapists enter the mental health system. The treating professional may offer extra confidentiality in terms of opening a file or setting a more private meeting place, keeping a special focus on a guided return to work and a future self-care plan (Goldberg et al., 2020). Creating pathways to accessible and affordable care for trainees and employees who need mental health consultations is a priority, but these are likely to be underused if stigma and other barriers to help-seeking are not addressed.

Role of Professional Associations in Supporting Self-Care

Professional associations have a crucial role in supporting the self-care needs of practitioners by offering a range of training opportunities focused on effective self-care strategies. Even short experiential self-care courses can empower practitioners to develop and apply essential skills intentionally (Guler & Ceyhan, 2020). Additionally, professional organizations should consider the responsibility of updating their ethical guidelines and competency frameworks to include concepts related to proactive self-care and the collective responsibility of both individuals and professional communities. Evaluating current professional guidelines regarding supervision and mentoring is crucial for understanding how self-care is incorporated and identifying potential areas for enhancement.

Conclusion

As therapists, it is important that we do not forget that we are also human beings. Caring for oneself begins with the recognition of this humanity and the understanding that the self sometimes requires attention and nurturance. It is important not to regard self-care as self-indulgence, ensuring that we do not deny ourselves the respite and replenishment we genuinely need. Engaging in reflective practice can significantly enhance a therapist's self-care, while dedicating time for self-care allows for deeper reflection on our work. As psychotherapists committed to the idea of positive mental health, we need to strengthen our own capacity to love, work and play (Jahoda, 1958).

References

Adams, M. (2014). *The myth of the untroubled therapist: Private life, professional practice.* Routledge/Taylor & Francis Group.

Bhola, P., Isaac, R., & Duggal, C. (2022). Psychological support for health care workers in India: Using a reflective lens. In H. Conniff (Ed.), *Psychological staff support in healthcare: Thinking and practice.* Sequoia Books.

British Association of Counselling and Psychotherapy. (2020). *Counselling skills competence framework.* Retrieved from https://www.bacp.co.uk/media/8890/bacp-counselling-skills-competence-framework-may20.pdf

Chow, D. L., Miller, S. D., Seidel, J. A., Kane, R. T., Thornton, J. A., & Andrews, W. P. (2015). The role of deliberate practice in the development of highly effective psychotherapists. *Psychotherapy, 52*(3), 337–345.

Ducar, D. M., & Cunningham, T. (2018). Honoring life after death: Mapping the spread of the pause. *American Journal of Hospice and Palliative Medicine, 36*(5), 429–435.

Figley, C. R. (2002). Compassion fatigue: Psychotherapists' chronic lack of self-care. *Journal of Clinical Psychology, 58*(11), 1433–1441.

Goldberg, M., Stanger Elran, R., Mayer, Y., & Lurie, I. (2020). The treatment of a patient who is also a mental health practitioner: Special considerations and recommendations. *Academic Psychiatry, 44*(5), 624–628.

Guler, D., & Ceyhan, E. (2020). Development of self-care behaviours in counsellors-in-training through an experiential self-care course: An action research. *British Journal of Guidance & Counselling., 49*(3), 414–434.

Hatcher, S. L., Kipper-Smith, A., Waddell, M., Uhe, M., West, J. S., Boothe, J. H., Frye, J. M., Tighe, K., Usselman, K. L., & Gingras, P. (2012). What therapists learn from psychotherapy clients: Effects on personal and professional lives. *The Qualitative Report, 17*(48), 1–21.

Haeyen, S. (2018). *Art therapy and emotion regulation problems: Theory and workbook*. Springer.

Hersey, T. (2022). *Rest is resistance: A manifesto by Tricia Hersey*. Little, Brown and Company.

Hochschild, A. R. (2003). *The managed heart: commercialization of human feeling. 20th Anniversary edition*. University of California Press.

Hou, J.-M., & Skovholt, T. M. (2020). Characteristics of highly resilient therapists. *Journal of Counseling Psychology, 67*(3), 386–400.

Jahoda, M. (1958). *Current concepts of positive mental health*. Basic Books.

Kessler, R. C., Bossarte, R. M., Luedtke, A., Zaslavsky, A. M., & Zubizarreta, J. R. (2020). Suicide prediction models: A critical review of recent research with recommendations for the way forward. *Molecular Psychiatry, 25*(1), 168–179.

Kissil, K., & Niño, A. (2017). Does the person-of-the-therapist training (POTT) promote self-care? personal gains of MFT trainees following POTT: A retrospective thematic analysis. *Journal of Marital and Family Therapy, 43*, 526–536.

Knight, C. (2013). Indirect trauma: Implications for self-care, supervision, the organization, and the academic institution. *The Clinical Supervisor, 32*(2), 224–243.

Knox, S., Burkard, A. W., Jackson, J. A., Schaack, A. M., & Hess, S. A. (2006). Therapists-in-training who experience a client suicide: Implications for supervision. *Professional Psychology: Research and Practice, 37*(5), 547–557.

Kottler, J. A. (2010). *On being a therapist* (4th ed.). Jossey-Bass.

Lubner, K., & Luca, M. (2019). A case study of a psychotherapists' narrative account of significant relationship breakdown and the perceived impact on his clinical work. *Journal of Psychological Therapies, 4*(1), 43–58.

Maslach, C., Schaufeli, W., & Leiter, M. (2001). Job burnout. *Annual Review of Psychology, 52*, 397–422.

McCann, L., & Pearlman, L. (1990). Vicarious traumatization: A framework for understanding the psychological effects of working with victims. *Journal of Traumatic Stress, 3*(1), 131–149.

McCormack, H. M., MacIntyre, T. E., O'Shea, D., Herring, M. P., & Campbell, M. J. (2018). The prevalence and cause(s) of burnout among applied psychologists: A systematic review. *Frontiers in Psychology, 9*, 1897.

Murray-Swank AB (2019) The cracks where the light gets in: Exploring therapist transformation following the loss of a family member to suicide. Journal of Psychotherapy Integration 29(2), 188-196.

Neff, K. D. (2011). *Self-compassion: Stop beating yourself up and leave insecurity behind*. Harper Collins.

New Zealand Psychologists Board. (2017). *Best practice guideline: Coping with a client suicide.* Retrieved from https://psychologistsboard.org.nz/already-registered/best-practice-documents-and-guidelines/

Pearlman, L. A., & Mac Ian, P. S. (1995). Vicarious traumatization: An empirical study of the effects of trauma work on trauma therapists. *Professional Psychology: Research and Practice, 26*(6), 558–565.

Posluns, K., & Gall, T. L. (2020). Dear mental health practitioners, take care of yourselves: A literature review on self-care. *International Journal for the Advancement of Counseling, 42*(1), 1–20.

Presley, V. L., Jones, C. A., & Newton, E. K. (2017). Are perfectionist therapists perfect? The relationship between therapist perfectionism and client outcomes in cognitive behavioural therapy. *Behavioural and Cognitive Psychotherapy, 45*(3), 225–237.

Råbu, M., Moltu, C., Binder, P., & McLeod, J. (2016). How does practicing psychotherapy affect the personal life of the therapist? A qualitative inquiry of senior therapists' experiences. *Psychotherapy Research, 26*(6), 737–749.

Rousmaniere, T. (2024). *Deliberate practice for psychotherapists: A guide to improving clinical effectiveness* (2nd ed.). Routledge.

Sanders, S., Jacobson, J. M., & Ting, L. (2008). Preparing for the inevitable: Training social workers to cope with client suicide. *Journal of Teaching in Social Work, 28*(1–2), 1–18.

Sandford, D. M., Kirtley, O. J., Thwaites, R., & O'Connor, R. C. (2020). The impact on mental health practitioners of the death of a patient by suicide: A systematic review. *Clinical Psychology and Psychotherapy, 28*(2), 261–294.

Simpson, S., Simionato, G., Smout, M., van Vreeswijk, M. F., Hayes, C., Sougleris, C., & Reid, C. (2019). Burnout amongst clinical and counselling psychologist: The role of early maladaptive schemas and coping modes as vulnerability factors. *Clinical Psychology & Psychotherapy, 26*(1), 35–46.

Skovholt, T. M., & Trotter-Mathison, M. (2016). *The resilient practitioner: Burnout and compassion fatigue prevention and self-care strategies for the helping professions* (3rd ed.). Routledge.

Stiles, J., & Fox, R. (2019). Taking care of business: Psychologist self-care in a neoliberal age. *The Australian Community Psychologist, 30*(2), 30–53.

Thériault, A., Gazzola, N., Isenor, J., & Pascal, L. (2015). Imparting self-care practices to therapists: What the experts recommend. *Canadian Journal of Counselling and Psychotherapy, 49*(4), 379–400.

Van Der Merwe, H. (2019). Emotional labour and the practicing psychologist: When the psychologist's professional emotions go awry. *European Journal for Qualitative Research in Psychotherapy, 9*, 27–40.

Waldman, J. (2003). New mother/old therapist: Transference and countertransference challenges in the return to work. *American Journal of Psychotherapy, 57*(1), 52–63.

Way, C., Lamers, C., & Rickard, R. (2019). An unavoidable bump: A meta-synthesis of psychotherapists' experiences of navigating therapy while pregnant. *Research in Psychotherapy: Psychopathology, Process and Outcome*. https://doi.org/10.4081/ripppo.2019.386

Whisenhunt, J. L., DuFresne, R. M., Stargell, N. A., Rovnak, A., Zoldan, C. A., & Kress, V. E. (2017). Supporting counselors after a client suicide: Creative supervision techniques. *Journal of Creativity in Mental Health, 12*(4), 451–467.

Yadav, S. (2023). *Women at leisure lie at the heart of feminist liberation*. Vogue India. https://www.vogue.in/culture-and-living/content/women-at-leisure-lie-at-the-heart-of-feminist liberation

Yang, Y., & Hayes, J. A. (2020). Causes and consequences of burnout among mental health professionals: A practice-oriented review of recent empirical literature. *Psychotherapy, 57*(3), 426–436.

Chapter 13
The Reflective Path: Integrating Reflection into Psychotherapy Training, Practice and Research

There are many ways of being reflective, and through the course of the book we have explored several models and pathways that can guide us in our journey to being reflective practitioners. The more comfortable we grow in using the reflective lens, the more flexible and adept we become at uncovering new ideas and methods to use in our work as therapists.

Pause and reflect…

What is the top lesson you will take away from the ideas in this book?

Have you found some methods of reflection to strengthen or change your therapeutic practice?

Keeping Our Head in the Air and Feet on the Ground

In some ways, reflective practice seems elementary, as it asks us to think about what we do in therapy. While reflective practice models make it appear like a systematic, rational cycle of thinking about our work, a meandering, uncharted process of discovery may be closer to the ideology of reflective work. Perhaps this is understandable given the inherent uncertainties, even contradictions, in human nature and in the psychotherapy process. Our engagement in reflective practice is a risk of sorts, a willingness to engage with uncertainty and open ourselves to vulnerability. There are several seemingly opposing perspectives on reflective concepts, methods and processes, and these dialectics are perhaps inherent in reflective practice:

P. Bhola et al., *Reflective Practice in Psychotherapy and Counselling*,
https://doi.org/10.1007/978-981-96-9732-8_13

- The art of being emotionally present and responsive vs the art of being intellectually reflective and analytical.
- The art of being spontaneous and authentic vs the art of delay and contemplation.
- Noting similarities and resonances with our client's story vs recognizing our differences and separateness.
- Thinking from inside out (based on our intuition, perspectives and strengths) vs thinking from outside in (based on the needs, priorities and feedback from our clients/multiple stakeholders).
- The value of exploration and discovery vs the power of repetition and mastery.
- Staying grounded in theories and models of therapy vs questioning our beliefs, assumptions and conceptual frameworks.
- Caring for others vs caring for ourselves.
- Accepting ourselves and our personal histories vs being open to change.

The energy of reflective practice can come from our awareness of and willingness to attend to both sides of these paradoxes in determining our immediate and long-term behaviours and choices. During the process of therapy, we may look through our clients' eyes but also through our own, shifting between imagining ourselves as similar to our clients *and* as foreign or different (Flaskas, 2009). Neither of these positions is more important or better—each can offer something that the other may not. In the same way, there is room for both affect and cognition, reflection during and after sessions, acceptance and questioning, privileging the self and privileging the other. During our therapeutic work, there are times we tilt in one direction, perhaps so invested in our client's well-being that we disregard our own emotional needs or so aligned with our own beliefs and theories that other truths have no place. This signals the need to redress the balance or find a way to connect with both aspects.

Curiosity can open many doors, and engaging with these dialectics can lead us to newer ways of thinking about and doin' reflective practice. There seems to be a constant quest for surprise, newness and originality in reflective practice. Therapeutic work can sometimes fall into a familiar rhythm—the sharing of difficult emotions, challenging a stuck behavioural pattern or moving towards an insight together. Moments of epiphany or transformation, in both therapy and reflective practice, are precious *because* they are rare. However, what seems repetitive still carries potential for learning and growth. Sometimes our reflection tells us to keep doing what we have always been doing, and this is also valuable.

Strengthening Reflective Practice in Training and Professional Development

Reflective practice lies at the core of being a psychotherapist, straddling domains of practice, training, supervision and research. Reflection can bring the strands of theory and practice together and help us crystallise when to go by the book and when to take a flight into the unknown. There are several opportunities and challenges in the process of honing reflective abilities as we strive to become more competent, ethical and effective professionals.

Although reflection and reflexivity are best nurtured from the training phase, these are not easy skills to teach and learn. The shift from an objective knowledge-based paradigm to a more subjective emotion-based paradigm can be challenging, as we let go of certainties and venture into less known territories. There is growing clarity and consensus around how reflection and reflective practice can be translated into skills and learning objectives for trainees and practitioners. A more nuanced understanding of the distinctions between reflection, critical reflection and reflexivity can aid the development of clear rubrics for the processes of training, learning and evaluation of these skills. We discuss methodologies that best build therapist confidence and competence, through engaging with crucial questions around how best to nurture reflection and how to express and evaluate this learning.

Making Room for Reflection

Reflective practice is considered a key professional competency which deserves legitimate space and allocation of resources within psychotherapy training frameworks. Organizations often place clinical work and the provision of client services as their top priority, viewing reflection as a luxury rather than a necessity. Perhaps the difficulty in capturing the impact of reflective practice initiatives on the development of other professional competencies and on client outcomes negatively affects organizational commitment and buy-in.

Training organizations have been exploring roadmaps for how to best integrate a reflective stance into training and workspaces. Stand-alone modules or courses are always useful, but this is not the only way. In fact, it may work better to embed reflective practice across lectures, academic presentations, discussions, supervision and therapy skills training. A range of reflective practice models can be presented as examples of a way of thinking, rather than as definitive steps to follow. Experiential exercises followed by reflective discussions to glean learnings about therapy, the self or the world are useful in introducing the value and flavour of reflection. Creative modes of self-expression and experience, using the imagination, art or movement can help to access layers of meaning and fresh perspectives. Trainees can be inspired by seeing reflection in practice, either through interacting with more experienced therapists or with psychotherapy training videos. Supervision has emerged as the primary space for scaffolded reflection. Supervisors also require support and training to strengthen their own skills in building reflective capacities in their supervisees. We see this as the next big step in growing reflective practice. Teaching and supervisory processes that allow trainees to pick up reflective skills at their own pace, giving them the room to explore ideas and set personalized goals, can increase personal engagement and a sense of ownership of the learning process.

Initially, it is the role of institutions and organizations to create and nurture reflective spaces for trainees. Budding psychotherapists then learn to keep time for reflection, incorporating it into their work day. As these trainees graduate to being professionals, they can create such spaces for others, eventually integrating the reflective stance across the profession of psychotherapy.

Creating a Sense of Safety

Reflective spaces are marked by uncertainty and trainees can get lost in the ocean of possibilities that the process opens up for them. All trainees will not be equally ready for the effort, openness and commitment that deep reflection requires. They can feel unsafe, become emotionally overwhelmed by their personal material and worry about exposing themselves to their peers and teachers. Trainer/supervisor attitudes and responses to trainees' nascent reflective attempts can be experienced as nurturing or blighting. A sense of safety is what frees trainees to go off the beaten path, take risks, make mistakes and explore new ideas. An ongoing relational process marked by gentleness, humour, the sharing of own experiences and doubts creates a safe place for such explorations. In guiding these explorations, supervisors can keep in mind that they are helping trainees learn 'how to be reflective' rather than look for a particular method or result from reflection.

Scaffolded feedback that evaluates where the trainee is at the present time and provides personalized suggestions for growth creates a positive learning atmosphere. The secure base that trainers provide also extends to the self of the therapist. We believe that an attitude of self-compassion is an essential nutrient for the growth of reflective capacities. Acknowledging that each reflective effort may not lead to a deep insight or a-ha moment, can help us enjoy and invest in the process of reflection with less anxiety and criticality. When we understand that it is human to have blocks, issues and blind spots and that *all* therapists make mistakes, there is greater openness to discovering ourselves as individuals and therapists.

Riding the Reflective Cycle

Training opens with a focus on *reflection in action*, where a supervisor supports an in-depth exploration of session content, experiences and processes. At this stage, the goal is to harness these reflections to deepen understanding of the client and the therapeutic journey, create hypotheses, and shaping the direction for the next session. This slow and supported consideration of what transpired in the therapeutic interaction sets the stage for *reflection in action*. Trainees gradually begin to develop the skills to think on their feet while the session is going on, allowing for micro course corrections and more responsiveness. Reflecting in real time can be a complex and demanding process, particularly when trainees are still growing into their therapist identity. Reflections to do with therapy skills (for instance, thinking that, I need to ask a more open-ended question here, as the client feels defensive and wary) can be easier to act on than reflections that have more to do with the self (for instance, noticing that, For some reason I feel threatened when this client talks about their previous therapist). Too much reflection-in-action can lead to emotional flooding that prevents action. Sometimes a functional choice is to put our reflections away to cope with the needs of the moment during the session, and flag them for later (Ferguson, 2018).

An intuitive felt process of being a therapist is nurtured by recursive loops of experiencing and reflecting both on and in action (Schön, 1991). When this habit is instilled during the training phase itself, this stays with us through our careers, becoming an intrinsic part of who we are as therapists. The shift from reflection-on-action to reflection-in-action happens gradually, in fits and starts. Therapists need to become comfortable with themselves, their presence with clients and basic session process before they will have the mental space to fully notice and act upon their reflections.

Titrating the Reflective Process

Some therapists can feel very drawn to the reflective process, but more reflection is not necessarily better. The temptation to go down the rabbit hole of reflective loops can leave less time to develop other skills and competencies. Theoretical knowledge and the development of practical skills need to grow side by side with reflective abilities. Our knowledge of theory creates a fertile ground for reflections to spring up from, and the application of our reflections to in-session skills keeps us grounded and connected to the underlying purpose.

The process of introspection and discovery can be challenging, as we let go of certainties and venture onto less known territories. The self of the therapist sometimes needs to be defended from the anxiety that constant reflective examination can bring. It can feel particularly overwhelming during times of concurrent stress, and we may need to turn off reflection to protect ourselves from getting trapped in a ruminative spiral. The recognition of the limits of our emotional tolerance helps us mark when we need a pause and a shift in focus. Having a specific focus and time duration for the reflective activity, asking particular questions or linking our reflections to an identified area of growth can help in keeping reflection meaningful.

Each of us develop a feel for when we need to slow down reflections, so that we can focus on action or defend the self; and when to intensify the reflective process to make sense of an experience or overcome a block. Exercising choice about what to reflect on and when, brings a sense of control that can ease us into the practice of reflection, reducing defensiveness and stress from the process. While there is no doubt that reflection can be most beneficial when we are busier and feeling stretched, we need to incorporate it into our regular routines in ways that are pragmatic and meaningful. Every action we take as therapists can be accompanied by some degree of reflection and over time, we might find a comfortable synergy between reflection and work.

Our reflective efforts will not always yield the fruit we were hoping for, and sometimes even after hours of effort, we can find that we neither understand ourselves nor our clients any better. Perhaps we are stuck in certain loops of thinking or keep finding ourselves hitting the same wall. Getting a fresh perspective from a colleague, using a more creative or non-verbal approach, or letting the issue lie fallow in our minds for some time, are ways we can try to overcome these blocks. It is also reassuring to recall that not all questions have answers, and sometimes, the result of our reflection might be to admit that I still don't know.

Reflecting in Shared Spaces

Reflection is often seen as a solitary and intellectual activity that is safely engaged with in the privacy of our minds, and this has its own rewards and comfort. The spaces of supervision and personal therapy offer opportunities to engage with many minds and voices and this engenders a different kind of return, deepening the reflective process as we encounter fresh perspectives and hear new voices. Sharing our worries and experiences can help us to feel less alone. Hearing other people's reflections on our experience can help us identify where we might have been rigid or blinkered and acknowledge that the way we view things is just one among many possibilities.

We advocate for therapists to actively seek opportunities for reflection with others in addition to their solitary explorations. While thinking along with those who are similar to us can deepen our understanding, thinking with those who are different can broaden perspectives. These reflections need not be centred on therapy experiences alone—reflective discussions and creative outputs around books, movies, journal articles, social trends and political events also fuel critical thinking. We are no longer limited to reflecting only with people who are geographically accessible, as opportunities for participating in online groups allow therapists to find their tribe from around the world.

There are various group processes that facilitate safety and structure for participants. As an example, Balint groups that keep a focus on the client rather than the presenter with clear cut guidelines for both presenting the case and running the discussion, offer a tried and tested methodology (Douglas & Feeney, 2017). Process groups that encourage the examination of group dynamics allow members opportunities to learn about how they impact others and are viewed by them. These insights into interpersonal patterns can enhance therapists' use-of-self in their work. Group members can also engage in a meaning-making process that tries to incorporate all the perspectives and emotions experienced. This can generate a more nuanced and contextual understanding of the issue being discussed, making the most of the many minds that one can access in a group. Of course, following an intense group experience, participants may need to retreat into the quiet of their own mind to chew on what they have learnt and derive a personal meaning that is relevant to them alone.

If not handled sensitively, reflective groups can encourage confirmation bias and groupthink, where group members agree with each other for fear of being excluded or out of shame about their reactions (Lyons, et al., 2019). The facilitator needs to create an openness towards dissent and disagreement, welcoming difference perhaps through a dialectical enquiry. Space for opposing positions can also be built by nominating a member to play devil's advocate and challenge group consensus. Group members can examine their reactions to hearing an outsider perspective, noting when they feel a defensive block rising and discovering what leaves them feeling more open to new ideas.

A Therapist Speaks: A Circle of Reflection and Kinship

Archana Ramanathan

I have often felt the need for a space to reflect with fellow therapists on topics that have impacted me. It is this desire that became a key motivator to start a reflective practice group - envisioned this as a space of holding and reflection, but unlike a supervision, training, or process group. Rather, I wished to explore therapy processes that elicited both the Therapist in our Self and the Self of the Therapist'.

The focus was on therapy processes that would be universal, across diverse therapeutic approaches. The topics for each session evolved from a self-reflective process and spanned relational experiences such as ruptures and repair and the navigation of values. I invited five therapists to form a closed group that met monthly for six months. We began each session with our reflections over the month, often stimulated by previous topics of discussion. I also provided an opening prompt for the day, which might be a question or a vignette from my own experience. For instance, "Think of a client you felt close to/distant from – what did you notice about your experience of empathy?" We then took the discussion to a deeper exploration of empathy, attachment and the therapeutic alliance.

The act of 'witnessing' and 'being witnessed' in the process of reflection stood out as one of the most emotionally significant experiences in the group. Group members appreciated the space to speak about deeply felt but more subtle experiences. Perhaps a difficult conversation with a client about cancellation fees, or a moment of distraction in a session - aspects which may not reach supervision, but still impact our work. One member described feeling like a 'vessel with residues' and it was helpful to acknowledge that as therapists, we become containers, and all experiences leave residues in us. We evolved metaphors to describe our (now shared) experiences better, noting that some clients felt like 'a child that was wailing' and others like a 'a child that did not cry at all.' This helped us acknowledge that sometimes the crying child got more attention from us in both supervision and reflection; while the 'quieter child,' may have felt less problematic and been overlooked. As we grew more comfortable with each other, the group became a space of holding, and we were able to share deeper vulnerabilities like the struggle to keep an empathic focus on the client when feeling triggered. As one member said, "the honesty and vulnerability of everyone helped to lower my own defences and I was able to introspect and share more deeply." I felt immensely moved by our reflections together on the connections that linked our personhood, the roles we play, our philosophy of life and how that influenced our work." It was also validating to hear one member comment that "this group was the perfect intersection of self in the context of work," which was very close to my intended goal.

Reflection was positioned as an intentional and purposeful activity, something we need to set time aside for. As the group progressed, members began to pay keen attention to their own practices of reflection. They were more observant of their here-and-now experiences or 'reflection-in-action,' and began developing their own practices of reflective writing and thinking. One member said, "I am beginning to notice a slight shift in the tone of my client as a micro-rupture and reflect on it." Another shared that, "I am noticing an urge to be liked by clients... on reflection, I realised that in some cases this can build alliance, and in other cases, it can prevent confrontation and progress." These words spoke of a deepening awareness and strengthening of our identity as therapists.

Our group created a safe space to share and reflect as a community - to become aware, express, attune, witness, hold, learn, support, and reimagine ways of working. It became possible to hold both similar and contrary views - finding kinship in the resonance and holding curiosity about the differences. One group member commented that "There are things that I don't know about myself, and sometimes it is just impossible to get there by reflecting alone." For me, this summarised the philosophy of building reflexivity together. I felt deep gratitude for the authenticity of the therapists in our group. Much like a weaver holding many threads, both the individual and collective, I marvelled at the rich tapestry of our collective meaning making experience.

Archana Ramanathan *is a therapist in private practice, in India. Her approach to therapy is integrative, culturally sensitive and queer affirmative. She uses media, art and play therapy approaches in her work with both children and adults.*

Assessing Reflective Capacities

One of the most common ways of assessing the level and quality of reflection during the training phase is through reflective journals or written assignments. These reflective portfolios allow trainees to crystallize and articulate their reflections within a defined space. Although the medium of expression is typically the written word, there is a welcome emergence of more creative ways of representing the reflective process. The use of varied modes such as art, drama, movement, digital diaries, photographs or voice notes to capture immediate experiences can encourage trainees to explore new pathways. Of course, the ability to write reflectively or even think reflectively cannot be equated directly with the ability to *act* in a reflective and effective manner (Eaton, 2016). As trainers, we can strengthen this link by actively connecting reflections with proposed action and subsequently reflecting on how the action was carried out. Asking what was learnt and how it was applied back to therapy is a crucial step in the reflective process. Written submissions are not the only way to assess reflective capacities and using methods like reflective role-play simulations can help trainers access capacities for reflection-in-action more directly.

The evaluative component can impact the way in which trainees engage with the process of writing. Trainees can feel under scrutiny and experience pressure to confess all their inner doubts, fears and vulnerabilities. A reluctance to do this, combined with a desire for better grades or faculty approval can hinder authentic reflection. Instead, trainees may play it safe and stick to writing that fits the expected reflective script. Compelling narratives often feature transformative journeys, where characters rise from adversity, celebrate triumphs or confront the harsh realities of failure. These stories can range from inspiring tales of redemption to cautionary accounts that reveal the emotional turmoil and negative outcomes following a crisis. However, reflective writing frequently overlooks those experiences that don't fit neatly into these categories, including moments that may have intensified biases or led to stagnation rather than growth (Hargreaves, 2004). It is essential to approach trainees' stories with a discerning eye, recognizing when they sound overly polished or idealized. Instead of glorifying successful outcomes, we should cultivate an environment where vulnerability is welcomed and the complexities of human experience are acknowledged.

Phased formative assessments paired with conversational feedback provide trainees with the opportunity to refine their emerging ideas, confront their anxieties and make necessary adjustments along the way. We support an adult learning paradigm where each trainee or practitioner brings their own motivations, expectations and goals to the table. Self-assessment is integral to this process, as it encourages therapists to set their own goals and clarify the methods they wish to pursue. This personalized approach increases their motivation to engage in reflective work and fosters a deeper commitment to their development and growth as practitioners.

Evidence for Reflective Practice: *Quo Vādis*?

Collective findings from trainees and practitioners showcase the varied ways in which intentional reflective practice can support personal and professional development. The emerging evidence base for reflective practice is skewed towards trainees and academic settings, with fewer studies involving practitioners and clinical settings (e.g., Carmichael et al., 2020). The tilt has been towards qualitative paradigms with relatively small sample sizes, with a focus on the Person of the Therapist (POTT) and Self Practice/Self Reflection (SP/SR) models. The encouraging evidence for the SP/SR approach has indicated positive impacts across a range of domains including self-awareness and acceptance, conceptual and technical skills related to cognitive-behavioural therapy and interpersonal skills to relate and communicate with clients more effectively (e.g., Bennett-Levy, 2019). Trainee CBT therapists described how an experiential SP/SR course helped them identify their self-schemas and create a reflective bridge between the personal' and professional allowing them to work more closely with their clients' emotions (Presley & Jones, 2024). Reflective accounts of trainees in a marital and family therapy programme revealed that a 9-month POTT course served to enhance awareness of their strengths, values and limitations and deepened their emotional awareness during therapeutic work. In the process, they grew to understand their own vulnerabilities and wounds and also experienced a sense of shared humanity with their clients. Perceived improvements in their clinical skills were accompanied by an evolving understanding of the role of therapy and their identity as therapists (Niño et al., 2015). Learning how to manage uncertainty and take risks within relationships are some of the most critical skills in the process of becoming a reflective practitioner, and these were among the key gains that trainees reported from a reflective practice programme (Woodward et al., 2015).

Reflective models that focus on building particular skills like countertransference awareness and management (Hayes et al., 2023), allow practitioners to be more intentional in how they choose to use reflection to further their professional development. Reflective practice can also protect therapists from burnout and attrition, through more mindful engagement with their work, and the development of coping strategies and self-care practices (Curry & Epley, 2020). In one of few studies that examined effective training strategies and processes, supervisors shared how a curious stance, use of humour and the creation of playful space were critical while building reflective skills among trainee clinical psychologists (Ooi et al., 2023). They pointed to the importance of a collaborative and non-directive atmosphere to foster reflection, one in which missteps and imperfections are an inevitable part of a therapist's developmental journey. More such process-oriented research can help build a body of knowledge on the content and process of delivering reflective practice programmes, ultimately linking these to specific therapist and client outcomes.

Improvements in the quality and quantity of research evidence are crucial to the long-term integration of the reflective approach within the field of psychotherapy. Limitations in the research designs of most studies with the lack of control groups, small sample sizes typically restricted to specific institutions or training programmes. Longitudinal designs can help examine the effectiveness of reflective practice initiatives of varying durations and trace the integration of all the learnings that might occur over time. The inclusion of client outcomes and feedback is important and this evidence can strengthen the support reflective practice competency frameworks within psychotherapy training. More nuanced approaches need to examine possible distress and negative outcomes as a result of participation in reflective practice initiatives. The identification of appropriate goals and effective reflective practice methods based on the stage of professional development is another potential focal area. We look forward to emerging clarity on the reflective skills and methods that are relevant across theoretical orientations and therapeutic modalities and those that are more specific. The evidence for training in critical reflection and reflexivity is particularly limited and we see this as a major lacuna.

Reflective practice brings close engagement with our personal identities and the systems that we are part of, and this cannot leave us or our work unchanged. These transformations are powerful and meaningful even when not quantified or documented, and it may be important to free the act of reflection from the kind of scientific and educational scrutiny that can stifle it. As therapists, we may often do something that feels right, without being able to articulate why. The emphasis need not be on teasing out every detail of knowledge or thinking, but rather accepting that everything need not be known.

Using a Reflexive Lens as a Therapist-Researcher

The person of the researcher—our values, beliefs, memories and needs, along with the contexts that have shaped our experiences, are inevitable influences on the research process. Our research questions could stem from something that intrigues us, something we have encountered in our therapeutic work or personal lives; or events in the world that have impacted us. Perhaps we are curious about the ways in which therapists' adverse early life experiences might impact their therapeutic interactions. We could wonder how home and recovery is imagined by women in long stay mental health facilities or feel increasingly interested in refugee mental health. A sense of personal connection can motivate and drive our engagement with the research process and direct our focus towards particular aspects of psychopathology, client experiences, the person of the therapist and the psychotherapy process. What is important is to locate where these research questions have emerged from, so we can also be aware of any expectations, ideologies, assumptions and biases that might accompany them. Who we are impacts both how we experience and conduct research - the methodology we choose, who our research participants are, how we relate to them and to their experiences, our analysis of the data and our presentation and discussion of the key findings. Without reflexive awareness, we could be drawn to find what we have already imagined, substantiating this through our choice of select quotes from interviews, or by highlighting certain statistically significant results and downplaying others.

We encourage researchers to engage with a series of prompt questions suggested by Jamieson et al. (2023). This can help embed reflexivity throughout the research process, inviting the researcher to consider the implications of the chosen method of analysis and examine the benefits of the study for both the researcher and the researched. One of the questions taps into the extent to which the researcher occupies an insider or outsider position vis-à-vis the identities and experiences of those invited to participate in the study. Such reflections can also show the researcher how they may be simultaneously insiders and outsiders, having both a sense of familiarity and distance with the participants. This interrogative reflexive process is ongoing, aided by the use of journaling and memoing as ways of documenting and processing emergent feelings, decisions and interpretation. Honest self-examination can also bring an awareness of beliefs and assumptions that might require being set aside or bracketed, so researchers have a more open authentic engagement with their research participants' experiences (Thomas & Sohn, 2023). This approach encompasses collective reflexivity by outlining a range of methods and processes that enable research team members to share and engage with diverse perspectives (Olmos-Vega et al., 2022).

Those who carry dual identities of therapist and researcher can find it challenging to keep the researcher hat on at all times. Although the training and experience as therapists can be an asset, bringing a certain wisdom and nuance to research explorations, strong tensions can surface between these two roles. The therapist self can evoke the desire to comfort, validate or help participants, even as the researcher seeks to remain objective and focused on the research question or method. It can be helpful for researchers to titrate the intensity of data collection, document their thoughts, feelings and experiences in reflective diaries, engage in self-care practices and access supervision regularly.

Each of us are located on a map of intersecting social identities, which extends beyond our therapist and researcher locations. Jacobson and Mustafa (2019) recommend that researchers engage in a reflexive process of identifying their social identities (e.g., age, gender, ability, relationship status, sexual orientation, class) on a *Social Identity Map*, before plunging into the research process. This can bring an understanding of how these positions operate to influence their lives, shape their values, feelings and actions and inevitably impact the research process. Reflections on the researcher's positionality vis-à-vis typical participant profiles spotlight the symmetries and asymmetries of knowledge and power and inform efforts to redress any power imbalances. This may be reflected in the thoughtful and sensitive use of language during the research process, closer attention to informed consent procedures and the transparency of the research process, as well as the inclusion of diverse perspectives from research colleagues and supervisors and people with lived experience. The co-production of research with space for the perspectives of diverse stakeholders, particularly potential research participants, can support the ethos of shared power and responsibility and yield new insights. In this way, we create reflective loops that help generate knowledge and outcomes that are often more meaningful. While the ethos of co-production is increasingly seen in large, funded research projects, we also advocate for the inclusion of lived experience perspectives in post-graduate and doctoral level research, making it an integral part of the research process.

A written reflexivity statement is a way to bring one's personal voice into the research process and enhances a reader's understanding of the research process and findings. There are few guidelines about writing such a deeply experiential account—one that can be viewed as an act of courage. The researcher could struggle to express their complex, often private emotions and experiences in words or even wonder if their narrative comes across as too self-indulgent and non-academic. While a researcher might seek clarity by reading statements from other doctoral work or published articles, ultimately it is their decision about how and how much they wish to share their stories. The research supervisor can discuss a basic framework but then take a step back and provide space for the researcher to own their narrative. More than what is written at the end of the research process, what is critical is the use of these reflections to inform decisions throughout the research journey. Time is needed for all the threads of reflection to coalesce towards the end of the research process, and a reflexivity statement is an effective way to bring these together.

The inevitable influences of researcher subjectivity and of the socio-economic-political-historical context are more often recognized in qualitative research paradigms while being relatively ignored in quantitative studies. In the future, we envisage that a reflexive lens will be increasingly used to engage with issues related to power and knowledge production across all research designs.

A Therapist-Researcher Speaks: (Working) Through the Looking Glass

Kanika Mehrotra

In the words of Margaret Atwood—we are all stories, in the end. Before I enter the stories of others, I must begin with my own story – about who I am, how I entered my doctoral research and how I left it.

I am a childfree, married, heterosexual, cisgender, female in the third decade of my life, from an upper middle-class, non-practicing Hindu, upper caste background in urban India. These multiple social belongings both inform and are informed by my practice as a psychotherapist and researcher. As I reflect on my research process, I imagine that perhaps a combination of these social and professional identities brought me to my research focus, i.e., the exploration of experiences of motherhood in persons with borderline personality features.

Initially, I was preoccupied with my outsider status, stemming from feminist critiques of who should study whom? Given that I neither had a diagnosis of borderline personality disorder (BPD), and nor was I a mother - was I the right person to research this topic? Reflecting on my anxieties about sameness and difference, I realised that researching the experience of motherhood as a childfree woman felt much more uncomfortable than researching the experience of persons with borderline personality vulnerabilities. On the one hand being a mental health professional and not carrying a label of a mental illness brought me privilege. On the other hand, I did not have access to the privileged social position afforded through motherhood. These intersecting identities informed my anxieties and spoke to the ideas of power inherent in the cultural scripts of mental illness and motherhood that were directing my attention in specific ways. Through this reflection I came to see that while I could never presume sameness or complete homogeneity with the participants, I could practice healthy humility and openness to their experiences.

We are a culture that tells its women not to be 'too vocal', 'too emotional', 'too selfish', 'too needy', 'too angry' or 'too sexual'. Borderline personality disorder as a deeply gendered diagnosis therefore (often) becomes the location for tensions between psychopathology frameworks, culture and power structures. This resonated with me both as a woman and a researcher as I sought to understand how my clients with borderline personality features experienced these intersections. Similarly, motherhood has also long since been hijacked by patriarchal ideas of the ideal mother, who is supposed to look and be experienced in a limited, specific way. This can often delegitimize the experiences of mothers who may fall 'outside' these strict categories. Being child free requires constant negotiation with the dominant narrative of successful womanhood. Along the way, I discovered unprocessed feelings of guilt and shame about being childfree. I noticed that these feelings would intensify when a participant shared her challenges of conceiving a child or spoke of her longing for motherhood. In this way, my own experiences acted as a compass to the ways in which messages of motherhood can be internalized.

I also discovered the power of unlearning through this process. Going into the study, my therapist ear was saturated with essentialised, problem focused stereotypes of what it means to be a mother with a BPD diagnosis. But to my surprise, my researcher ear found many stories of joy, meaning, and strength instead. Today, I find myself much more sensitive to the ways in which borderline personality disorder and the mother–child relationship is portrayed in research literature and in psychotherapy. I believe that bias can be insidious. We may have moved past the times of the refrigerator mother, but realities such as the deficit-focus in current research or the label of the difficult patient for persons with a BPD diagnosis indicate that we still have a long way to go.

Through locating and reckoning with all my intersecting identities- therapist, researcher and woman, I was able to connect with the humanity of my participants. It is a powerful experience to work on research that is a natural extension of one's personal principles. I believe that this helped me find greater clarity and authenticity within myself- my values, life choices, roles as researcher and therapist all feel more aligned. While the process of constantly examining and re-examining myself was sometimes challenging, this work has reinforced my belief in the need for women's stories and voices to occupy space in popular discourse and has imbued my professional identity with a deeper sense of purpose and meaning.

Dr. Kanika Mehrotra *is a clinical psychologist, psychotherapist and researcher, trained at NIMHANS, India and the University of Rhode Island, USA. She uses a social justice informed, relational lens in her clinical work and currently practices in India.*

The Question is the Answer: Unpacking Critical Debates in Psychotherapy Practice

These are some questions that have stayed with us, stirred us and sometimes left us stymied during our journeys as clinicians, teachers and supervisors. We bring them into this shared space for collective reflection.

A Rose by Any Other Name? The Place and Meaning of Diagnoses

What's in a diagnosis? When we first meet a client, our conversations and observations come together to create an understanding what has brought them to therapy. Problem formulations, working models, representations, diagnoses—these are diverse ways of making meaning of each client's story. Although the identification of signs and symptoms and the use of diagnostic names is deeply embedded in the communicative discourse of mental healthcare, this approach has encountered criticism for being incomplete, inaccurate and even invalidating.

When we explore the evolving landscape of psychiatric classification and nomenclature, it is clear that diagnostic categories are not written in stone. There have been huge changes related to the understanding of sexual orientation and gender identity, with the removal of ego-dystonic homosexuality from the diagnostic lexicon, and the replacement of transsexualism and gender identity disorder with more affirming terms like gender incongruence. These shifts have not always been in step with changes in the social, political and legal firmament, and a recent apology letter to LGBTQ + communities from Division 39 of the American Psychological Association acknowledges the impact of former pathologizing theories, diagnoses and practices (LeRoy & Tummala-Narra, 2020). There are ongoing pushes and pulls related to diagnostic frameworks, apparent in the controversy around the inclusion of prolonged grief reaction as a new category, and the inconsistencies related to dimensional and categorical approaches to personality functioning in the DSM-5 and ICD-11.

This process of naming can be both clarifying and limiting. While it shines the spotlight on one set of human experiences, other aspects may be left in the shadows. An ICD or DSM diagnosis can offer a route into a person's world and create pathways to care, but these are not the only paths. We forefront two frameworks as exemplars of alternate or complementary approaches; the psychodynamic diagnostic manual (PDM-2, Lingiardi & McWilliams, 2017) and the power-threat-meaning framework (PTMF; Johnstone and Boyle, 2018). The PDM-2 offers a way of thinking about the matrix of emotional, cognitive, interpersonal and social experiences and functioning that is grounded in psychodynamic clinical models and theories. This person-centred approach allows us to move between the uniqueness of the person and the recognition of personality patterns and commonalities, bringing these together to create a comprehensive picture of the person's inner life. The assessment includes both adaptive and maladaptive aspects of functioning and has room to include subjective experiences of both client and therapist. The power-threat-meaning framework shifts the question from "what's wrong with you?" to "what happened to you?" (Blue Knot Foundation, 2012, p.14). Biological factors are just one part of an interlinked web of influences that include negative operations of interpersonal and structural power in a person's life. Symptoms are reframed as emerging from efforts to survive in the face of past and present threats. Psychotherapist and client together explore the personal meaning ascribed to these difficult experiences and co-construct a more hopeful narrative. While the PDM-2 and PTMF represent different approaches, both frameworks recognize how the experience of individual distress shapes and is shaped by interactions with culture and context, including factors such as poverty, unemployment, trauma and marginalization. When therapists experiment with different ways of engaging with diagnoses, there is a greater appreciation of what each approach has to offer. One might veer from one approach to the other, based on the client's needs, the demands of the work setting and evolving personal inclinations. The effort is to find a meeting ground between the lived and living experience of the client and the diagnostic classificatory systems. There are times when it is hard to match client experiences with existing diagnostic categories, and while some therapists might consider using a not yet diagnosed placeholder, others may prefer to engage therapeutically without using a diagnostic framework at all.

Pause and reflect....

Are there some diagnoses that seem more difficult to name and share with your clients?

Reflect on the possible reasons for your hesitation or discomfort?

Even when we are certain of the frame and the diagnosis, sharing this information with clients can be a complex process—one that is part science, part art and part ethics. As we engage in dialogic meaning-making to build a shared understanding of our client's often intangible experiences, the measured use of language becomes salient. Even as we draw from terminology used in established nosological frameworks, both connotation and nuance can be lost (or added) in translation when we work in languages other than English or practice in diverse cultural contexts. Some of our wariness regarding conversations about diagnoses may stem from our worries about the potential negative impact on the client and the desire to protect them. The what, how and when of this process can be particularly challenging when we feel pessimistic about the course or outcome of the illness. Our decisions may also reflect, sometimes unacknowledged, biases regarding particular diagnoses. A reflexive awareness of our own attitudes and behaviours can help us understand the reasons why we sometimes use euphemistic alternatives, delay difficult discussions or just wait for the client to bring in their questions.

A diagnosis has implications for the client's self-image and can get embedded into the story of their lives in different ways. Mental health practitioners are used to holding knowledge and power close, so it can feel natural to be the one deciding when and how to share information about diagnoses. This could reflect paternalistic systems of care, where the therapist retains power 'for the good of the client'. However, we must not forget that a clinical label carries deep significance for our clients who have the right to know, question, explore and revisit this 'name' that encapsulates their experiences. We might imagine that diagnosis will be stigmatizing, but the client may experience both the name and the process of naming process as useful and validating. There is no way to know for sure how each client may respond during the process of sharing the diagnosis. Research on what persons with lived experience of borderline personality vulnerabilities think about the diagnostic process indicates that some appreciate the binary, finding it empowering and seeing it as a way to make sense of their experiences and access mental healthcare. The feeling that their experiences are not inexplicable, that they are shared and recognized by others can open pathways to change and recovery. On the other hand, some individuals also report finding the label stigmatizing and instead connect better with a more complex fluid and evolving language (Tedesco et al., 2024). Reflective therapists can become more sensitive to the language that an individual client finds acceptable. We suggest engaging in a joint curious exploration of what the symptoms and experiences mean, how they connect to the diagnostic label and what the client wants to do about and with them. In this way, the therapist and client can together make meaning of the diagnosis within their relationship. Understanding that this is a very individual preference can guide therapists to reflect on the particular meaning that being viewed through a diagnostic lens carries for the client. This understanding can help us decide whether we diagnose at all, and of course when and what we share. If diagnosis-making is seen as a process of formulating our client's story, and indeed as a therapeutic intervention in itself, it can strengthen the alliance and guide the therapeutic journey.

At their worst, diagnostic categories can be a reductionist way to capture complex human experiences, obscuring as much as they reveal, and trapping both clients and therapists into narrow definitions of who we are and what we do. At best, a name can offer a framework, space and language to create a shared understanding of human experience and the potential for change. A nuanced, critical engagement with the history and evolution of diagnostic frameworks can be illuminating. Reflecting on our own experiences further helps clarify our relationship with diagnoses and understand how this process of naming can sometimes silence or exclude our clients' realities.

Inside Out or Outside in? Navigating Intersections Between Psychotherapy and Politics

Ensconced in the therapy room, therapist and client can imagine themselves sitting in neutral or at least non-aligned territory and view therapy as an apolitical enterprise. Even a cursory look at the history of psychotherapy reveals complex and enduring intersections between the psy-disciplines and politics. Some of the best-known theories of human experience and related therapies have emerged from the crucible of socio-political forces. Viktor Frankl's belief in man's search for meaning amid the personal and collective trauma in the Nazi concentration camps, and the subsequent emergence of logotherapy, reminds us of the intimate links between psychotherapy and politics. Theories and therapies have clearly reflected the gender politics of their time. When women were denied the right to vote and had little political participation, their experiences and realities also found limited representation in several psychological theories.

Psychotherapy has itself been used as a political weapon of conformity and oppression, with psychiatrists and psychologists not just quietly complicit but engaged in active support of several political regimes. When we revisit historical accounts, there is clear evidence of mental health practitioners' alignment with Nazi ideology and their involvement in the identification, detention and extermination of persons with mental health conditions (Strous, 2007). In a compelling exploration of the Bolivarian revolution, Llorens (2020) details the ways in which psychiatry and psychology was used to curb dissidence against the political regime in Venezuela. There were deliberate efforts to seek ideological solidarity from mental health practitioners, enlisting their support in labelling opposition leaders with psychiatric diagnoses and incarcerating dissidents in mental health wards. Not all mental health practitioners complied, and there were serious consequences for those who expressed dissent in the politically polarized society. Too often, these problematic (and very interesting) parts of the history of psychotherapy are often left out of training curricula, and we see this as a lost opportunity. A more honest and complete engagement with forces that have shaped psychotherapy in the past can help us to determine how we wish to interact with these forces in the future.

Pause and reflect...
The personal is political and the political is personal.

This slogan speaks of the connections between personal experience and larger social and political structures. This can mean different things to different people.

Reflect on your response to this slogan and what it means to you—both as a person and in your work as a therapist.

Politics is not just knocking at the door of the therapy room but is already inside—as part of the experiences, struggles and lives of both client and therapist. As conversations around political affiliations and events are increasingly being initiated by our clients, we are learning to listen, engage in dialogue and navigate the terrain of differences and similarities. In this process, there is much to learn about our client's wishes and fears around safety, power, belongness and exclusion.

What does politically informed and responsive therapy look like in an increasingly fractured world? While we may not have immediate answers or solutions, we can offer a space for clients to engage with difficult questions and find ways of sitting with dilemmas and diverse perspectives. There is much power in the act of bearing witness and in the process of keeping mind in mind—it is often in the telling and the listening that healing and transformation can begin. There are wonderful possibilities for psychotherapists to provide a holding space to listen to silenced stories and to make the invisible visible. Llorens reminds is that "to conduct political psychotherapy is not to 'open space for the political' or 'discuss political issues in sessions', but to recognize that life and the therapeutic relationship are inevitably immersed in power relations" (Llorens, 2020, p.179). As reflective therapists, we can explore different ways of engaging with the interface between power, politics and psychotherapy. We are being political when we recognize the impact of inequalities and injustice in our clients' stories, and see how it is more difficult for some clients to find employment, use public transport or move to a different neighbourhood. Prejudice, violence, terrorism and oppression can enter and pervade our inner worlds in both subtle and overt ways. When we recognize that suffering is embedded within a broader socio-political, economic, ecological and technological matrix, it impacts how we formulate a client's distress. Understanding that anxiety or paranoia are not always be irrational, and that the fragility of social systems can mirror the fragility of the minds we encounter, informs the resources we offer and where we situate the need for change.

There is a world outside that needs healing, and there have been urgent calls to turn the therapy room into a cell of revolution (Hillman & Ventura, 1992). The field of psychotherapy is perhaps still more focused on inner revolutions and less on changing laws, policies or the world. There is a notable increase in conversations and debates around the praxis of a politically aware psychotherapy although some of this needs to move beyond armchair activism and black badges on Instagram. While some therapists have moved beyond the therapy room in their bid to alleviate suffering, engagement in advocacy for social change and social justice is still an individual choice and not a collective mandate for psychotherapists. It can be easier when one is invited to the table, to be part of policy consultations for education reforms, disability benefits or laws around child sexual abuse. But sometimes need to be part of the resistance, drawing attention to problems that governments and systems do not wish to recognize. Such engagement requires commitment and could involve personal risk in certain environments, prompting us to reflect on how much we are truly willing to invest. Political action calls for the development of new skills such as media interface, network building or policy decoding and can take time away from other valued responsibilities. As we embrace more concrete roles in advocacy, we must remain cautious not to pressure clients into taking strong positions or actions that they are not ready for. As always, therapists' needs and passions should not supersede those of the client.

Psychotherapists need a grounded and sensitive training process to help them understand how to engage with complex issues related to diversity and inequity. Llorens (2020) recommends a range of questions to help therapists to expand their reflective repertoire and create space for the political and social. Opportunities for open dialogue in classroom, small group and supervision spaces can mirror the possibilities for diverse voices and shared meaning that we are eventually hoping for in the therapy room. We could initiate conversations on political viewpoints and controversies, while inviting trainees to reflect on any personal experiences of poverty, war, discrimination or displacement. Examining passionately held truths and generational shifts in perspectives on issues like gender, religion and sexuality can help therapists recognize the familial and cultural influences shaping their own beliefs. Questions about pioneers, rebels or politically active family members can open interesting avenues for discussion. This needs to be done sensitively, appreciating that trainees can be differently triggered by such questions. When therapists are encouraged from the training stage to recognize how politics shapes expectations around how we live, love, work and seek help, they have the opportunity to develop their own understanding of the intersections between the personal, the political, and the psychotherapeutic. This can strengthen psychotherapy's potential to serve as a fulcrum for meaningful change toward a better world.

What Can We Learn from Each Other? The Power of Cross Pollination

In a letter to 'John', displayed at the Freud Museum in London, Anna Freud shares her thoughts about psychoanalysts and their development. She exhorts them to have wide-ranging interests spanning sociology, religion, history and literature across countries and cultures, in order to expand their outlook on their patients. To quote her, "In the great literary figures you will find people who know at least as much of human nature as the psychiatrists and psychologists try to do".

In their essence, both the psychotherapeutic profession and reflective practice straddle diverse disciplines that explore what it means to be human. Exploring through the varied lenses of art, history, philosophy, physics, technology and economics can deepen our understanding of ourselves, our clients, relational processes and the contexts that we all live in. Philosophy has much to teach us about fallacies in thinking, economics illuminates the ways in which human needs are met, and the field of memory studies offers newer insights into the processes and reasons for remembering and forgetting. The frictions and synergies, both within and outside the mental health disciplines, can stimulate the transfer and integration of knowledge as well as catalyse innovations and change. The pitfalls of working in silos are not unknown, but we still tend to align with other mental health practitioners when planning practice and research initiatives. Interventions to improve the mental health of rural children would be more effective if they are integrated with initiatives that address issues related to poverty and other resource inequalities, access to education, primary healthcare, juvenile justice and other relevant public health policies. Curiosity and cross-sectoral learning can deepen our knowledge of key theoretical constructs and strengthen our mental health interventions and research. Methods that are integral to other disciplines, e.g., immersive ethnographic approaches drawn from anthropology, can bring in nuance, complexity and a critical gaze, enriching our research questions and processes. Newer changes and challenges, such as the digital revolution and climate change, demand crosspollination and collaborations for us to potentiate meaningful and sustained impacts. The footprint of mental healthcare is expanding with the emergence of new interdisciplinary fields such as *neurourbanism* which spans the intersections of mental wellbeing, neuroscience and the urban disciplines including urban planning, architecture and sociology (Adli et al., 2017). Whether it is the gamification of digital therapy modules or the increasing use of somatic movement interventions, many recent developments in psychotherapy have been derived from our engagement with other disciplines. It is in this creative ferment that we can continue to grow and stay relevant in an increasingly complex human world.

We want to bring particular focus to the importance of philosophy and anthropology—two disciplines once deeply intertwined with psychology and psychotherapy. The early architects of psychotherapy engaged seriously with philosophical questions of the self, freedom, suffering and meaning. Anthropological inquiry highlights how distress is never experienced in a vacuum. Rather, it is shaped, named and responded to through cultural scripts, kinship structures, spiritual beliefs and sociopolitical histories. Suffering and healing are both culturally mediated, and clients are seen as meaning-makers embedded in complex world. These disciplines offer both critique and compass, helping us navigate the relational and ethical terrain of therapy. Our call for integration is not a nostalgic return to past practices but a response to contemporary clinical realities where clients continue to bring in moral injuries, existential uncertainties and culturally shaped narratives of distress that defy neat diagnostic categories. Integrating these perspectives into psychotherapy requires a rethinking of how we train clinicians going beyond curriculum content to cultivate modes of inquiry that value uncertainty, pluralism and reflexivity. Rebuilding legitimacy for a broader, interdisciplinary approach takes courage—the courage to embrace complexity, to name what resists quantification and to show how attending to meaning, culture and ethics makes our work more responsive, humane and socially relevant.

We envision psychotherapy as a space of possibilities that extend far beyond the confines of the therapy room, with windows wide open to new ideas and perspectives. Collective human experiences, such as the historical trauma among Aboriginal people or the violent partition of India in 1947, have left deep psychological scars with ripple effects across generations. These impacts are not only felt by individuals but are also visible in the frayed fabric of society. Such profound histories cannot be fully engaged with or healed within the therapy room alone. Art, film, literature, politics, post-colonial studies, museum studies and collective movements carry tremendous potential to create space for what is not easily acknowledged or articulated.

Pause and reflect…

Eyes of Stone is a film about spirit possession, faith and healing, situated at the temple of goddess Bhankya Mata in rural India. The filmmaker, Nilita Vachani, adopts a feminist lens to explore Shanta's journey of faith and healing. Shantha is a 19 year old woman from a village in Rajasthan, married at age 10 and mother to two surviving children. Her persistent experiences of headaches, fever, fatigue and a sense of disconnection from the world is punctuated by states of possession and trance—all attributed to the evil gaze of the 'dakan[1]'. Her story shows us how it is often the dispossessed who are possessed. It is during the moments of possession that women find the space to speak about what is often unspoken within rigid patriarchal systems.

Think about possible collaborations across various disciplines and the methods you might like to use if you wanted to understand the phenomenon of possession more deeply as a psychotherapist.

[1] Evil spirit.

Conclusion

Reflective practice arose as a response to the needs of professionals, but reflection itself is a tool that is beneficial to humanity at large. We believe that the complexities of a changing and multilayered world, where competing worldviews and realities constantly jostle for attention, can only be met through ongoing reflection and adaptation. We envision the development of more reflective societies and structures, including schools and community organizations, that encourage dialogue and critical thinking.

In the best part of the tradition of reflective practice, we would like to question everything, including reflective practice itself. When reflective practice becomes the convention rather than an anti-establishment movement, does it lose some of its potency? The more we research, structure, teach and evaluate reflection, the more it becomes canon, and perhaps engenders less original thought. We hope that a critique of reflective practice, along with a recognition of its transformative potential, will guide its ethical and effective applications and keep the field vibrant and evolving.

References

Adli, M., Berger, M., Brakemeier, E. L., Engel, L., Fingerhut, J., Gomez-Carrillo, A., Hehl, R., Heinz, A., Mayer, J. H., Mehran, N., Tolaas, S., Walter, H., Weiland, U., & Stollmann, J. (2017). Neurourbanism: Towards a new discipline. *The Lancet Psychiatry, 4*(3), 183–185.

Bennett-Levy, J. (2019). Why therapists should walk the talk: The theoretical and empirical case for personal practice in therapist training and professional development. *Journal of Behaviour Therapy and Experimental Psychology, 62*, 133–145.

Blue Knot Foundation. (2012). *Practice guidelines for treatment of complex trauma and trauma informed care and service delivery*. http://www.blueknot.org.au/ABOUT-US/Our-Documents/Publications/Practice-Guidelines

Carmichael, K., Rushworth, I., & Fisher, P. (2020). 'You're opening yourself up to new and different ideas': Clinical psychologists' understandings and experiences of using reflective practice in clinical work: An interpretative phenomenological analysis. *Reflective Practice, 21*(4), 520 533.

Curry, A., & Epley, P. (2020). "It makes you a healthier professional": The impact of reflective practice on emerging clinicians' self-care. *Journal of Social Work Education, 58*(2), 291–307.

Douglas, L., & Feeney, L. (2017). An established practice in new surroundings: Concepts, challenges, pitfalls and guidelines for NCHD Balint Groups. *Irish Journal of Psychological Medicine, 34*(1), 1–5.

Eaton, C. (2016). "I don't get it",—The challenge of teaching reflective practice to health and care practitioners. *Reflective Practice, 17*(2), 159–166.

Ferguson, H. (2018). How social workers reflect in action and when and why they don't: The possibilities and limits to reflective practice in social work. *Social Work Education, 37*(4), 415–427.

Flaskas, C. (2009). The therapist imagination of self in relation to clients: Beginning ideas on the flexibility of empathic imagination. *Australian and New Zealand Journal of Family Therapy, 30*, 147–159.

Hargreaves, J. (2004). So how do you feel about that? Assessing reflective practice. *Nurse Education Today, 24*(3), 196–201.

Hayes, J. A., Cartwright, C. C., & Zhao, F. (2023). Training therapists to manage countertransference via reflective practice. In L. G. Castonguay & C. E. Hill (Eds.), *Becoming better psychotherapists: Advancing training and supervision* (pp. 127–147). American Psychological Association.

Hillman, J., & Ventura, M. (1992). *We've had a hundred years of psychotherapy & the world's getting worse.* Harper & Row.

Jacobson, D., & Mustafa, N. (2019). Social identity map: A reflexivity tool for practicing explicit positionality in critical qualitative research. *International Journal of Qualitative Methods.* https://doi.org/10.1177/1609406919870075

Jamieson, M. K., Govaart, G. H., & Pownall, M. (2023). Reflexivity in quantitative research: A rationale and beginner's guide. *Social and Personality Psychology Compass, 17*(4), e12735. https://doi.org/10.1111/spc3.12735

Johnstone, L. & Boyle, M. with Cromby, J., Dillon, J., Harper, D., Kinderman, P., Longden, E., Pilgrim, D. & Read, J. (2018). *The Power Threat Meaning Framework: Overview.* British Psychological Society.

LeRoy, M., & Tummala-Narra, U. (2020). *Letter of Apology to LGBTQ+ Communities and APA Division 39 Members (past and present).* On Behalf of the Board of Directors, APA Division 39 - Society for Psychoanalysis and Psychoanalytic Psychology. https://div39members.wildapricot.org/LGBTQ-Apology

Lingiardi, V., & McWilliams, N. (2017). *Psychodynamic diagnostic manual*, Second Edition: PDM-2. Guilford Publications.

Llorens, M. (2020). *Politically reflective psychotherapy: Towards a contextualized approach.* Springer International Publishing.

Lyons, A., Mason, B., Nutt, K., & Keville, S. (2019). Inside it was orange squash concentrate: Trainees' experiences of reflective practice groups within clinical psychology training. *Reflective Practice, 20*(1), 70–84.

Niño, A., Kissil, K., & Apolinar Claudio, F. L. (2015). Perceived professional gains of master's level students following a person-of-the-therapist training program. A retrospective content analysis. *Journal of Marital and Family Therapy, 41*, 163–176.

Ooi, S. M., Coker, S., & Fisher, P. (2023). Clinical psychologists' experience of cultivating reflective practice in trainee clinical psychologists during supervision: A qualitative study. *Reflective Practice, 24*(4), 481–495.

Olmos-Vega, F. M., Stalmeijer, R. E., Varpio, L., & Kahlke, R. (2022). A practical guide to reflexivity in qualitative research: AMEE Guide No. 149. *Medical Teacher, 45*(3), 241–251.

Presley, V. L., & Jones, G. (2024). 'Crossing the reflective bridge': How therapists synthesise personal and professional development from self-practice/self-reflection during CBT training. *The Cognitive Behaviour Therapist, 17*, e18. https://doi.org/10.1017/S1754470X24000175

Schön, D. A. (1991). *The reflective practitioner: How professionals think in action.* Ashgate Publishing Ltd.

Strous, R. D. (2007). Psychiatry during the Nazi era: Ethical lessons for the modern professional. *Annals of General Psychiatry, 6*, 8. https://doi.org/10.1186/1744-859X-6-8

Tedesco, V., Day, N. J. S., Lucas, S., & Grenyer, B. F. S. (2024). Diagnosing borderline personality disorder: Reports and recommendations from people with lived experience. *Personality and Mental Health, 18*(2), 107–121.

Thomas, S. P., & Sohn, B. K. (2023). From uncomfortable squirm to self-discovery: A phenomenological analysis of the bracketing experience. *International Journal of Qualitative Methods.* https://doi.org/10.1177/16094069231191635

Woodward, N., Keville, S., & Conlan, L. (2015). The buds and shoots of what I've grown to become: The development of reflective practice in trainee clinical psychologists. *Reflective Practice, 16*(6), 777–789.

MIX
Papier aus verantwortungsvollen Quellen
Paper from responsible sources
FSC® C105338

If you have any concerns about our products,
you can contact us on
ProductSafety@springernature.com

In case Publisher is established outside the EU,
the EU authorized representative is:
Springer Nature Customer Service Center GmbH
Europaplatz 3, 69115 Heidelberg, Germany

Printed by Libri Plureos GmbH
in Hamburg, Germany